Dynamic Contrast-Enhanced MRI Atlas of Prostate Cancer

Robert L. Bard

Dynamic Contrast-Enhanced MRI Atlas of Prostate Cancer

With 614 Figures

Springer

Robert L. Bard, MD, DABR, MACR
121 East 60th St.
New York NY 10022
USA

ISBN 978-3-540-78422-7 ISBN 978-3-540-78423-4 (eBook)

DOI 10.1007/978-3-540-78423-4

Library of Congress Control Number: 2008938342

Cover design: Frido Steinen-Broo, eStudio, Calamar, Spain

Printed on acid-free paper

9 8 7 6 5 4 3 2 1

springer.com

Dedication

To my patients,
whose courage showed me possiblity.

To my wife, Loreto,
whose vision generated reality.

Foreword

In the United States there were an estimated 218,890 new cases of prostate cancer in 2007 and an estimated 27,050 deaths from the disease. According to these figures, in the United States, prostate cancer is the most common cancer in men, accounting for almost 30% of all new cancers, and also the second leading cause of cancer death in men.

A number of interesting and critically important issues need to be addressed in relation to prostate cancer, including: the reason why the disease is so frequent and ubiquitous; the role of PSA-based screening programmes; the utility of immediate versus delayed management of early cases; the rationale for surgery versus radiotherapy; and the optimal use of medical treatments.

During the past decade, major improvements in staging have occurred as a result of new imaging approaches, such as MRI and PET. At the same time, treatments have evolved, with novel approaches in surgery (coelioscopic interventions, robotic-assisted prostatectomy, and alternative endoscopic resections), radiotherapy (conformational irradiation, IMRT), and systemic therapies (docetaxel as first-line chemotherapy in the hormone-refractory setting).

It is well recognized that, while 60% of men aged 60 will be carrying small cancers in their prostate and the overall lifetime risk of developing prostate cancer is currently 1 in 7 and rapidly increasing, the chance of dying from the disease in the Western world is only 3.5–4%. These figures underline the potential risk of over-detection and over-treatment. This is why it is so important to better understand the pathogenesis, the evolution, and the natural history of the disease, as well as the impact (both positive in terms of cure/remission rate and negative in terms of morbidity/mortality) of all the therapeutic tools that we have in our armamentarium.

In this context, the contribution of Dr. Robert Bard's textbook on prostate cancer is tremendous. He clearly describes the diagnostic processes that can contribute to screening and permit the early detection of prostate cancer. He also clarifies the indications for and the limits of their use in most clinical settings. Later, he describes the different stages of the disease, from purely intraprostatic tumors to truly generalized ones. Interestingly, one chapter specifically addresses the treated prostate, in which exploration is not always very easy. Finally, through a number of case studies, Dr. Bard helps readers to become more familiar with the most common pitfalls that oncologists face in the management of prostate cancer.

Prostate cancer is going to be one of the most interesting and difficult challenges of modern medicine. It has a close relationship with aging and has both a direct and an indirect impact on the health economy of most developed countries. Furthermore, empowered patients who are well informed about the disease and its treatment are becoming increasingly influential. These factors make prostate cancer the perfect example of a disease that needs to be managed by professionals who, throughout their careers, maintain an appropriate level of skills and knowledge in order to achieve the best possible results for the patient himself as well as for the entire community.

David Khayat
Paris, France

Prologue

Screening for prostate cancer with digital rectal examination (DRE) and prostate-specific antigen (PSA) has met with controversy during this decade. The 2008 position statement of the American College of Preventive Medicine concludes: "...there is insufficient evidence to recommend routine population screening with DRE or PSA" (Lim et al., Am J Prev Med 2008;34(2):164-70).

Medical imaging with high-resolution ultrasound, elastography, and power Doppler has proved clinically useful. 3-D sonography differentiates between cancer and inflammation by documenting the capsular effacement/penetration that occurs with malignant tumors.

As with many imaging modalities, the use of MRI to detect prostate cancer was met with initial euphoria (Schnall et al., *Radiology* 1991;178:797-802) followed by wise reticence. Dr. May (May et al., BJU *International* 2001;87:66-69) stated that "treatment should not be altered based on endorectal coil (EC) MRI findings". Presentations of dynamic contrast enhanced (DCE) MRI showed improved results for the diagnosis of local disease and extension of tumor for staging purposes. Difficulties in gray-scale perception of abnormalities led to the introduction of computer-aided diagnosis with colorized representations of malignant findings that significantly improved the detection of major pathologies, with subtle imaging features imperceptible to the human eye.

The following is a brief presentation of current clinical MRI techniques, including DCE-MRI and magnetic resonance spectroscopy (MRS), and their respective advantages and disadvantages.

Standard MRI at 1.5 Tesla

T1-weighted in the axial plane with 4-mm slices with a large field of view (FOV): T1-weighted imaging is necessary to detect hemorrhage in the prostate bed, which will appear as signal loss on T2.

T2-weighted in three planes with 2.5- to 4.0-mm slices with a small FOV: T2-weighted imaging shows tumor as signal loss; however, false positives occur in hemorrhage, calcification, fibrosis [postinflammatory, postoperative, posthormonal (ADT), postradiation, or following thermal ablation treatment], and inflammation. False negatives occur in the presence of infiltrating nonfocal tumors and massive benign hyperplasia. While some tumors (20%) are not visible, cancer may be differentiated from prostatitis by the focality of signal loss and distinctness of the border. Small tumors (less than 0.5 cc) may not be imaged, and transitional zone tumor is difficult to distinguish from benign hyperplasia.

Extracapsular extension is denoted by focal growth beyond the capsule, infiltration of the periprostatic fat, and asymmetry of the neurovascular bundles. Seminal vesicle invasion is detected as enlargement and loss of signal.

DWI-MRI

DWI-MRI uses diffusion-weighted imaging analysis of Brownian movement of water. Apparent diffusion coefficient (ADC) is a variation of this sequence. Initial results from its application to prostate disorders have been mixed. This older technology is being replaced by DCE-MRI imaging.

EC-MRI

EC-MRI uses an endorectal receiver coil which improves the signal to noise ratio and spatial resolution. However, patient discomfort and deformation of the prostate alter the information gathered. Also, motion artifacts due to the endorectal coil (patient or bowel) may increase. Due to pressure alteration of prostatic shape, EC-MRI images are not used for radiation treatment planning.

MRS

MRS measures the in vivo levels of the metabolites citrate, creatine, and choline. Cancer has a high choline content. The large sample field means that small tumors might not be sampled and thus may be missed in the final data collection. MRS is inoperative in the fat, limiting the potential diagnosis of extracapsular extension. Inflammation and post-treatment artifacts produce false positives. The low overall specificity for detection of low grade cancer at 44% (Lemaitre et al, *J Radiol* 2008: 89: 1053-1064) precludes this as a screening modality .

3-Tesla MRI

The higher field strength improves the signal to noise ratio as well as the spatial resolution and may decrease the imaging time and allow for imaging without an endorectal coil. However, increased magnetic and chemical artifacts and lack of signal detection from tissue distant from the endorectal coil antennae may limit the accuracy. High magnetic field strength may pose a danger to patients with metallic devices. Indeed, patients with unrecalled ophthalmic injuries or postoperative metallic implants are forced to stop the high field strength examination owing to pain in the affected area. Special 1.5-T protocols are often as accurate as 3-T images, with the possible exception of the posterior prostatic capsule and rectal wall. However, this region is well visualized by 18-MHz sonography.

Perfusion or DCE-MRI

DCE-MRI uses intravenously injected gadolinium chelate contrast, which has few side-effects, and the presence of intravenous flow reduces patient movement. Tumor angiogenesis induces immature blood vessels that are both heterogeneous and leaky. These characteristics can be demonstrated by measuring the perfusion parameters with MRI with T1-weighted dynamic imaging.

Signal enhancement with time is measured qualitatively and quantitatively. Visually on T1-weighted images this appears as increased white on the dark background. The many variables include: time of appearance of enhancement (enhancement delay), time to peak, slope of enhancement, intensity of peak, and wash out.

Pharmacokinetic parameters include permeability surface area product per unit volume of tissue, lesion leakage space (extravascular extracellular space per unit volume of tissue), and contrast exchange rate. The acquisition time should be 10-30 s. There has been no consensus as to the optimal protocol, and trials with whole mount pathology have been designed to correlate imaging findings with tumor volume and aggression. Standard DCE MRI has limited resolution, but most vascular homogeneous tumor nodules enhance early and discretely.

Perfusion can also be assessed without injecting a contrast agent by using arterial spin labeling techniques, diffusion MRI, or BOLD (blood oxygen level dependent) MRI. However, these latter methods are limited by a low signal to noise ratio and problems with quantification. The main indication for perfusion MRI is assessment of antiangiogenic and antivascular treatments (Huwart et al., *J Radiol* 2007;88:331-338) since the blood flow of a successfully treated tumor decreases before the morphology and size change. While it may take 6 weeks for PSA to drop below 1 ng/mg, hyperemia reduction may be observed immediately after thermal treatments and within days following other therapies. Tumor recurrence in a treated gland is often missed with MRI without contrast enhancement owing to the overall signal loss directly related to the therapeutic modality.

fTP MRI

fTP MRI was developed to improve on the limitations of MRS and standard DCE-MRI by affording better visual conspicuity and more useful pharmacokinetic data. This modality has increased the yield of positive biopsies, improved staging, and facilitated the success of image-guided therapies (Rouviere et al., *Journees Francaises de Radiologie*, Paris, 2007). The Harvard Medical School team reported 96% accuracy with this technology at the 2008 Medical Imaging and Computer Assisted Intervention Meeting in New York. While lymph node metastases are best diagnosed by Combidex lymph node MRI, hypervascular foci that have responded to treatment with decreased vascularity have been documented by standard fTP MRI on nodes measuring 3x3 mm and greater in size. fTP imaging has highlighted bladder cancers found incidentally during prostate imaging, allowing for life-saving early intervention in patients with low-grade prostate cancers. This modality is uniquely suited to detect recurrent cancer following focal treatment, thermal ablation and radiation therapy.

Robert L. Bard
New York, September 2008

Acknowledgments

I thank Loreto Bard, Executive Director of the Biofoundation for Angiogenesis Research and Development, for her assistance in coordinating international multidisciplinary medical exchanges that advanced the concepts developed in this book. I wish to thank members of: the Prostate Cancer Research Institute; Drs. Duke Bahn, Stanley Brosman, Arthur Lurvey, Mark Scholz and Charles Myers; members of the Catholic University Hospital in Rome, Italy, Drs. Giuseppe Brisinda, Federica Cadeddu and Giorgio Maria: members of the Mayo Clinic Foundation, Drs. Thayne Larson, Benjamin Larson and Lance Mynderse: member of the Academic Hospital of Bicetre, Dr.Francoise Giuliano: members of The Prostatitis Foundation, Drs. Susan Keay and John Warren: members of the NY Roentgen Society, Drs. Richard Stock, Lincoln Pao, Michael Zelefsky, Alan Pollack, Shalom Kalnicki: members of the Societe Francaise de Radiologie, Drs. Guy Frija, Olivier Helenon, JF Moreau, Olivier Rouviere and JM Correas; members of the Instituto Radiologia, Policlinico Umberto I, Rome, Drs. Plinio Rossi, Roberto Passariello and Vito Cantisani: members of the Groupe Hospitalier Necker-Enfants Malades, Paris, France, Drs. Bertrand Dufour, N. Thiounn, JM Correas and Y. Chretien; members of the Imperial College of Medicine, London, Dr. David Cosgrove and Sir Richard Sykes; members of the American Urological Association, Drs. Carl Olsson, William DeWolf, Edward Messing, Louis Denis, Eric Rovner, Ernest Sosa, Alexis Te, Michael Manyak, Michael Marberger, Joseph Smith, Jr, Harris Nagler, J. Fracchia, Peter Scardino, M. Droller, P. Schlegel, S. Kaplan, H. Lepor, M. Grasso, N. Romas, A. Melman, I. Grunberger, R. Macchia, M. Choudhury and Patrick Walsh; members of the New York Cancer Society, Drs. Marvin Rotman and Howard Hochster. Dr. Jelle Barentsz, president of the International Cancer Imaging Society, for developing lymph node detection technology and disseminating awareness throughout the medical profession. Special thanks to Drs. Catherine Roy, Francois Cornud, Olivier Helenon and Peter Scardino whose books have provided new hope for cancer victims and further advanced medical knowledge. Finally, input from Dr. John Melnick and Dr. Mark Liebeskind and support from members of my staff Niurka Achury and Mary Ann Sta. Rita were indispensable in the timely publication.

Contents

Chapter

1 Anatomic Variants and Benign Conditions

Fig. 1.1 a–e

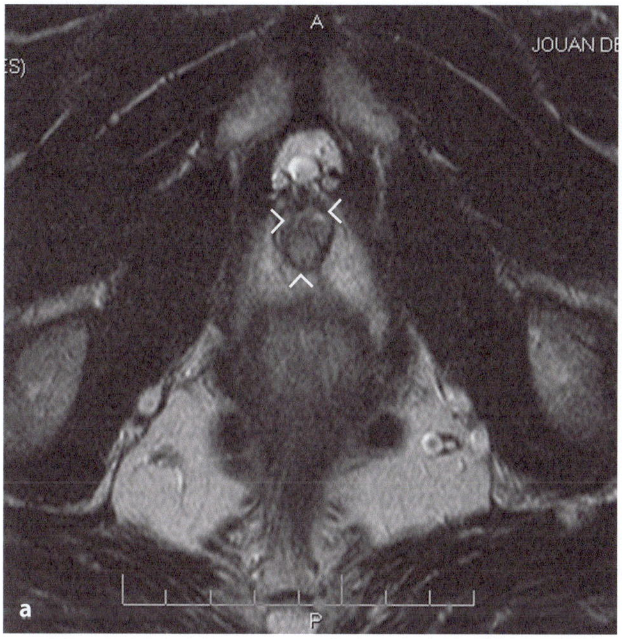

Fig. 1.1 a Normal prostatic apex-note white crescent shaped peripheral zone due to greater signal from high fluid content of the glandular structures and darker rounded heterogeneous central zone due to lesser signal from lower fluid containing more fibrous tissues.

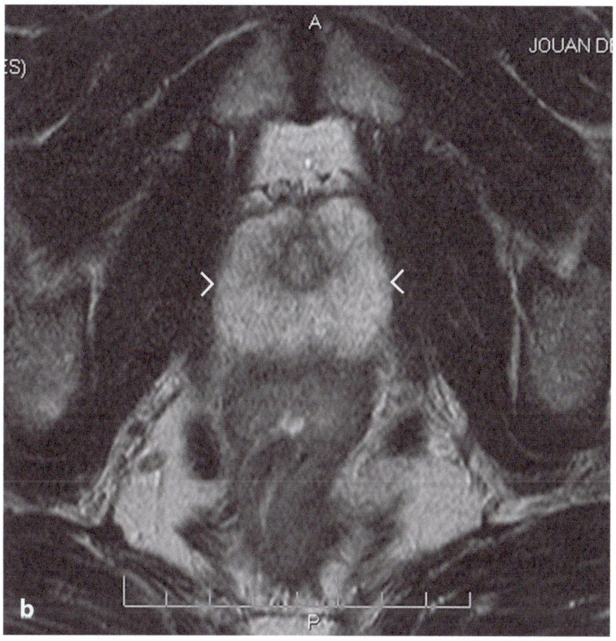

Fig. 1.1 b Normal prostatic midgland-peripheral zone is white.

Fig. 1.1 c, d

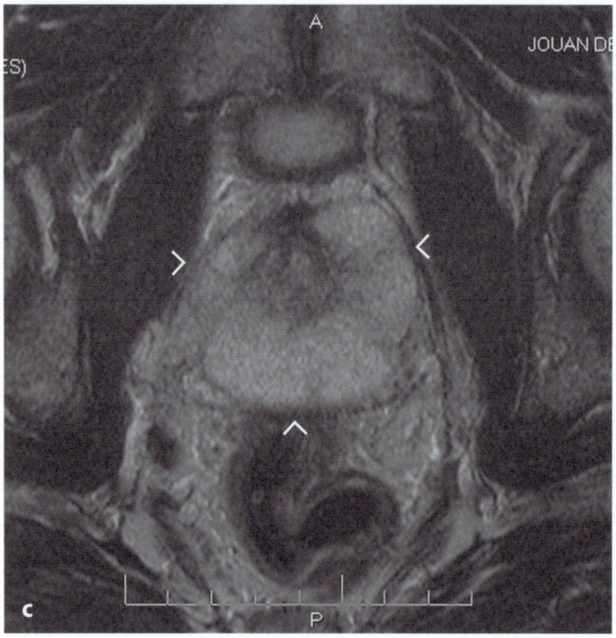

Fig. 1.1 c Normal prostatic base-peripheral zone is white.

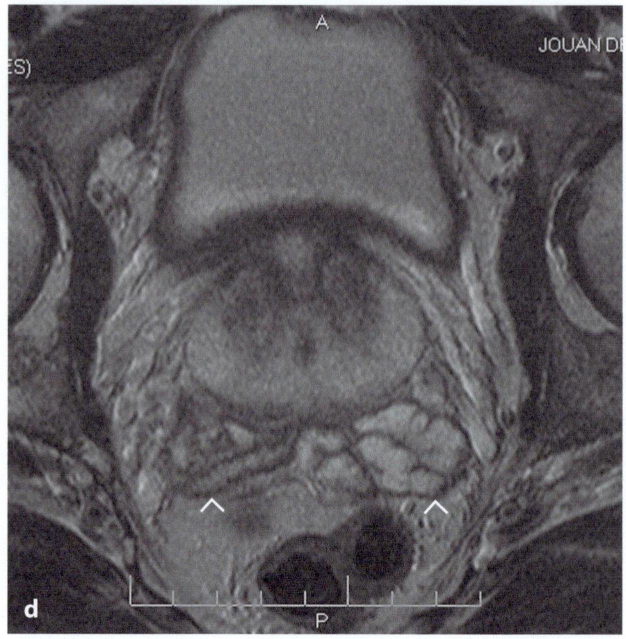

Fig. 1.1 d Normal seminal vesicles-note serpiginous dark septations

Fig. 1.1 e

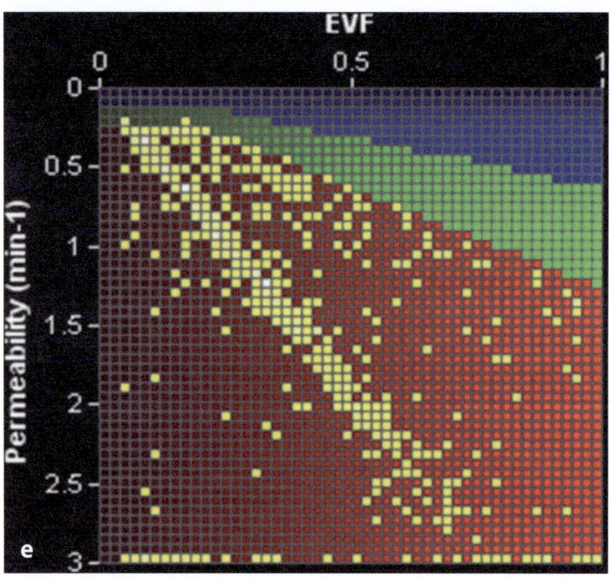

Fig. 1.1 e Enhancement chart: blue = benign / red = malignant / green = suspicious

Fig. 1.2 a–j

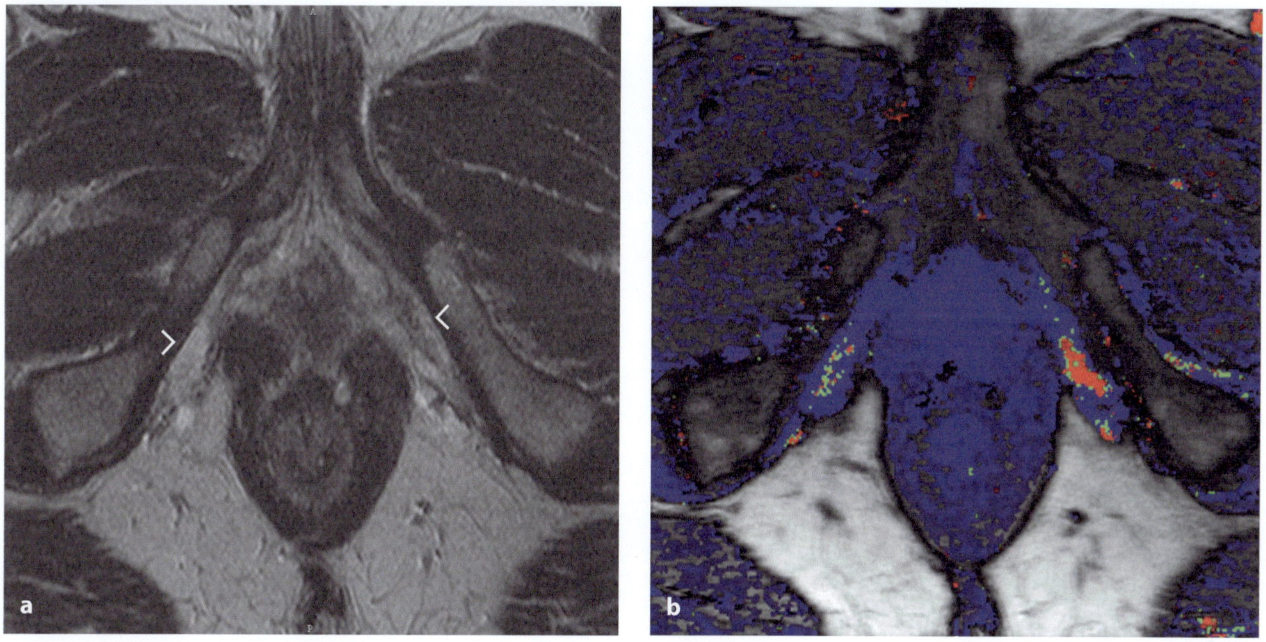

Fig. 1.2 a, b Perineal veins/bilateral signal voids with vascular flows

Fig. 1.2 c, d

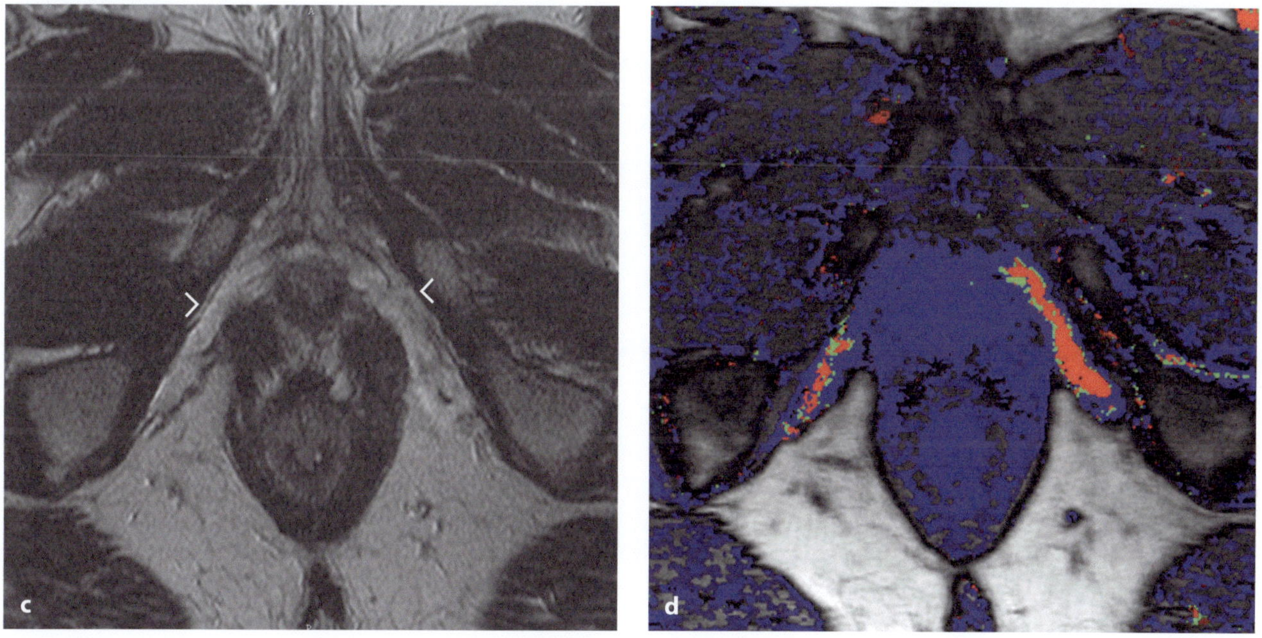

Fig. 1.2 c, d Periapical pelvic veins/signal voids with vascular flows

Fig.1.2 e, f

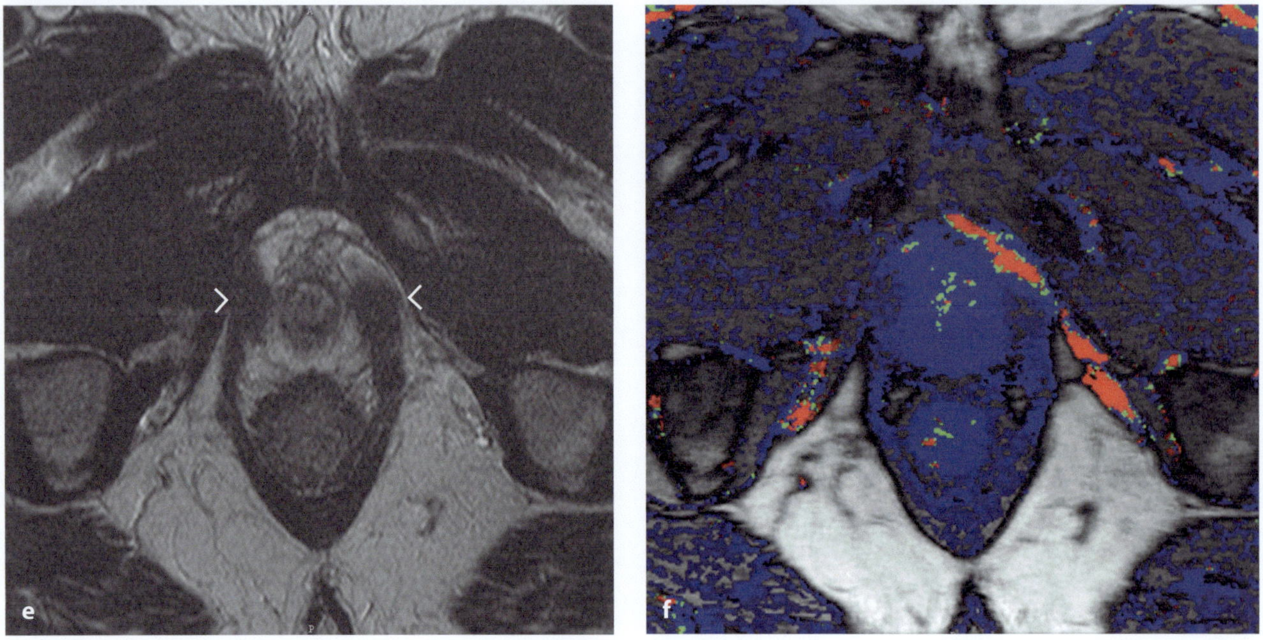

Fig. 1.2 e, f Apex pelvic veins/signal voids with vascular flows

Fig.1.2 g, h

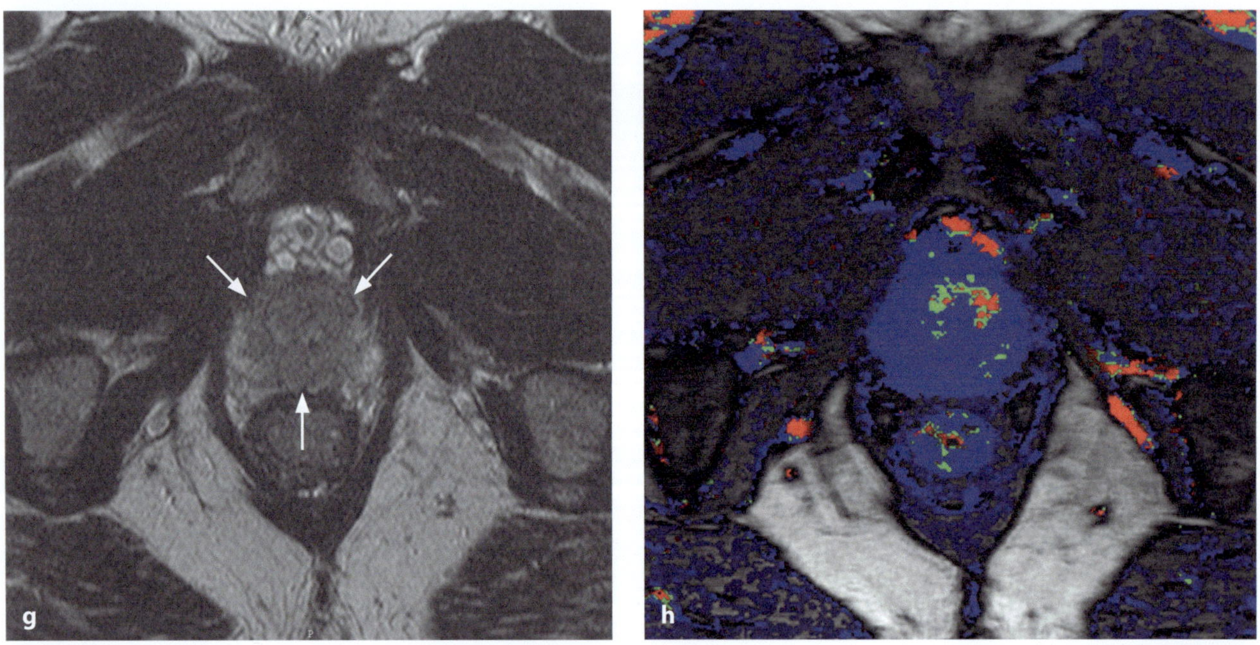

Fig. 1.2 g, h Midgland pelvic veins/signal voids with vascular flows. Note central benign hypertrophy with mainly blue background

Fig. 1.2 i, j

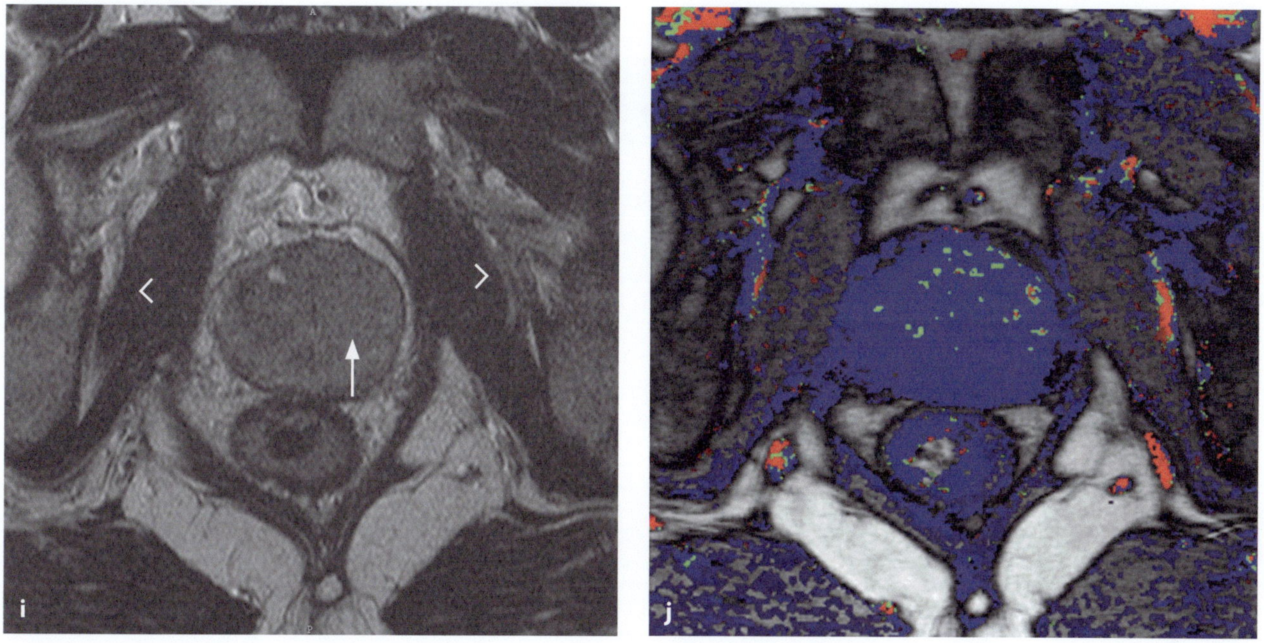

Fig. 1.2 i, j Levator sling veins/signal voids with vascular flows/note diffuse vascular flow in hypertrophic areas demonstrated

Fig. 1.2 k, l

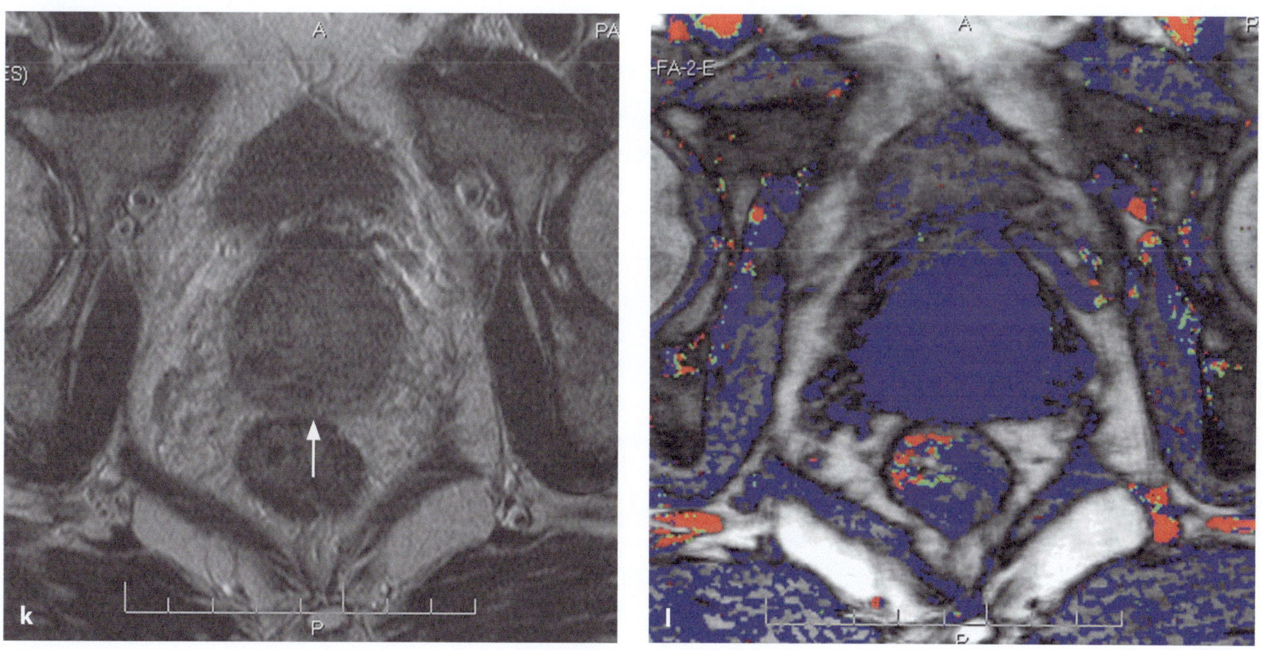

Fig. 1.2 k, l Base peripheral zone thinned by avascular central hypertrophy/note symmetric vascular pattern

Fig. 1.3 a–f

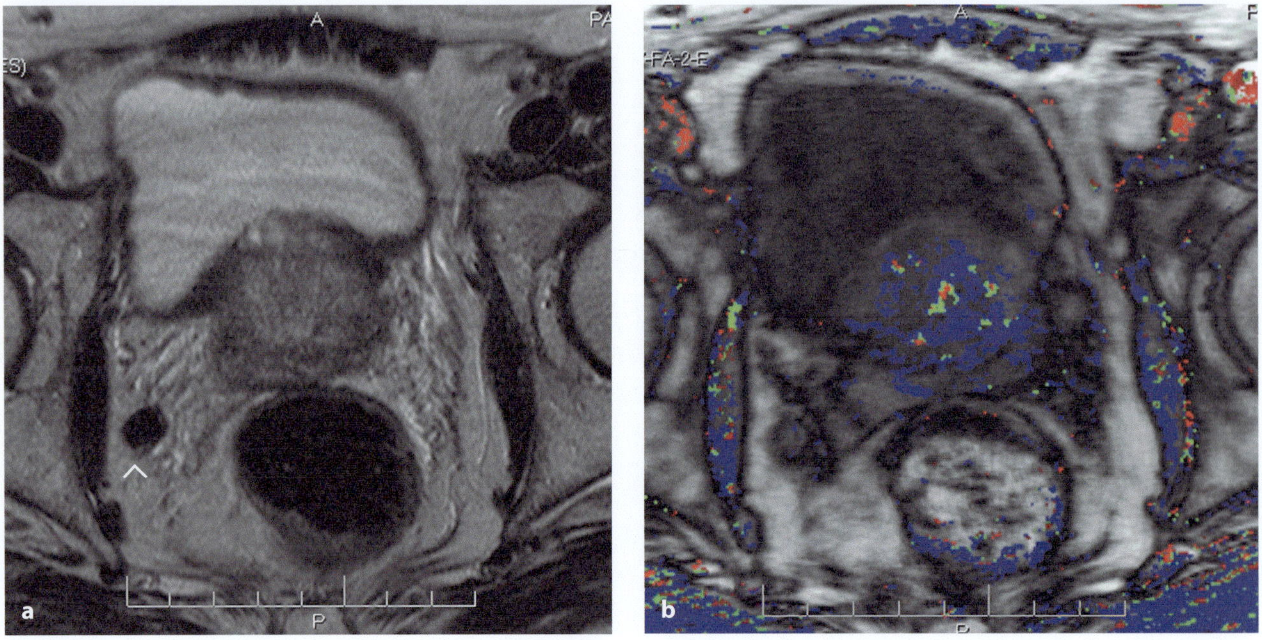

Fig. 1.3 a, b Phlebolith/right rounded avascular focus lateral to seminal vesicle without vascular flow

Fig. 1.3 c, d

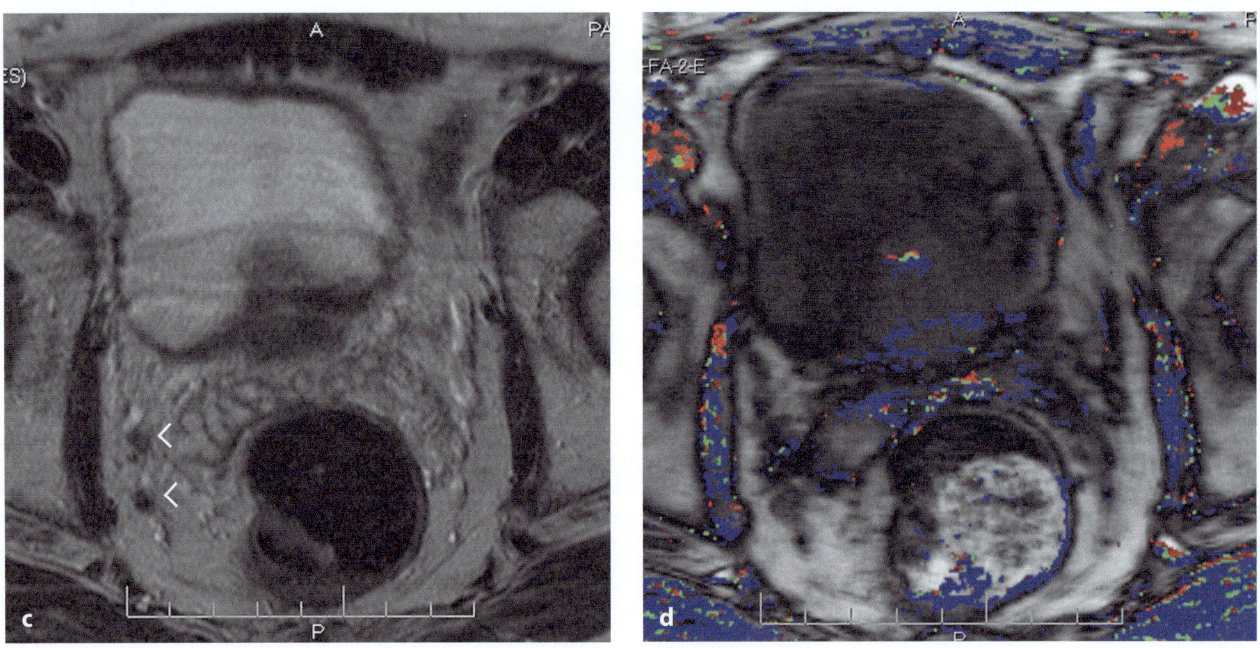

Fig. 1.3 c, d Phleboliths/two smaller black regions without vascular flows

Fig. 1.3 e, ff

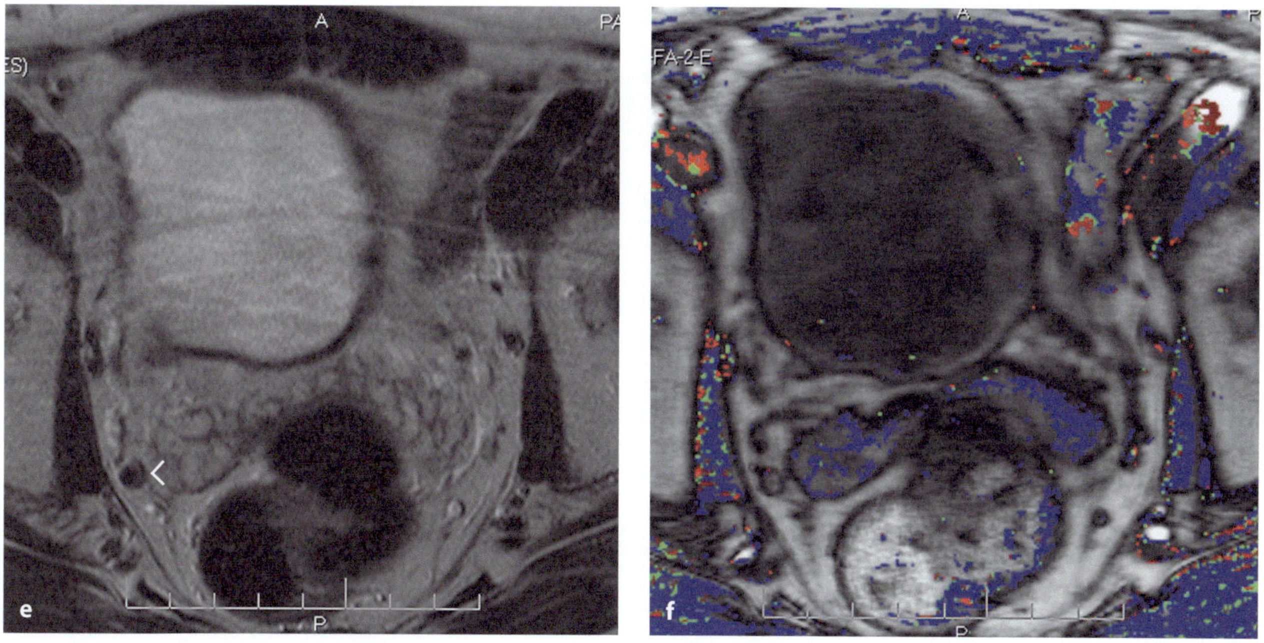

Fig. 1.3 e, f Phlebolith/ right side with trace vascular flow

Fig. 1.4 a, b

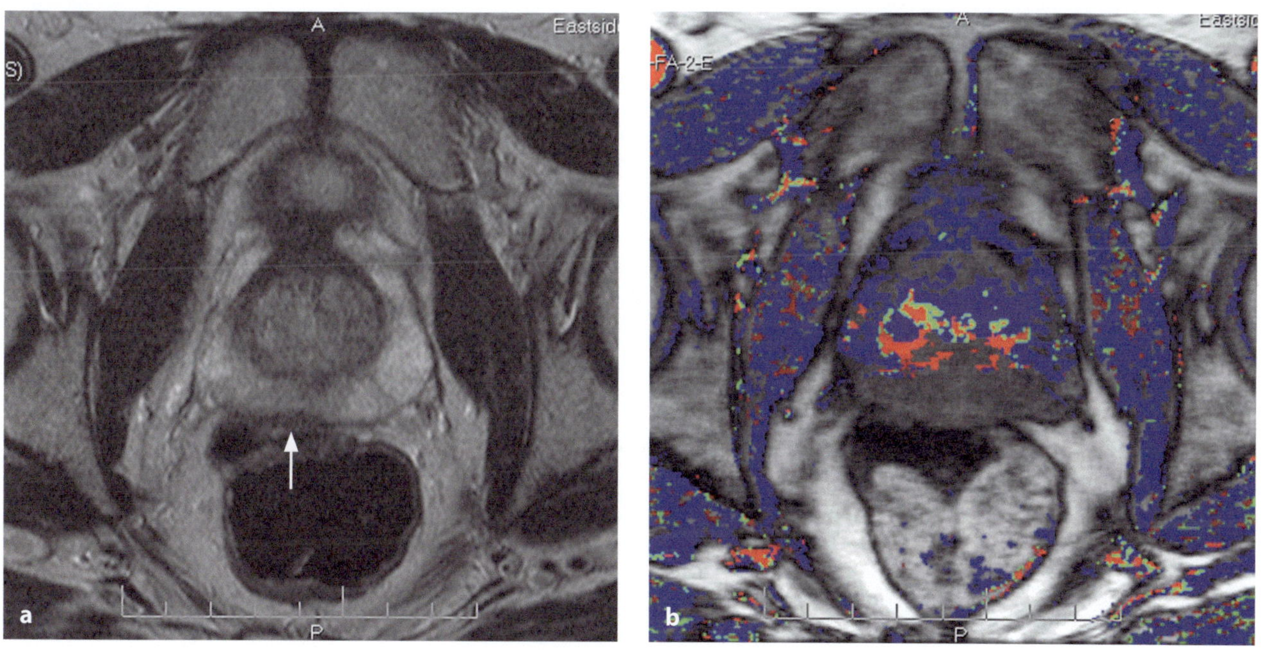

Fig. 1.4 a, b Artifactual flow void posterior midgland due to fibrosis and atrophy secondary to multiple previous biopsies

Fig. 1.5 a, b

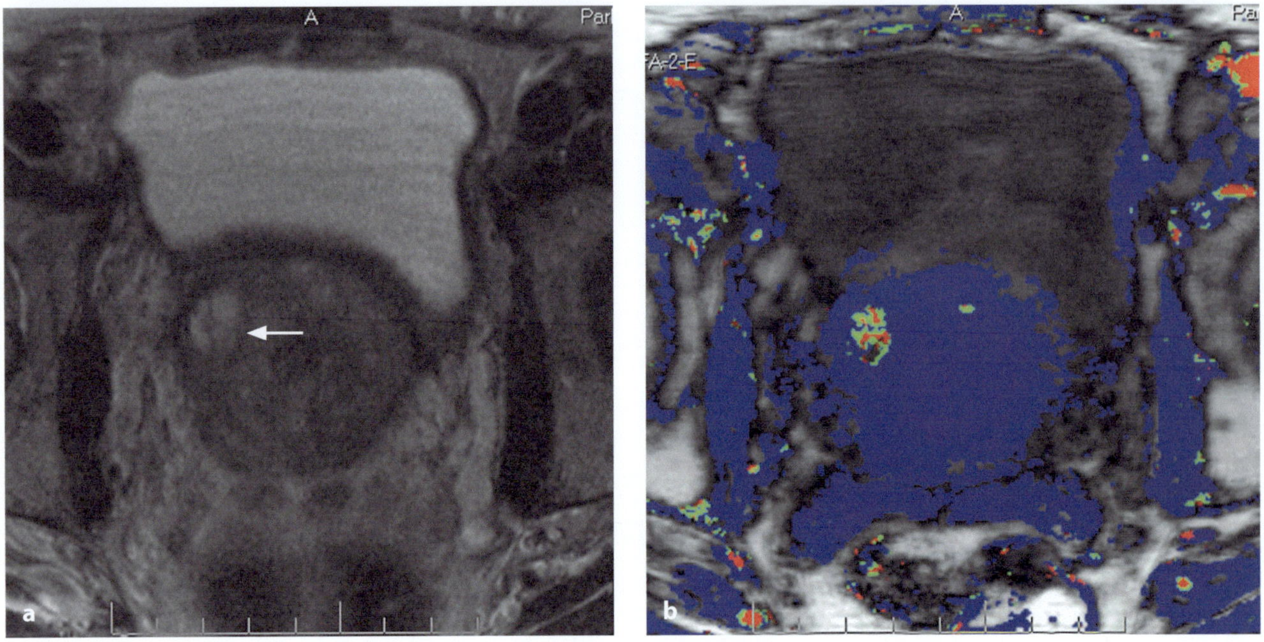

Fig. 1.5 a, b Right anterior base focal benign prostatic hypertrophic (BPH) nodule simulating tumor

Fig. 1.6 a, b

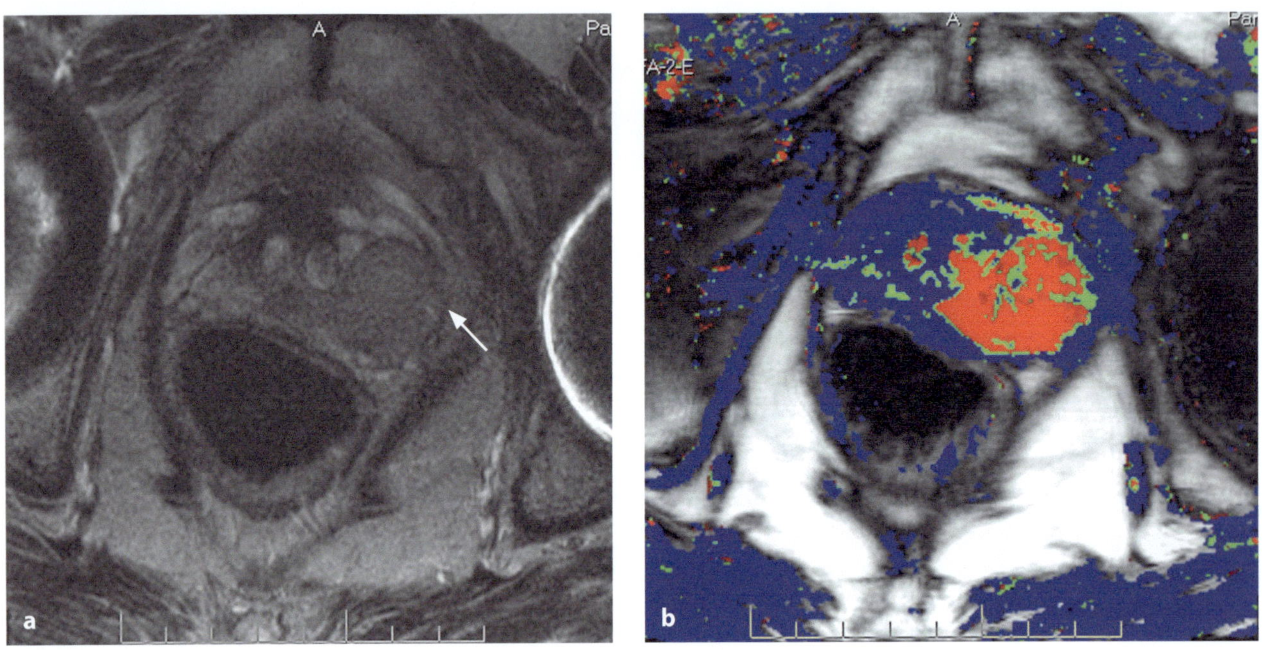

Fig. 1.6 a, b Left midgland BPH nodule simulating tumor by pushing through peripheral zone-noted intact capsule suggesting benignity

Fig. 1.7 a, b

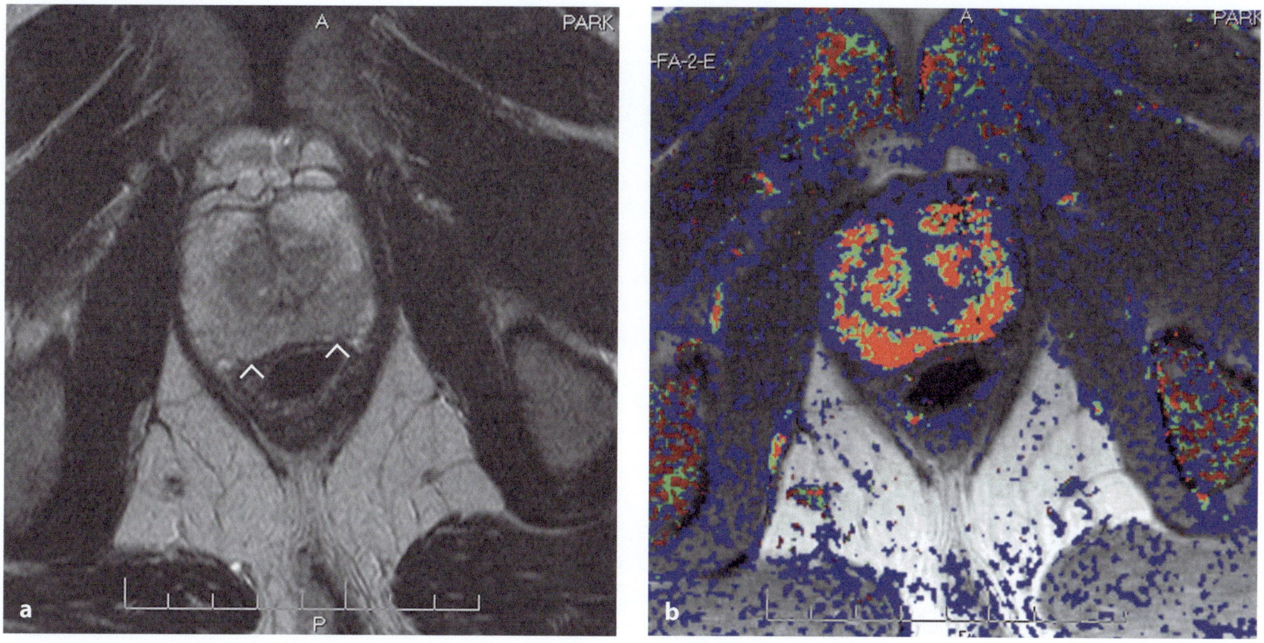

Fig. 1.7 a, b Prostatitis/midgland symmetric hyperemia follows peripheral zone

Fig. 1.8 a–c

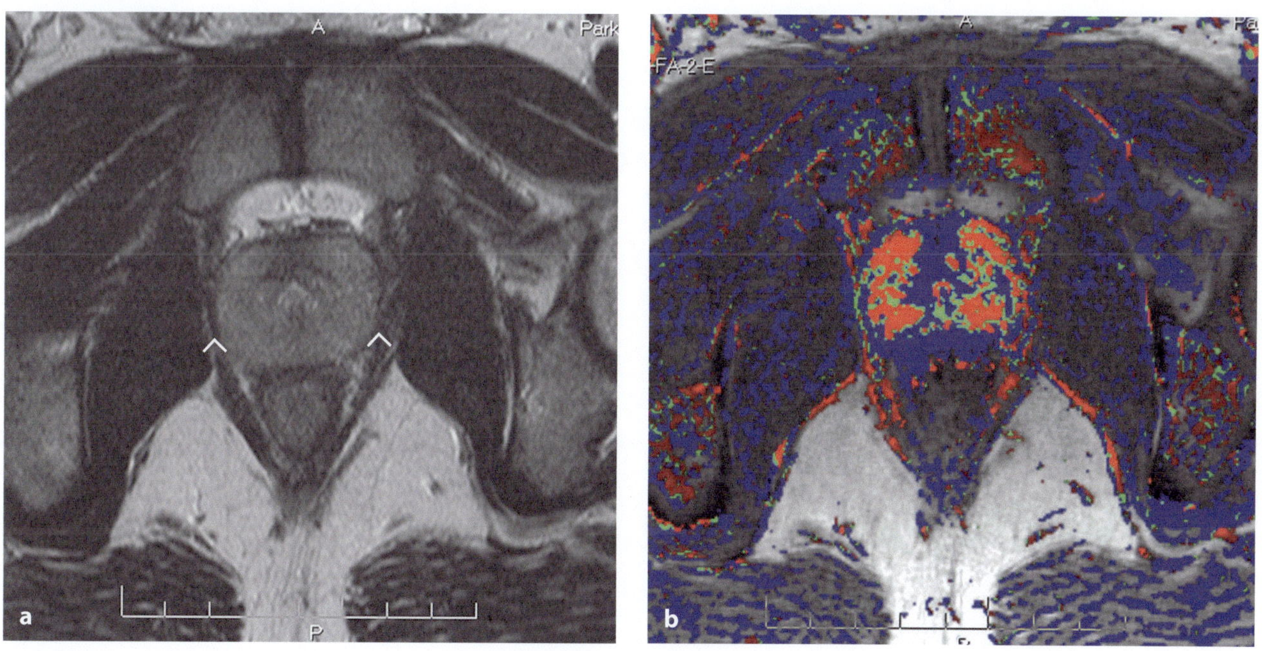

Fig. 1.8 a, b Prostatitis/apex symmetric hyperemia follow peripheral zone

Fig. 1.8 c, d

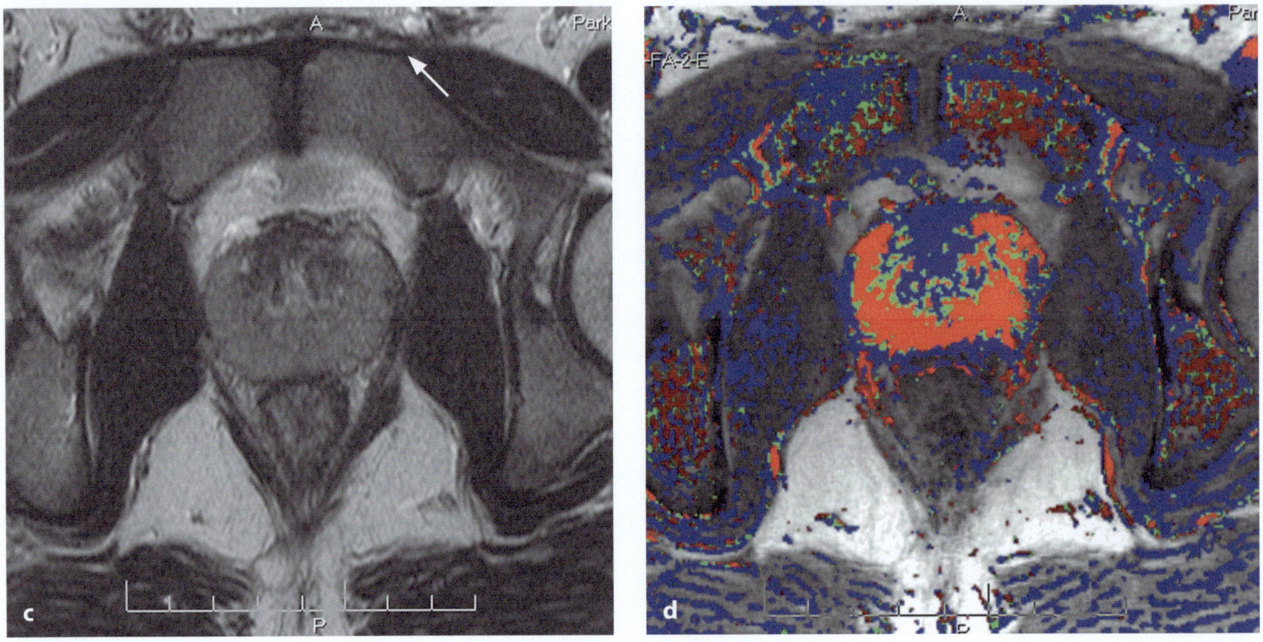

Fig. 1.8 c, d Midgland symmetric hyperemia-note artifactual color in bone due to patient motion-note: boney cortex has no blood vessels thus color in the cortex proves findings are of artifactual nature

Fig. 1.8 e, f

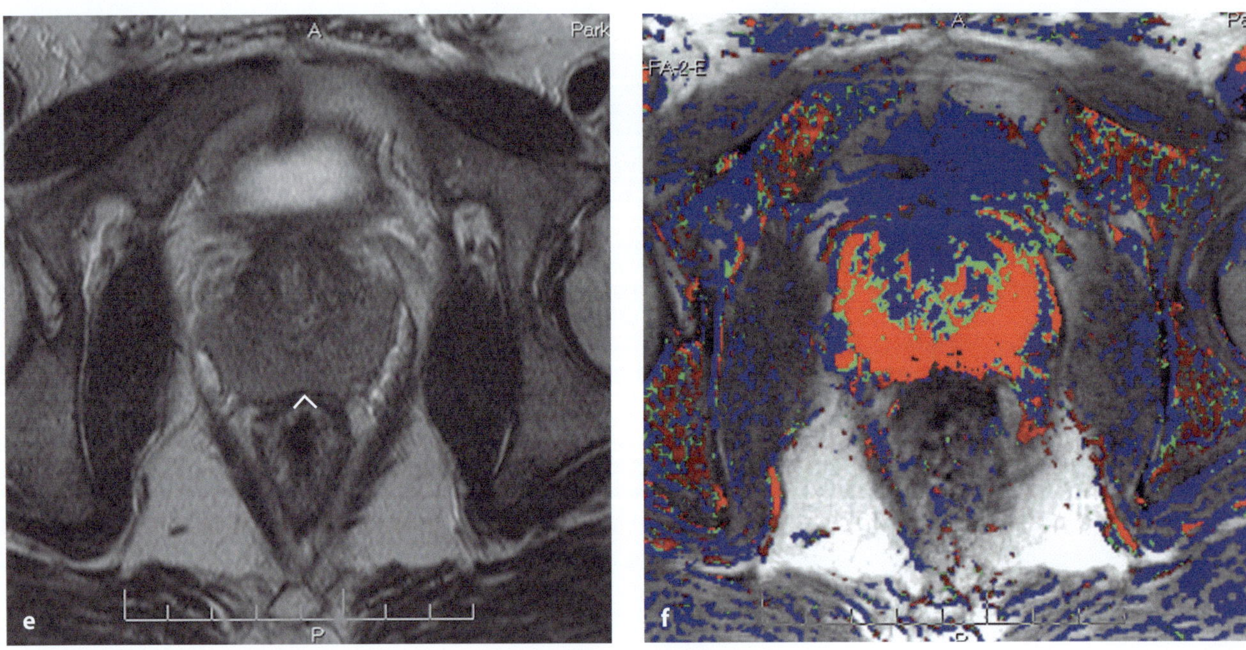

Fig. 1.8 e, f Proximal midgland-symmetric peripheral zone hyperemia

Fig. 1.8 g, h

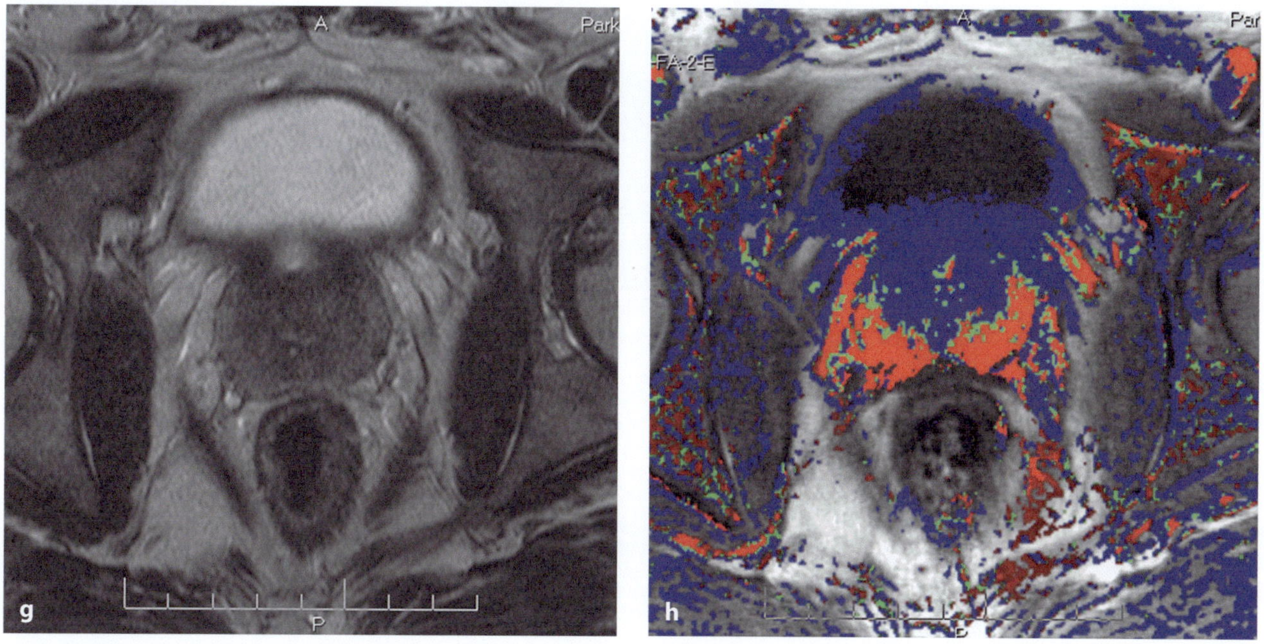

Fig. 1.8 g, h Base-symmetric peripheral zone hyperemia

Fig. 1.9 a, b

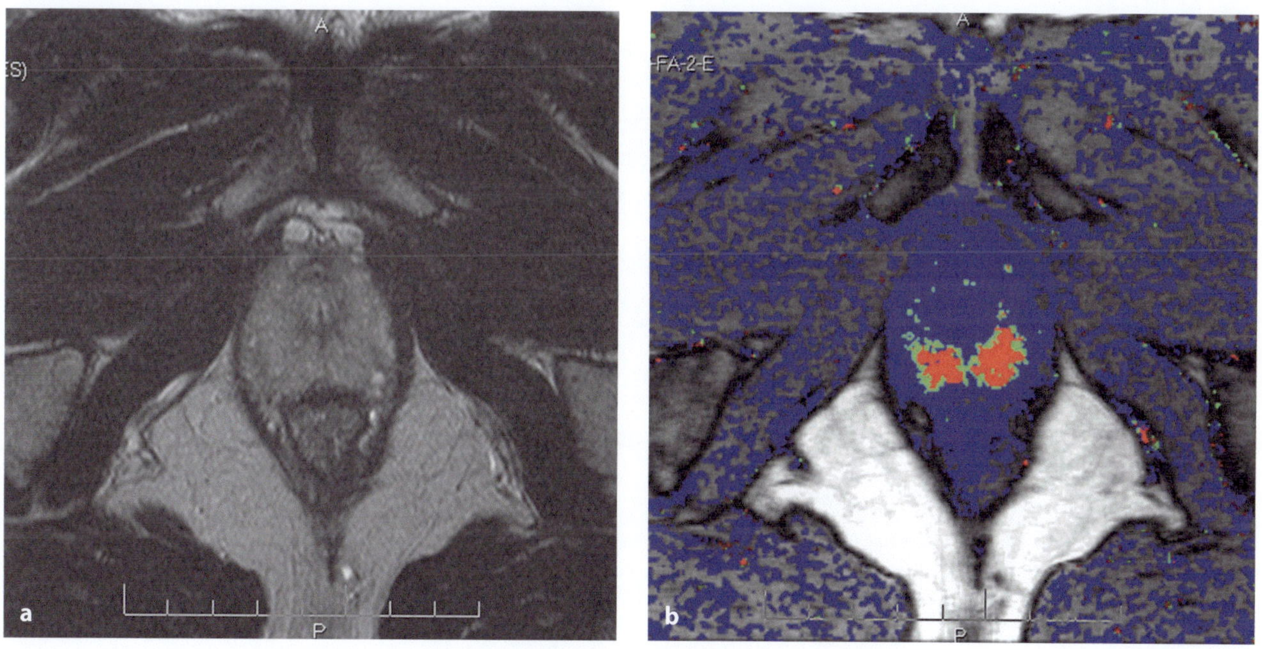

Fig. 1.9 a, b Prostatitis/apex symmetric hyperemia in peripheral zone

Fig. 1.10 a,b

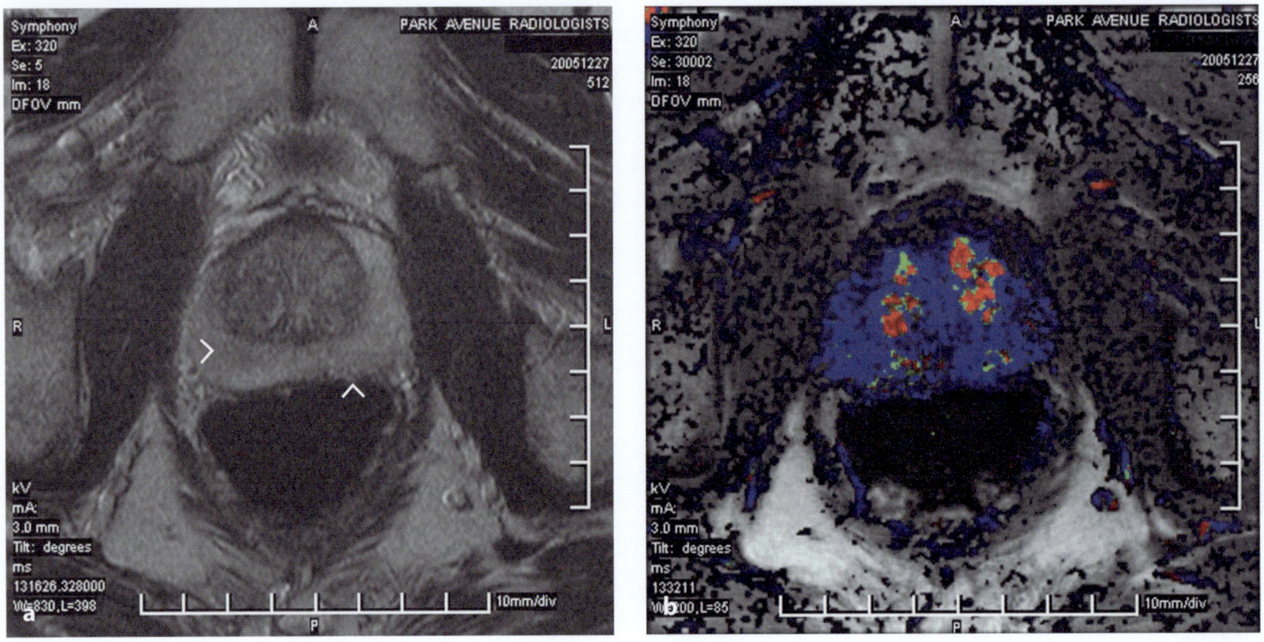

Fig. 1.10 a, b Prostatitis/midgland symmetric central zone hyperemia with trace posterior midgland symmetric peripheral zone hyperemia

Fig. 1.11 a,b

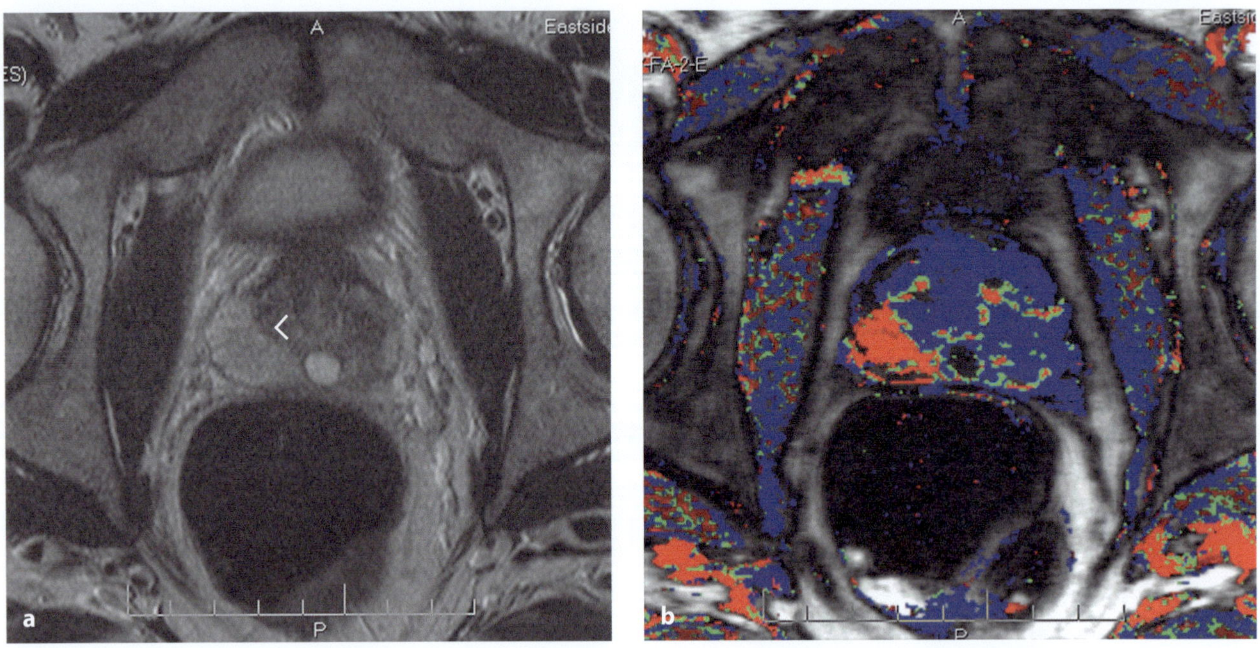

Fig. 1.11 a, b Prostatitis/right midgland inflammation with midline cyst and left sided atrophy and fibrosis

Fig. 1.12 a,b

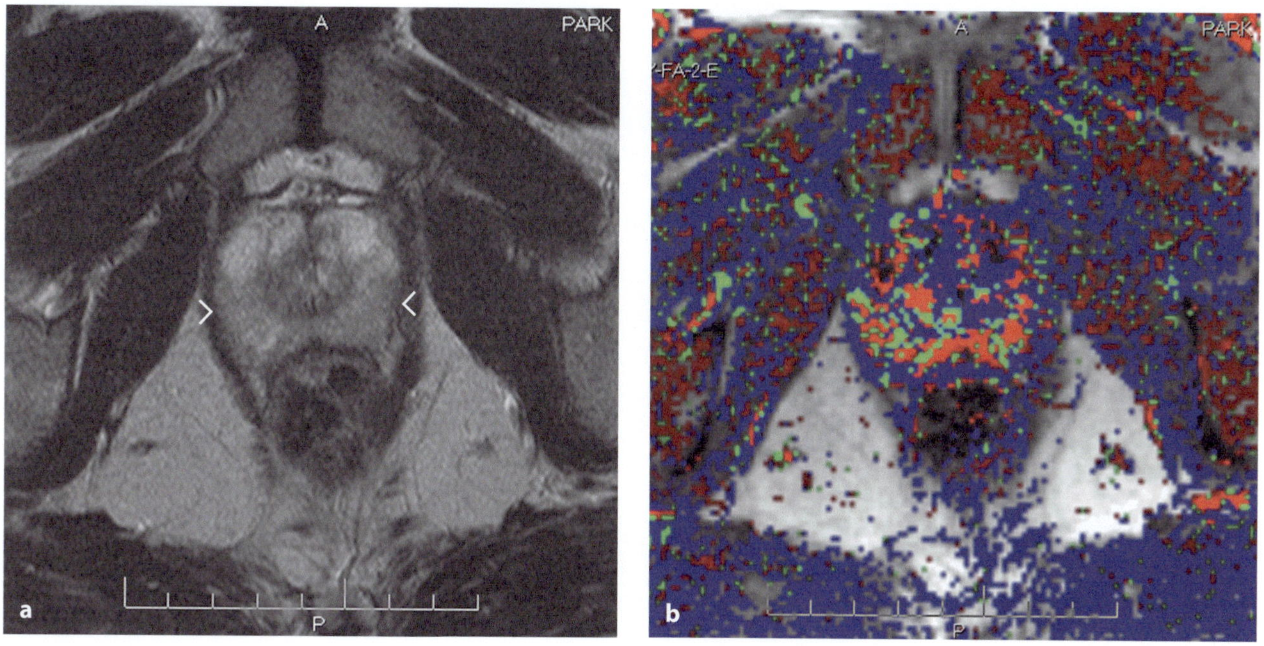

Fig. 1.12 a, b Prostatitis/midgland symmetric hyperemia "butterfly pattern"

Fig. 1.13 a,b

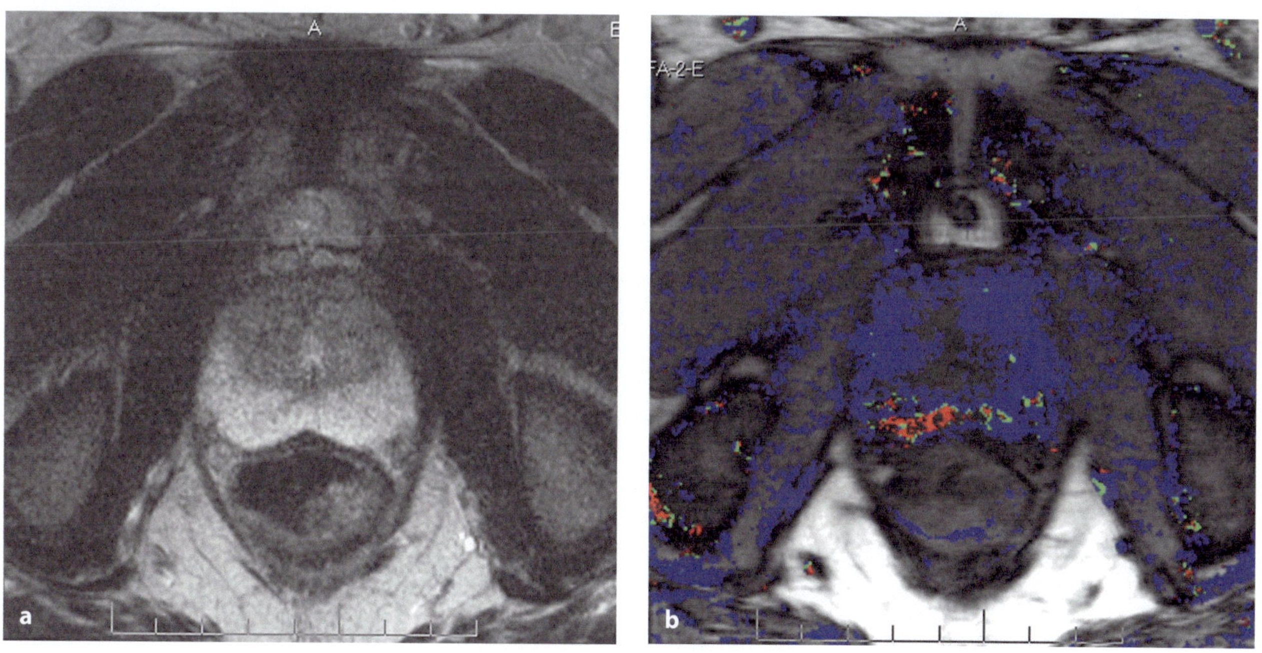

Fig. 1.13 a, b Prostatitis/asymmetric right midgland discoid hyperemia

Fig. 1.14 a–h

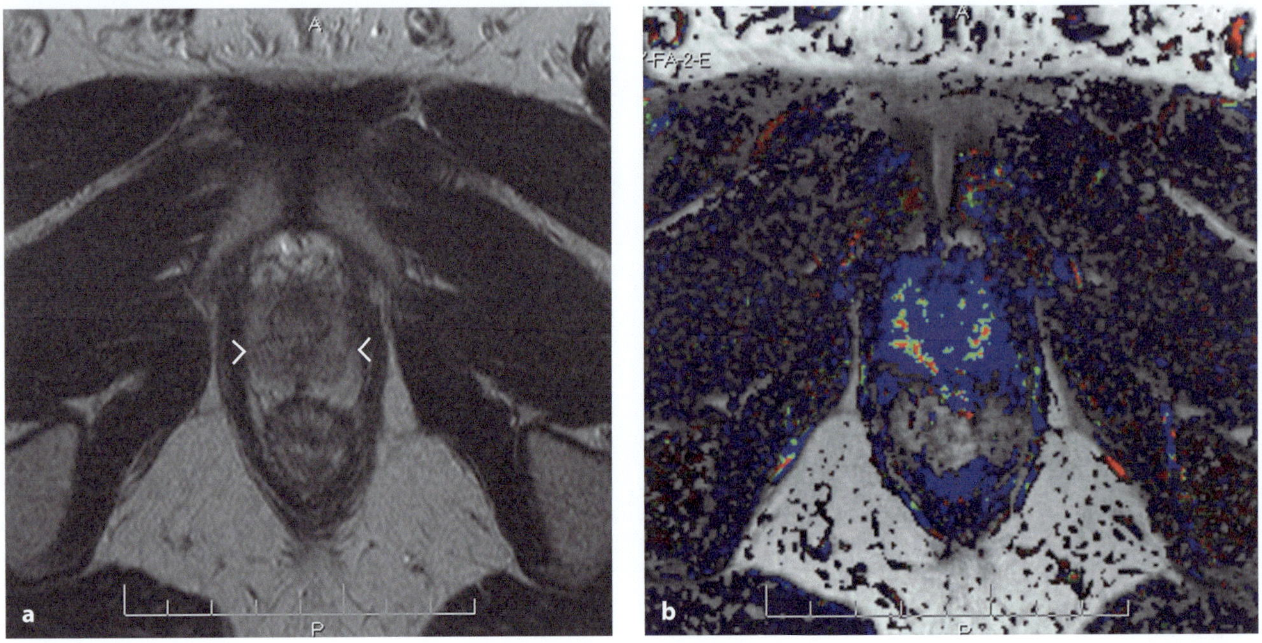

Fig. 1.14 a, b Prostatitis/apex symmetric hyperemia

Fig. 1.14 c, d

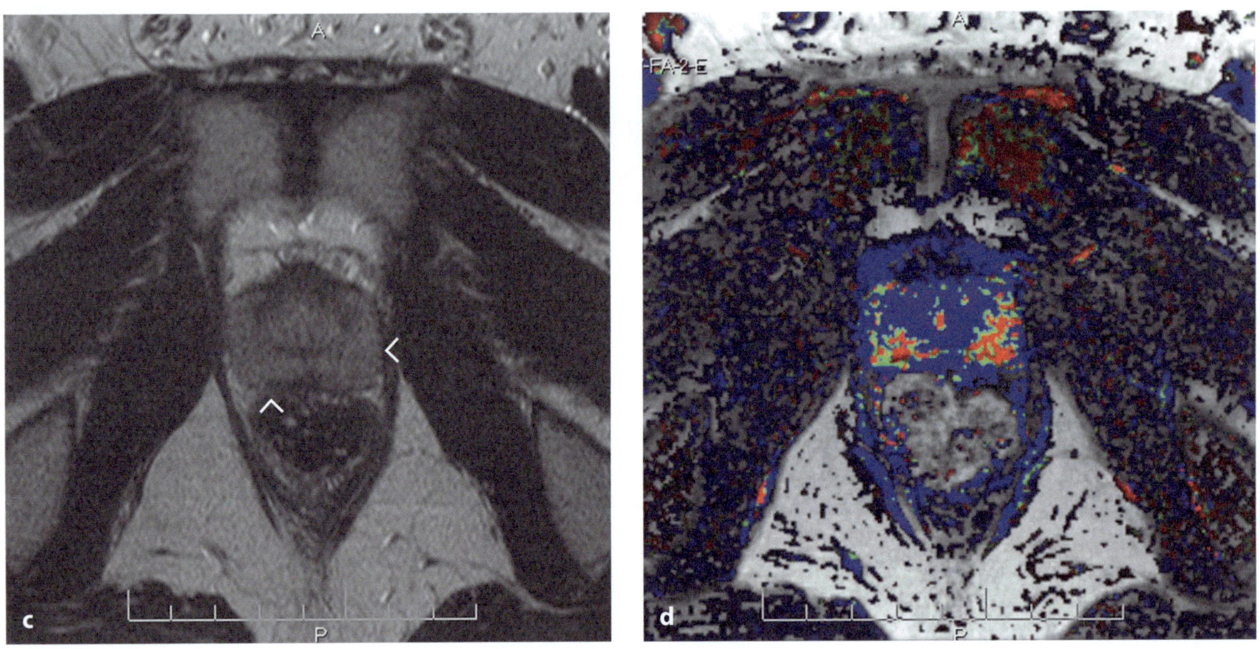

Fig. 1.14 c, d Extending to midgland with symmetric hyperemia

Fig. 1.14 e,f

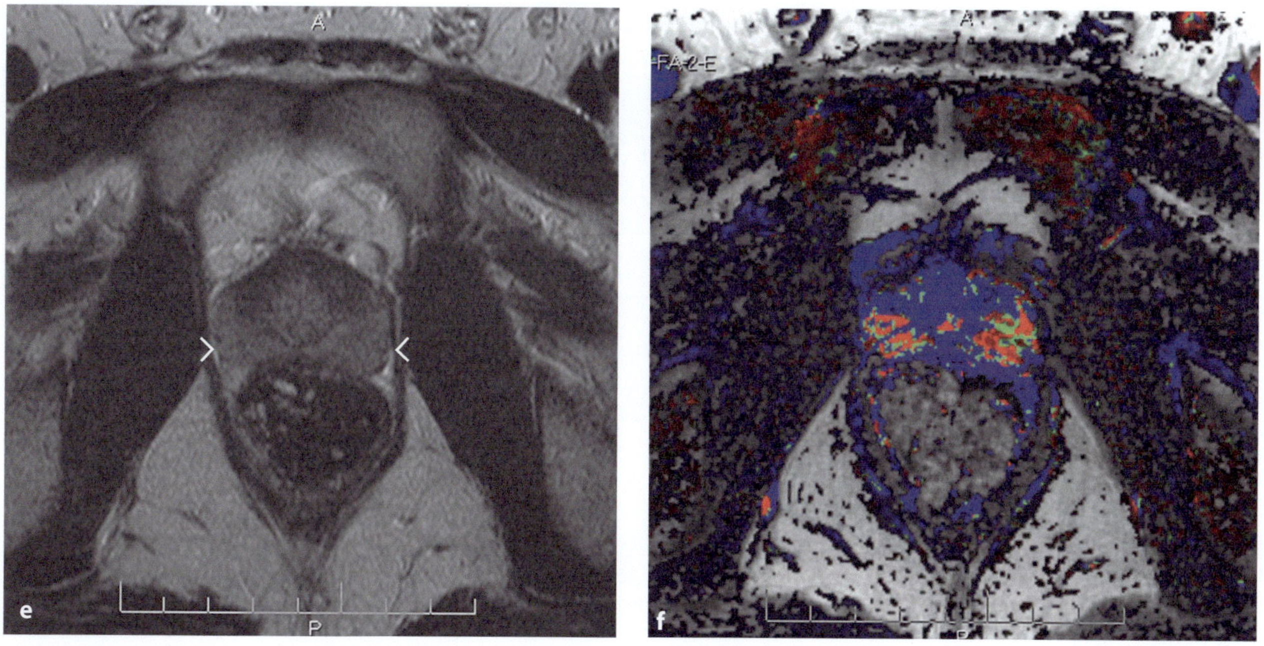

Fig. 1.14 e, f Extending to base with symmetric hyperemia

Fig. 1.14 g, h

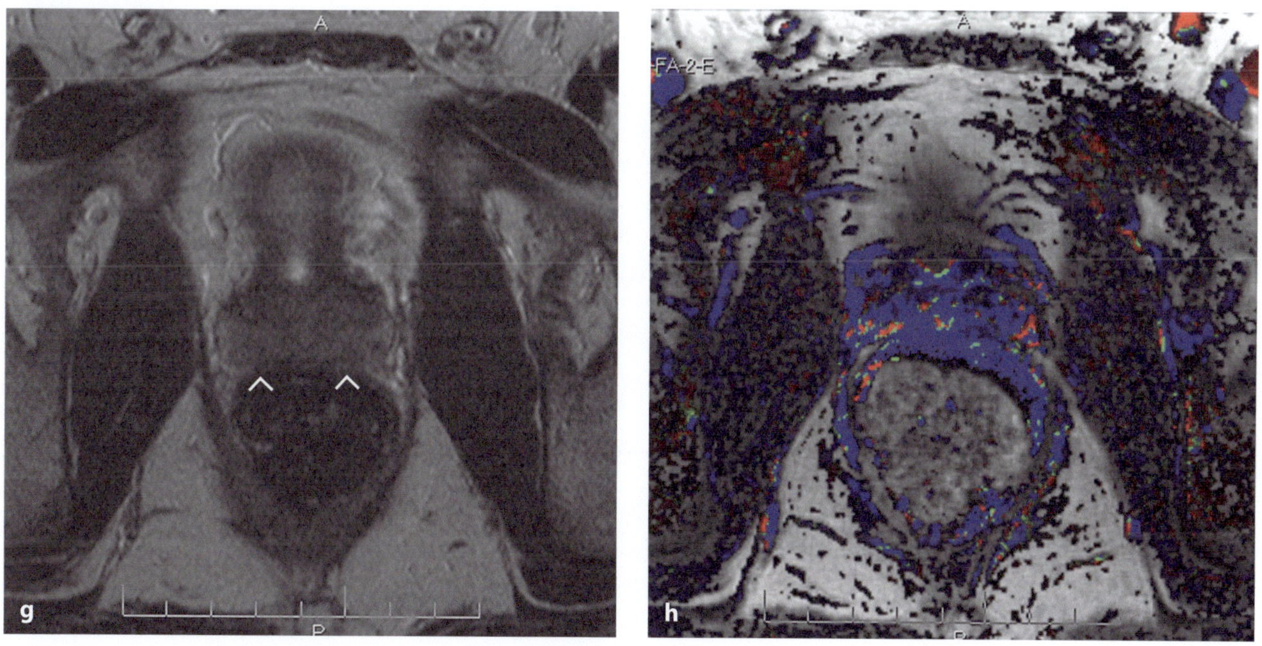

Fig. 1.14 g, h Extending to seminal vesicles with patchy hyperemia

Fig. 1.15 a, b

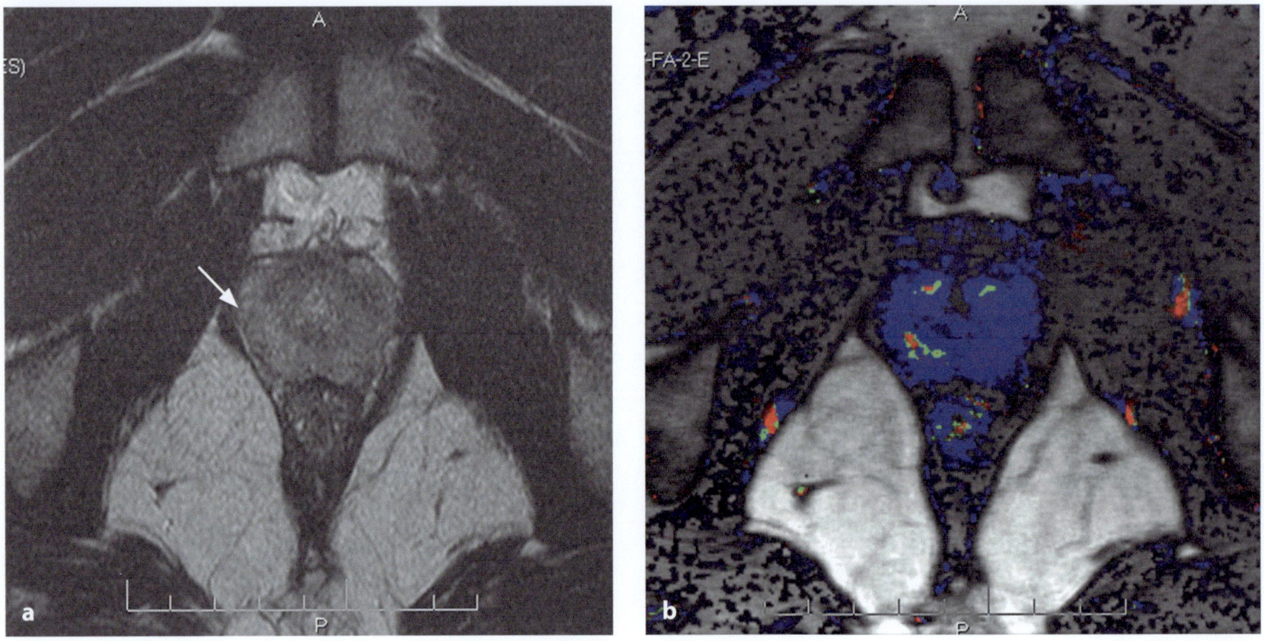

Fig. 1.15 a, b Sarcoid/asymmetric right midgland hyperemia

Fig. 1.16 a, b

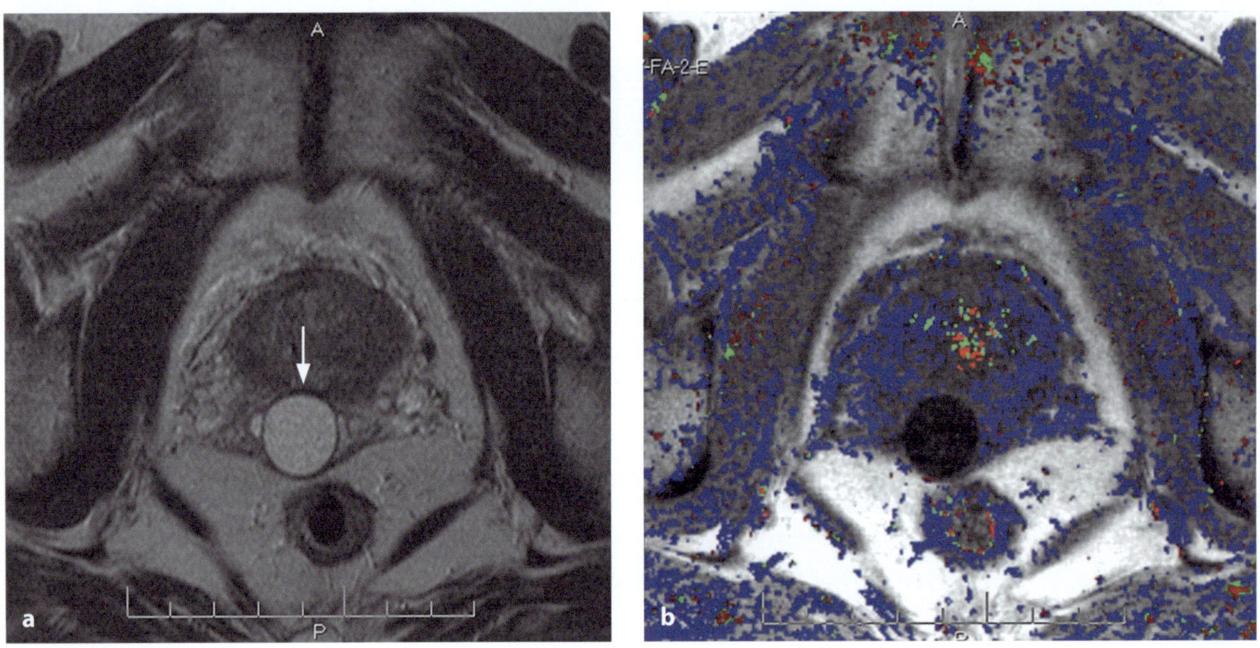

Fig. 1.16 a, b Congenital cyst/midline base avascular region

Chapter

Intraprostatic Cancers

2

Peripheral zone cancer often appears as focal low signal (dark) areas on T2 weighted images although a significant percentage appear homogeneous within the gland and are only imaged by DCE-MRI.

Central and anterior tumors are harder to detect on T2 weighted images and most often appear as darker homogeneous regions of signal loss.

Fig. 2.1 a, b

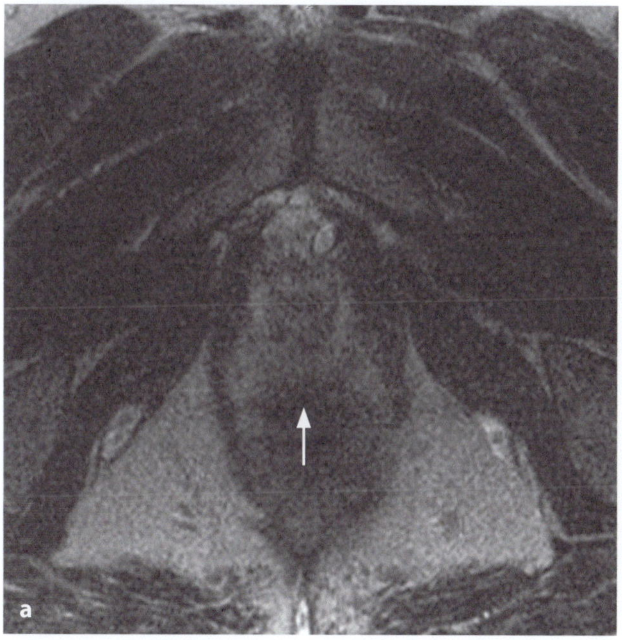

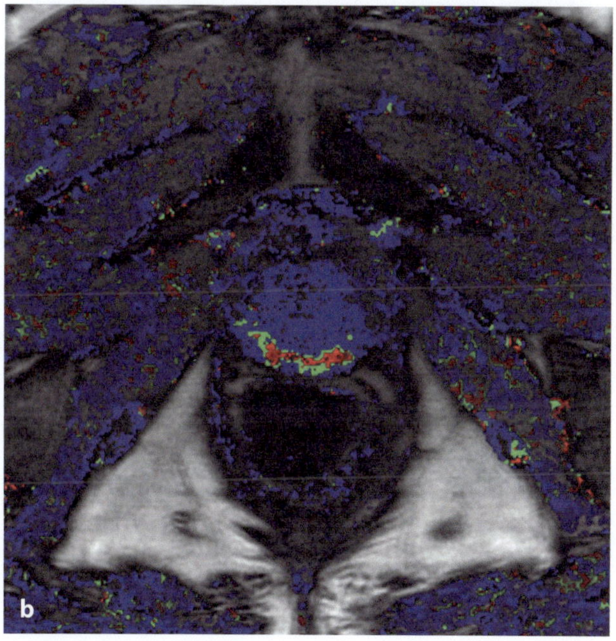

Fig. 2.1a, b Apical posterior linear lesion

Fig. 2.2 a, b

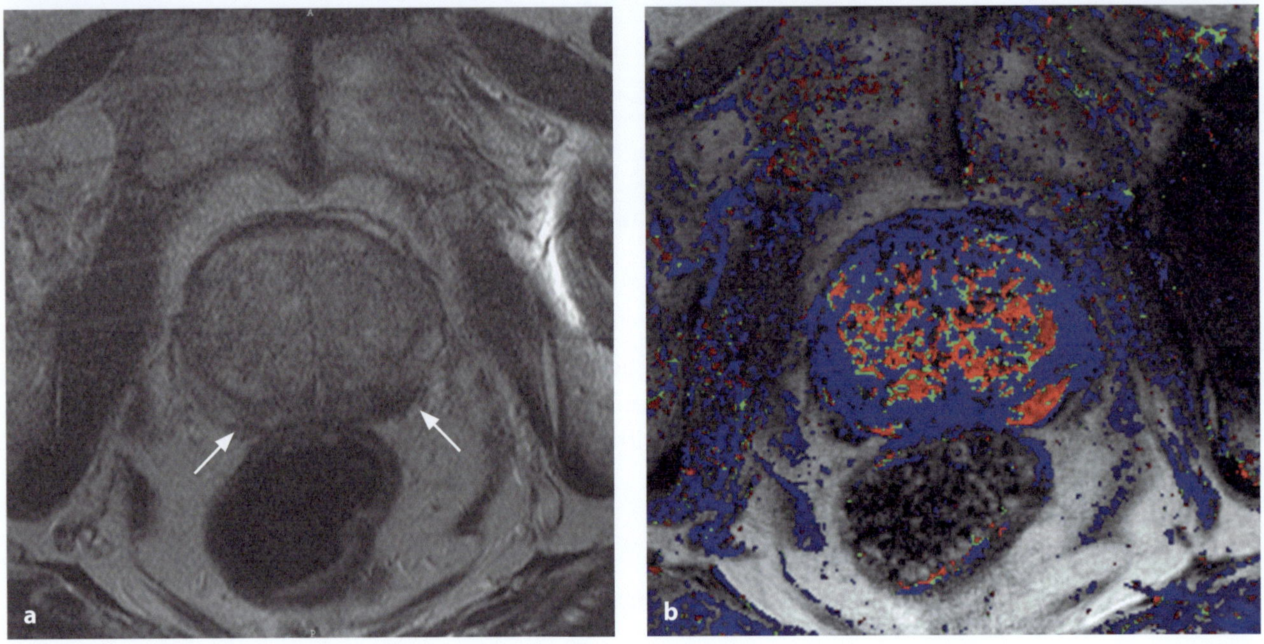

Fig. 2.2a, b Midgland right/left lateral posterior linear lesions

Fig. 2.3 a, b

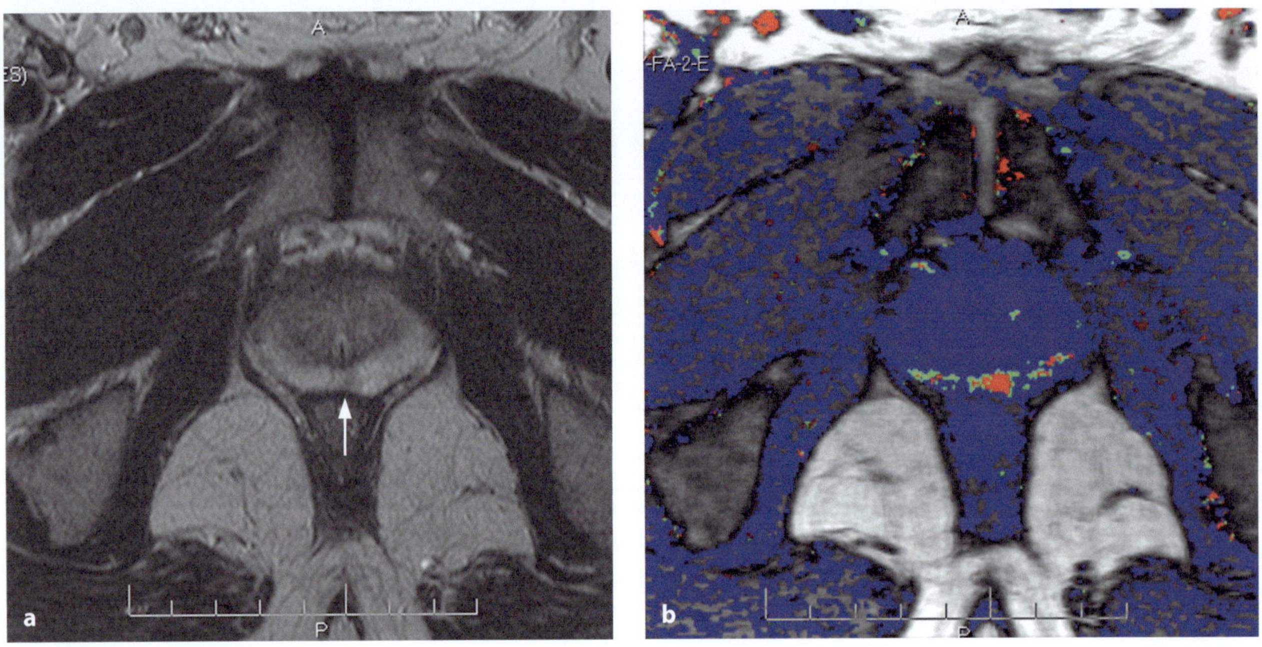

Fig. 2.3 a, b Apical posterior linear lesion

Fig. 2.4 a, b

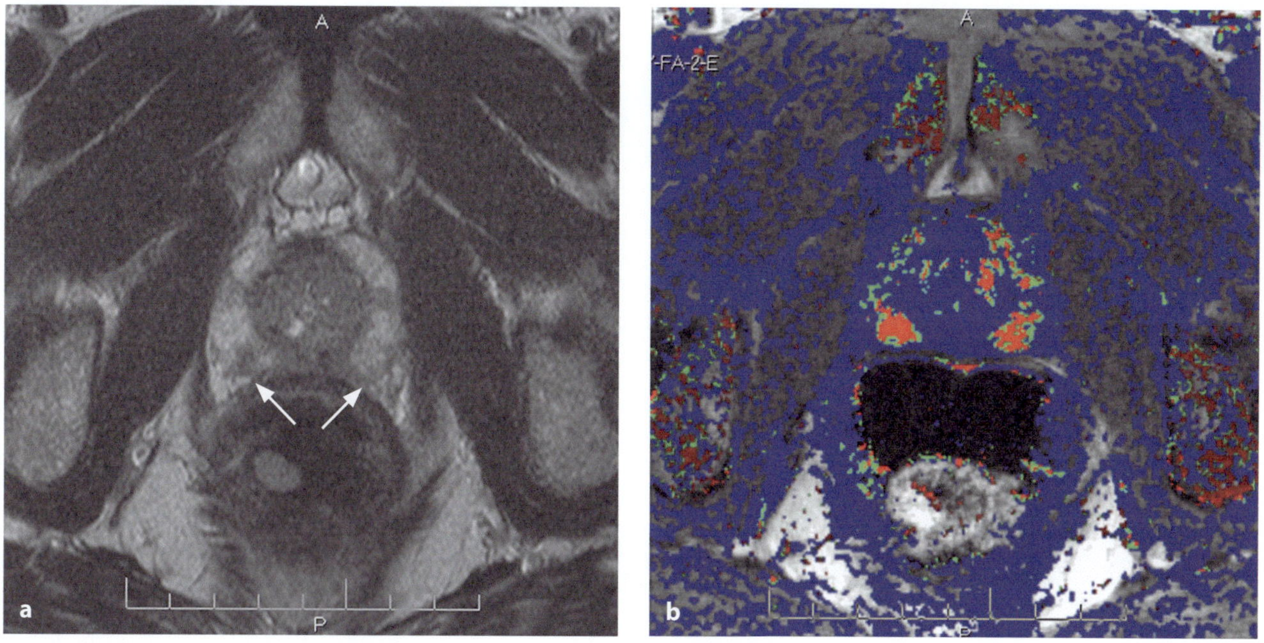

Fig. 2.4 a, b Midgland right and left posterior and left anterior focal lesions

Fig. 2.5 a, b

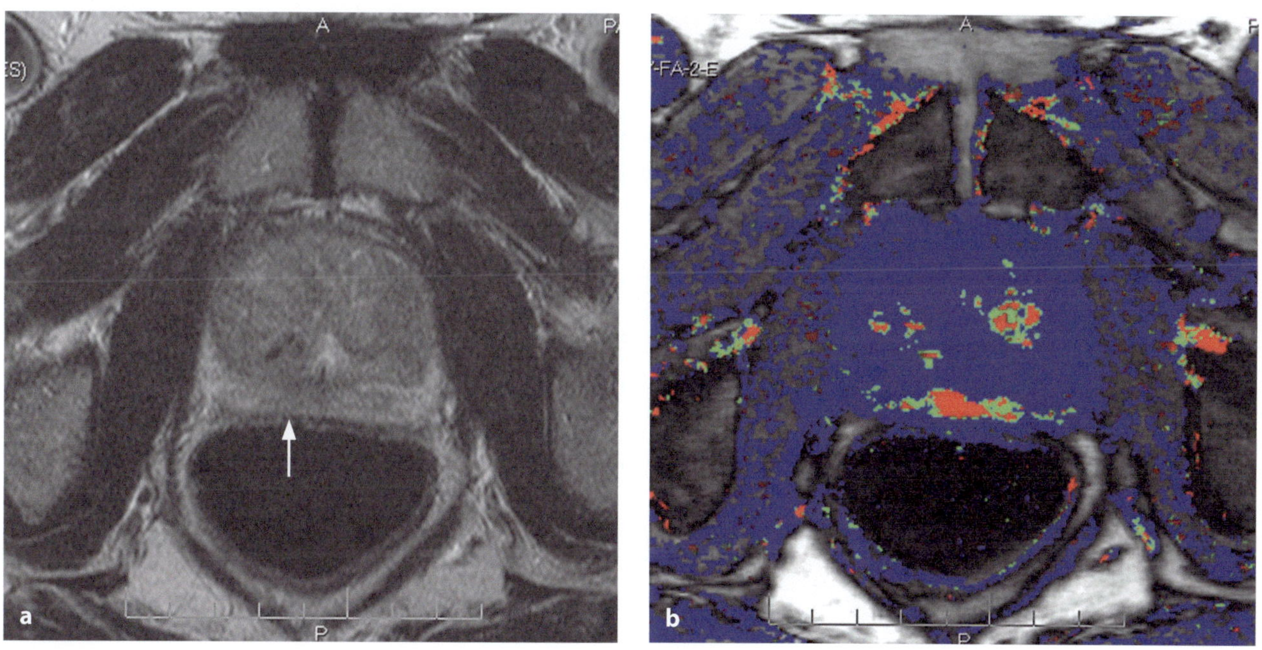

Fig. 2.5 a, b Midgland posterior focal lesion

Fig. 2.6 a, b

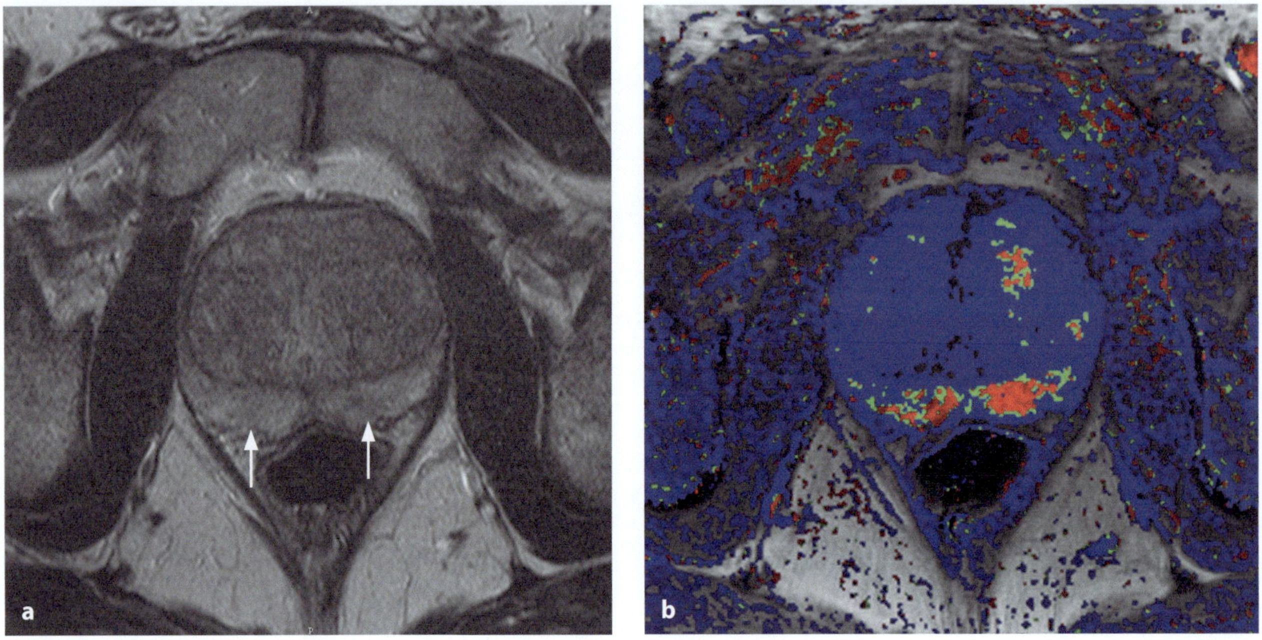

Fig. 2.6 a, b Midgland right and left posterior focal lesions

Fig. 2.7 a, b

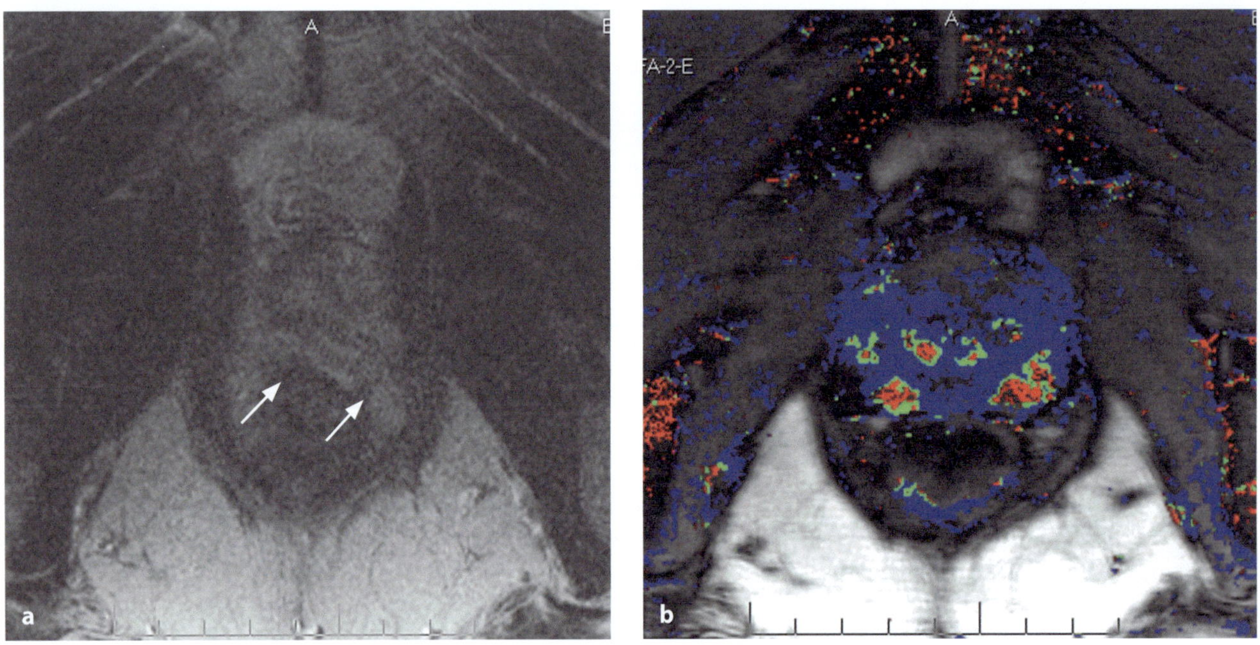

Fig. 2.7 a, b Midgland right and left posterior focal lesions

Fig. 2.8 a, b

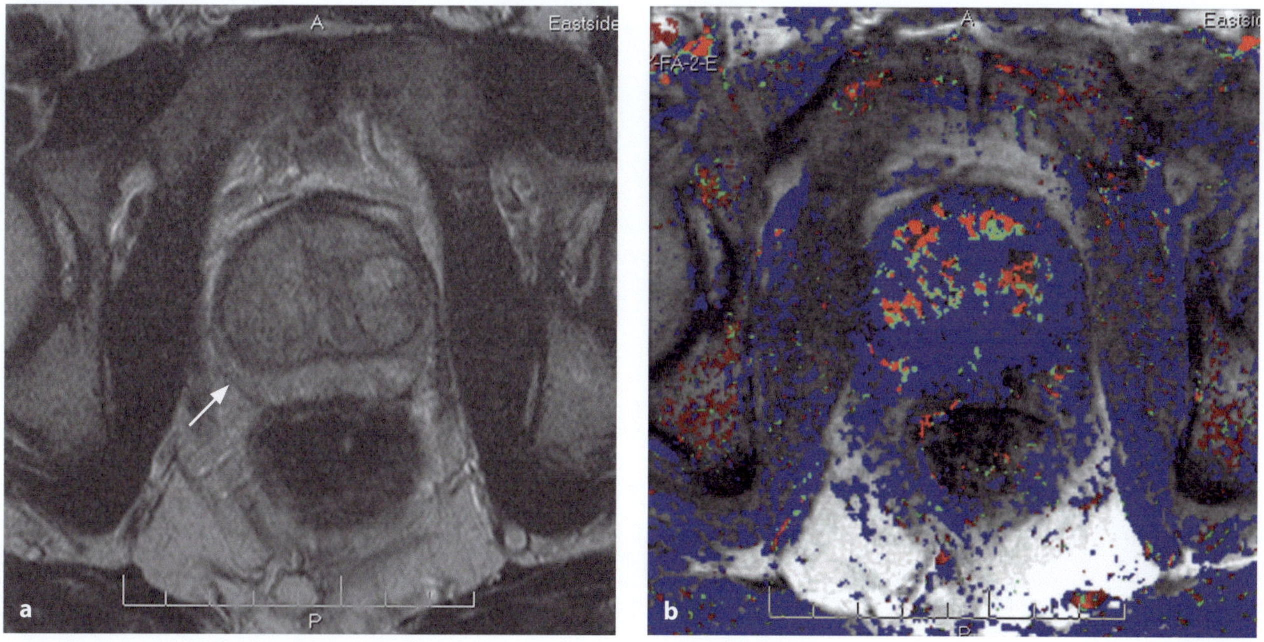

Fig. 2.8 a, b Midgland right lateral diffuse lesion

Fig. 2.9 a, b

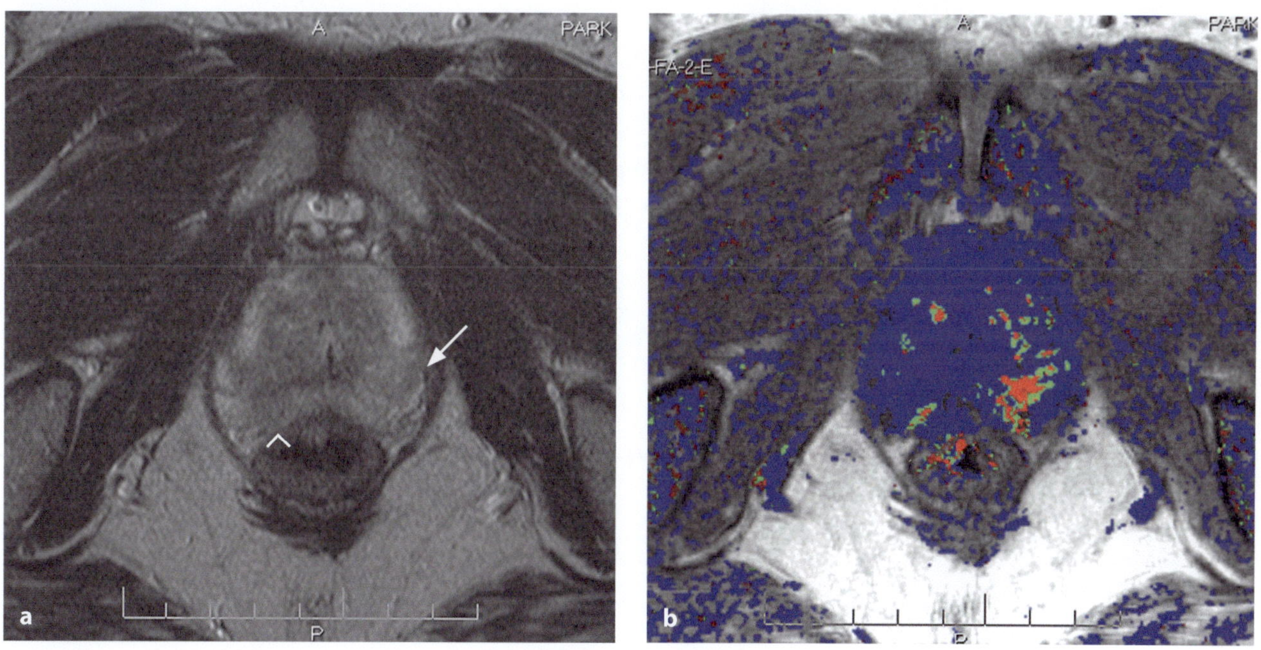

Fig. 2.9 a, b Midgland left focal lesion-note right fibrosis as low signal

Fig. 2.10 a, b

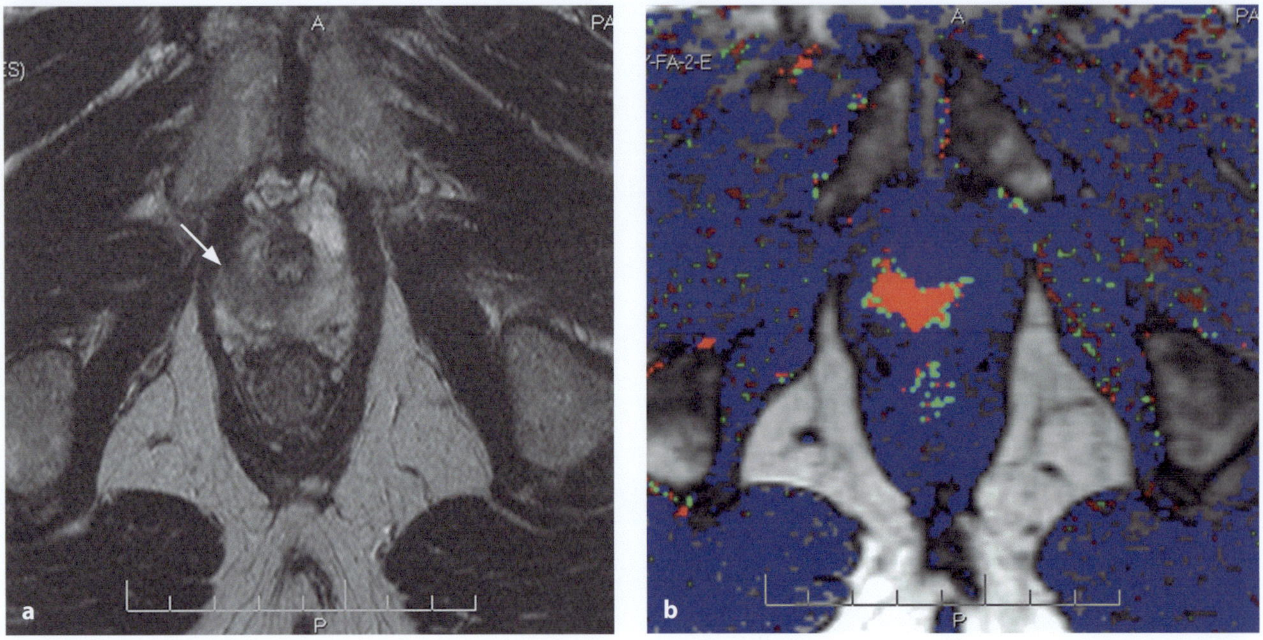

Fig. 2.10 a, b Apical right focal lesion

Fig. 2.11 a, b

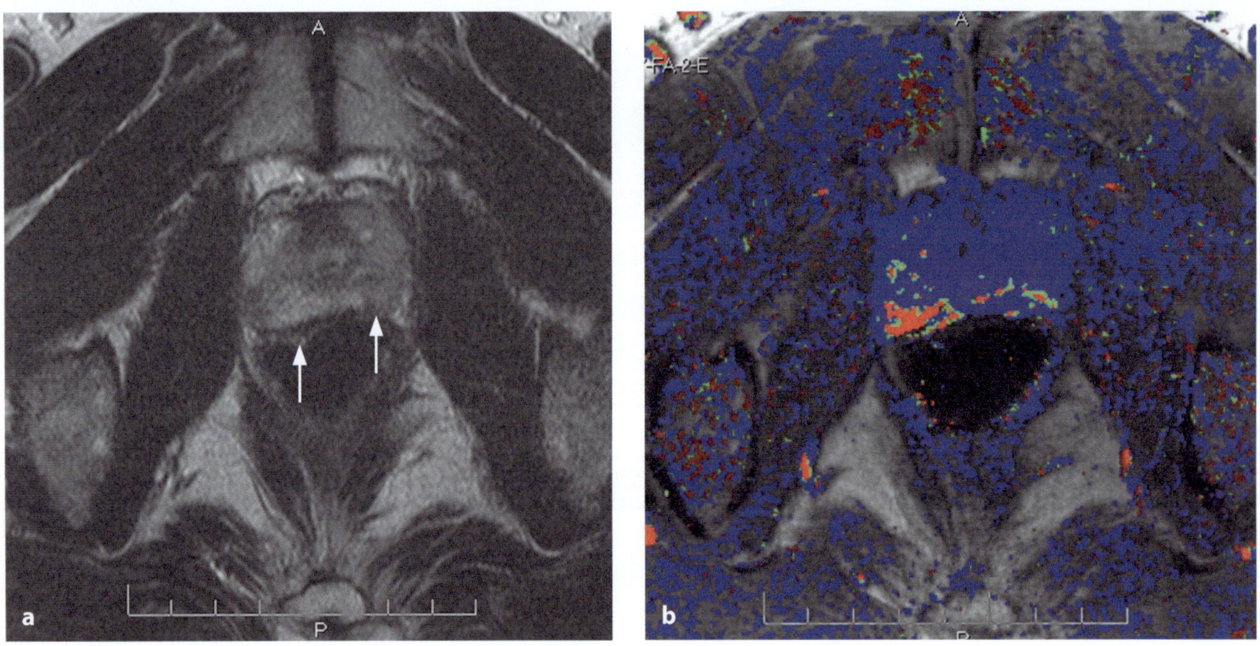

Fig. 2.11 a, b Midgland right and left linear lesions

Fig. 2.12 a, b

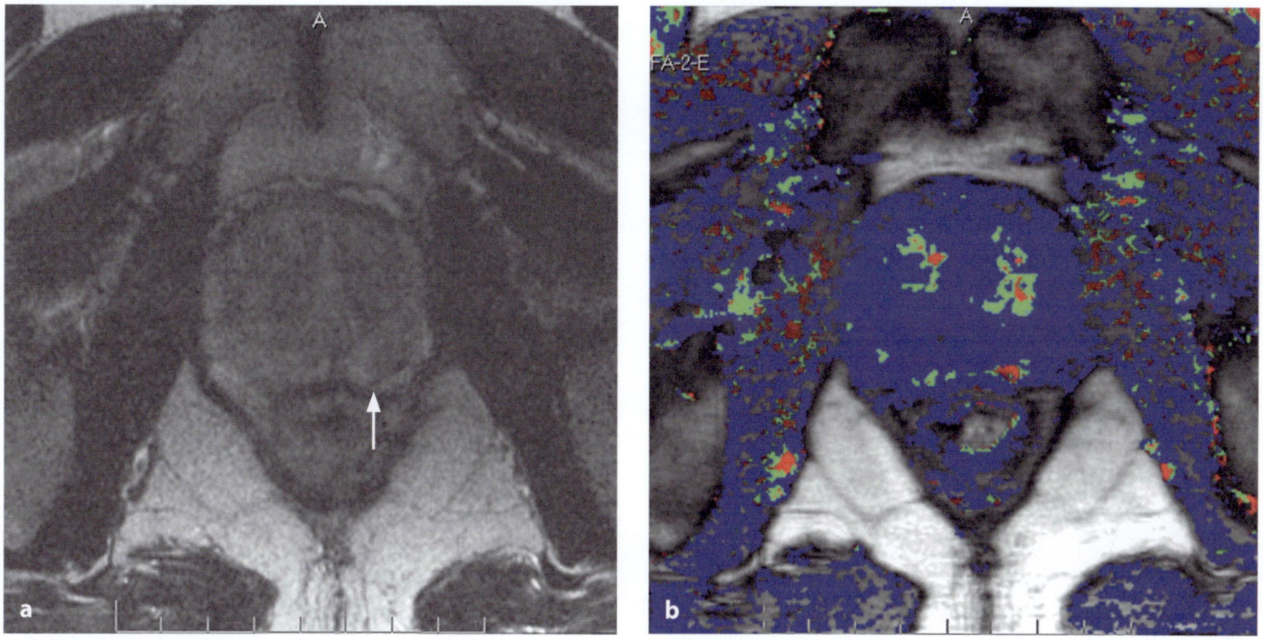

Fig. 2.12 a, b Midgland posterior focal lesion

Fig. 2.13 a, b

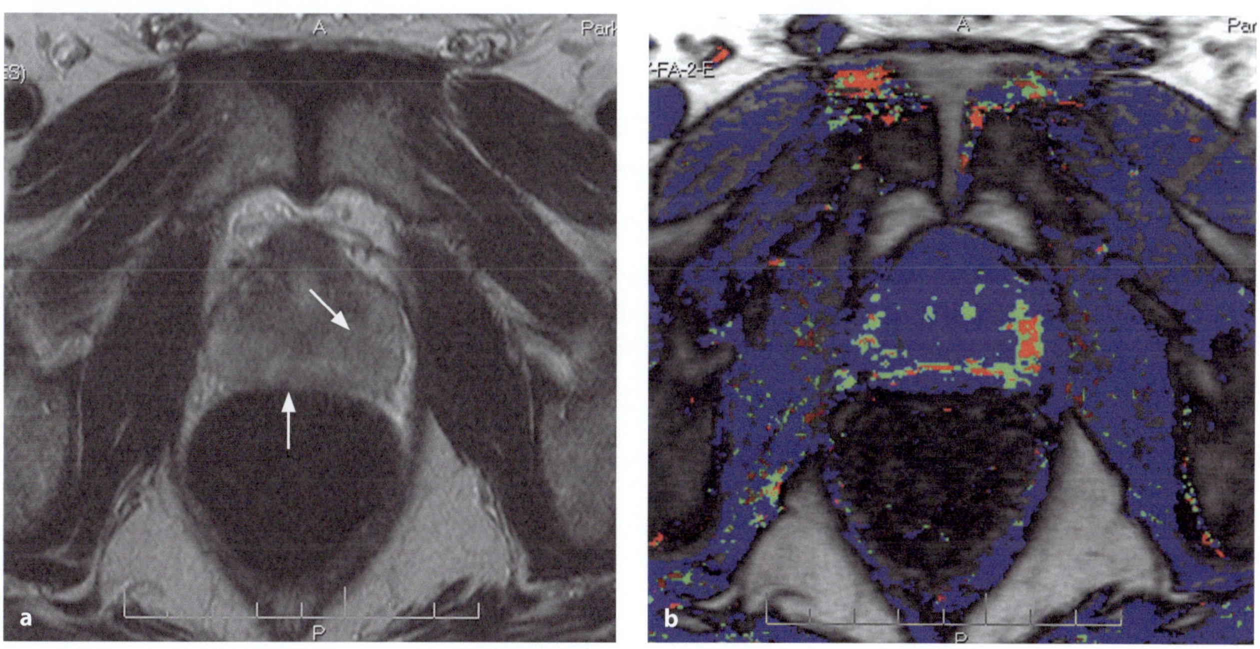

Fig. 2.13 a, b Midgland posterior linear/left lateral focal lesions

Fig. 2.14 a, b

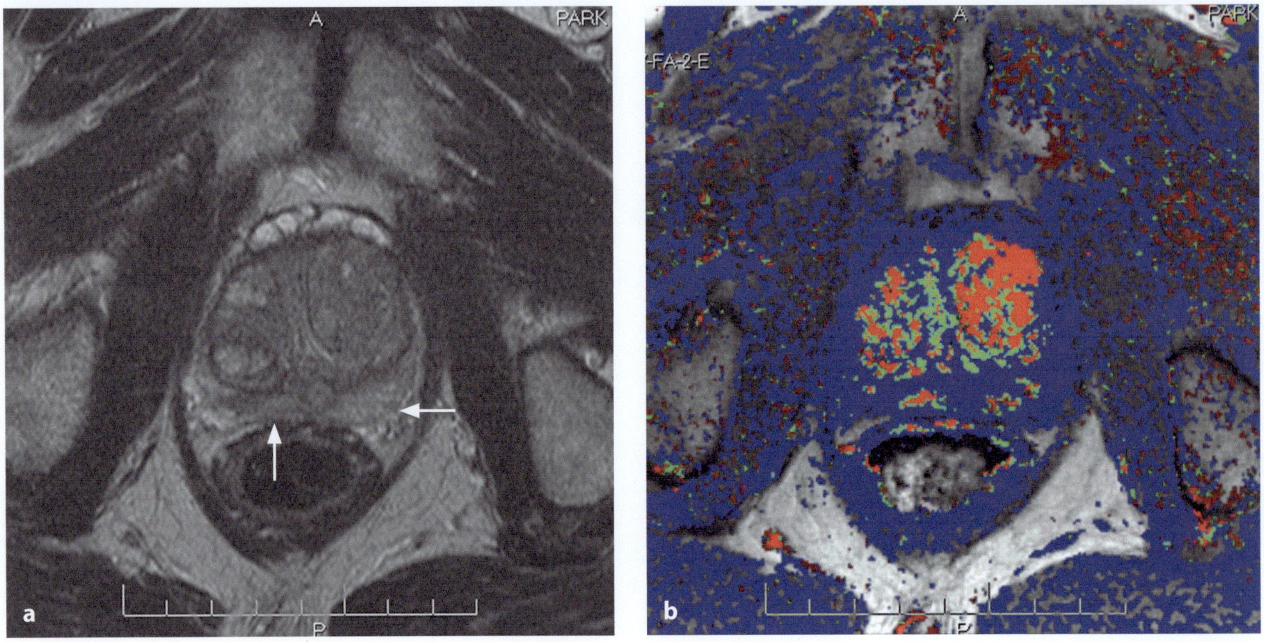

Fig. 2.14 a, b Midgland posterior focal lesions with bilateral fibrosis

Fig. 2.15 a, b

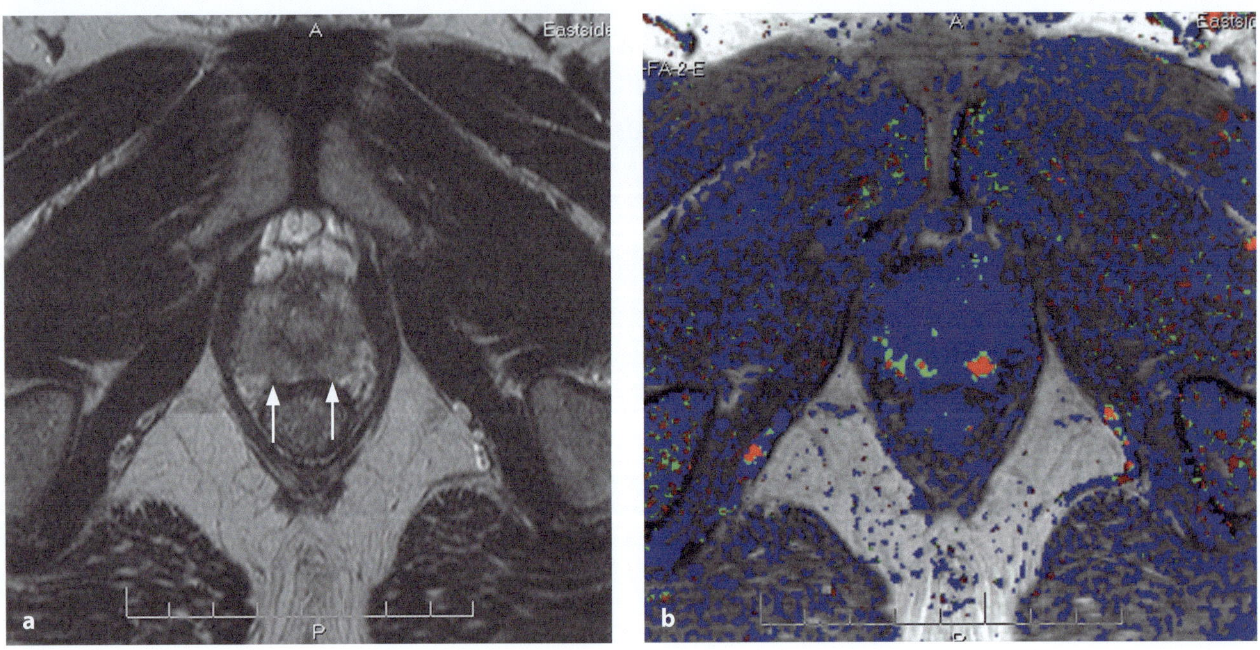

Fig. 2.15 a, b Apical right linear lesion and left focal lesion

Fig. 2.16 a, b

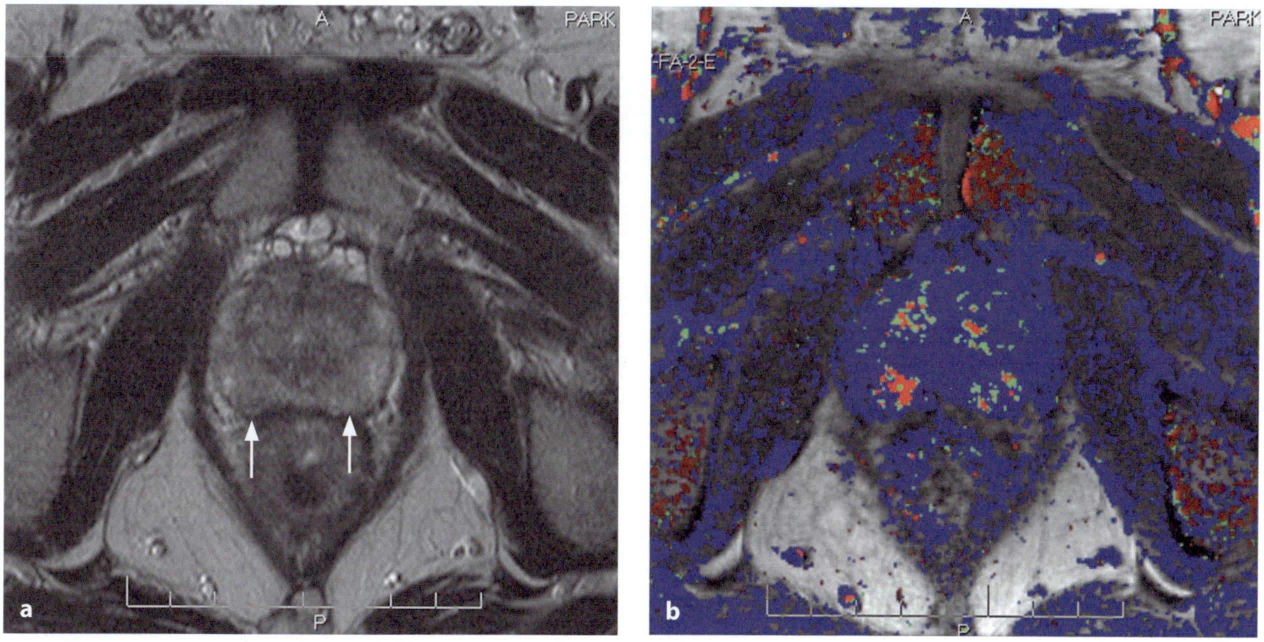

Fig. 2.16 a, b Midgland right focal and left diffuse posterior lesions

Fig. 2.17 a, b

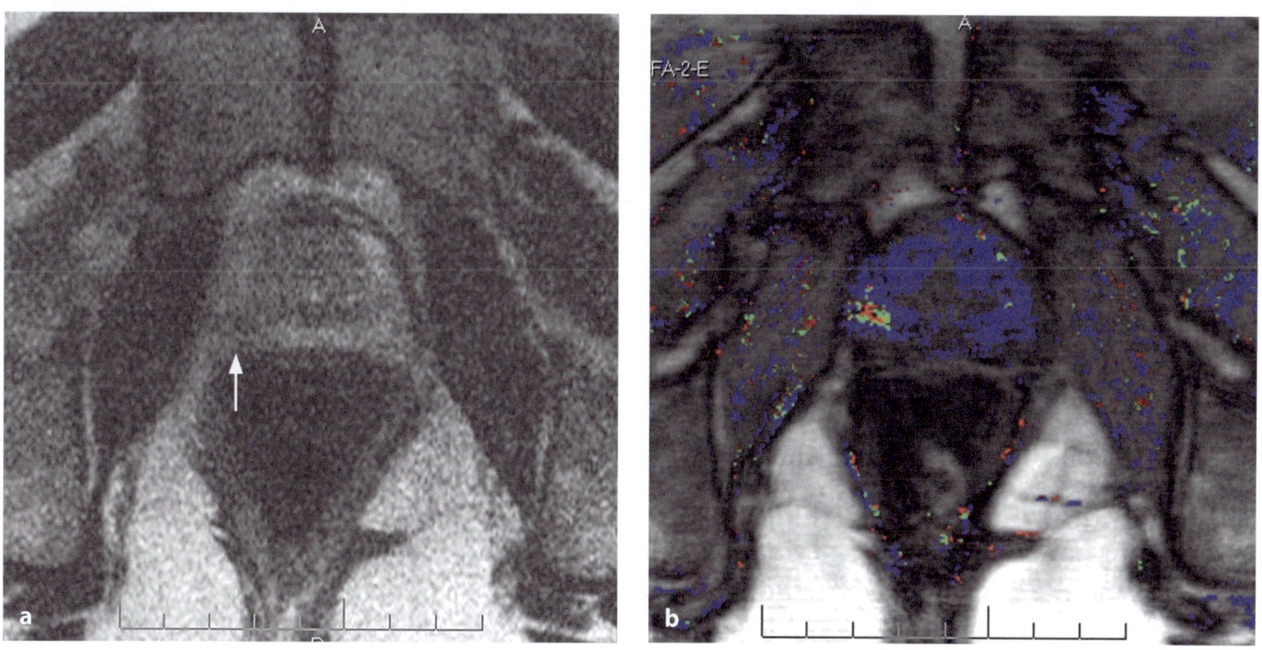

Fig. 2.17 a, b Midgland right posterior focal lesion

Fig. 2.18 a, b

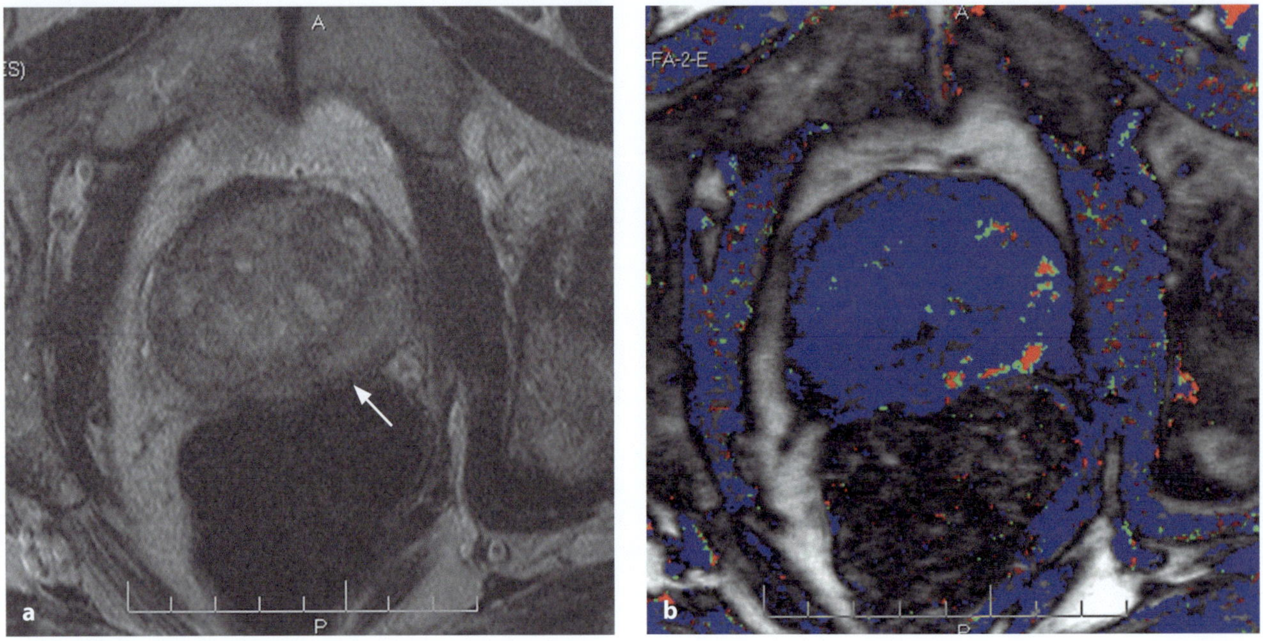

Fig. 2.18 a, b Midgland left posterior linear lesion

Fig. 2.19 a, b

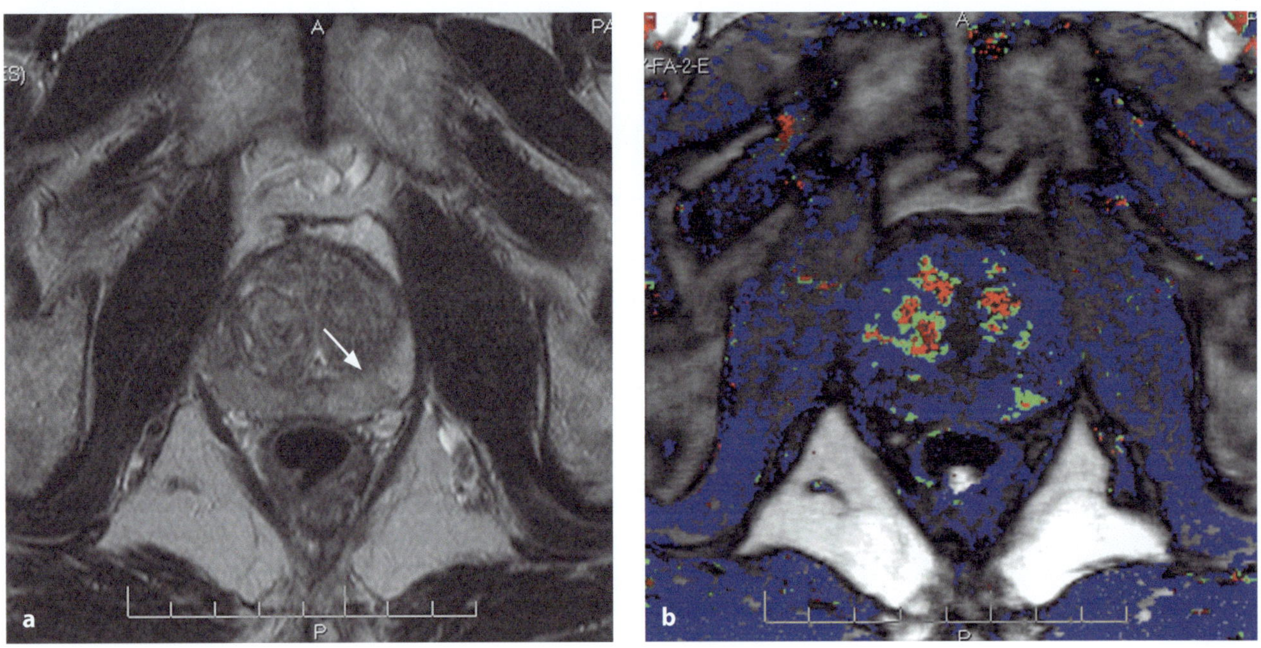

Fig. 2.19 a, b Midgland left posterior focal lesion

Fig. 2.20 a, b

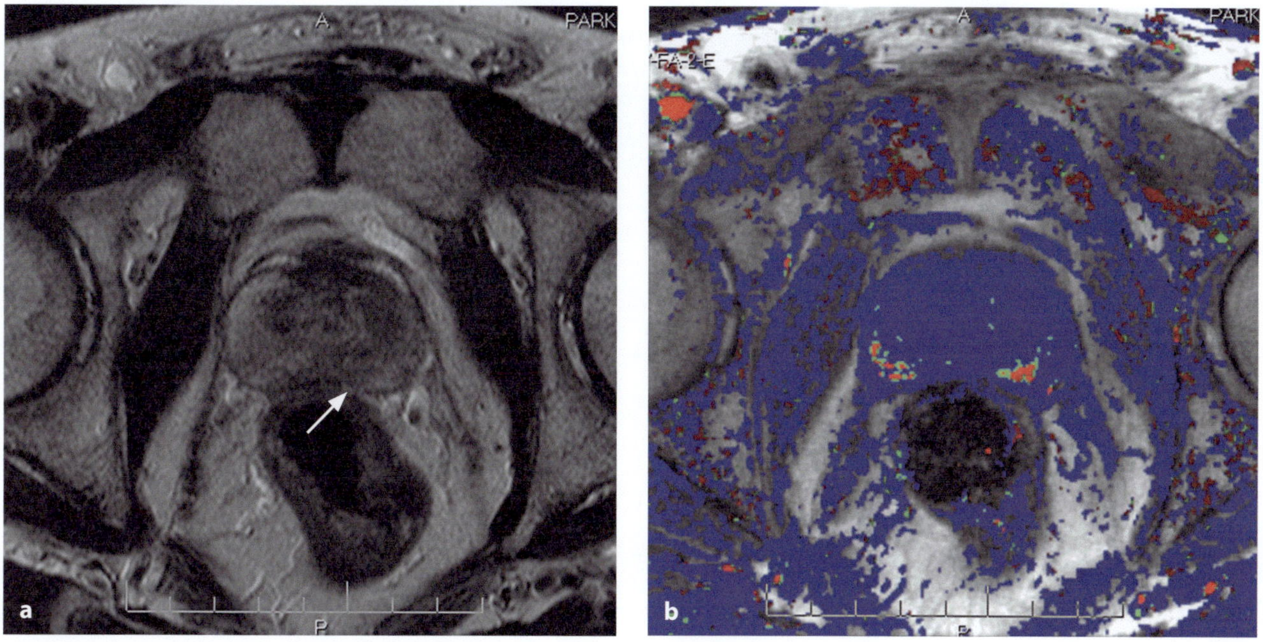

Fig. 2.20 a, b Midgland left posterior focal lesion

Fig. 2.21 a, b

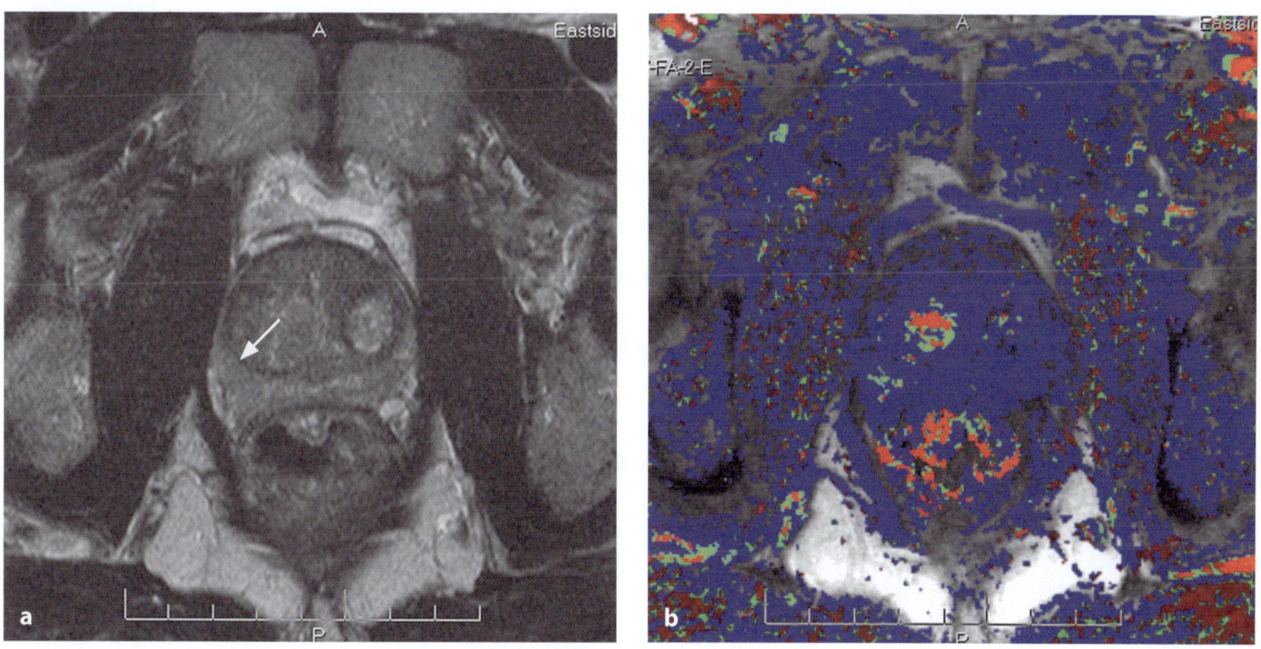

Fig. 2.21 a, b Midgland right posterior lateral focal lesion

Fig. 2.22 a, b

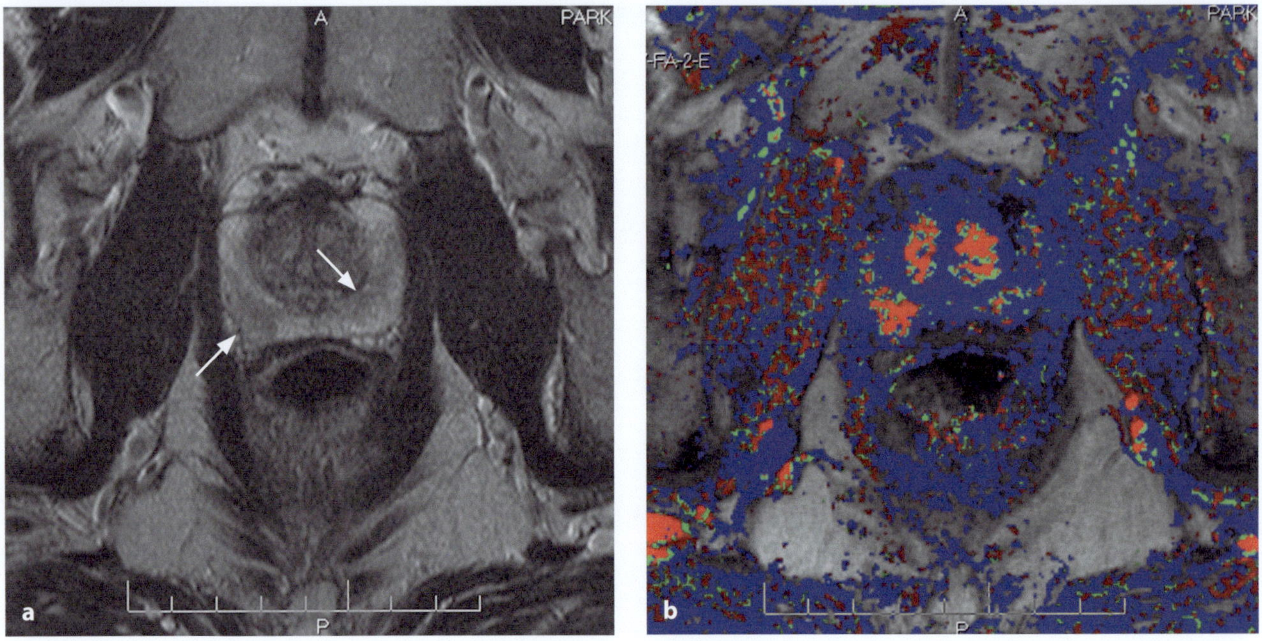

Fig. 2.22a, b Midgland right posterior focal and left posterior diffuse lesions

Fig. 2.23 a, b

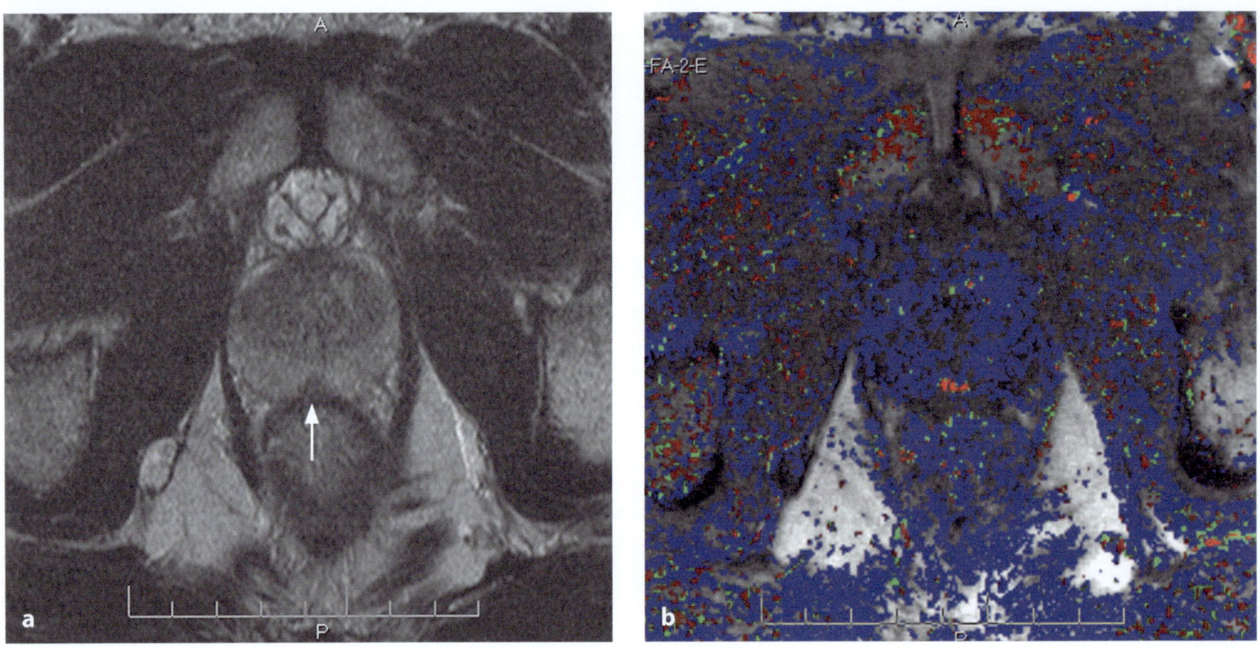

Fig. 2.23 a, b Midgland posterior focal midline lesion

Fig. 2.24 a, b

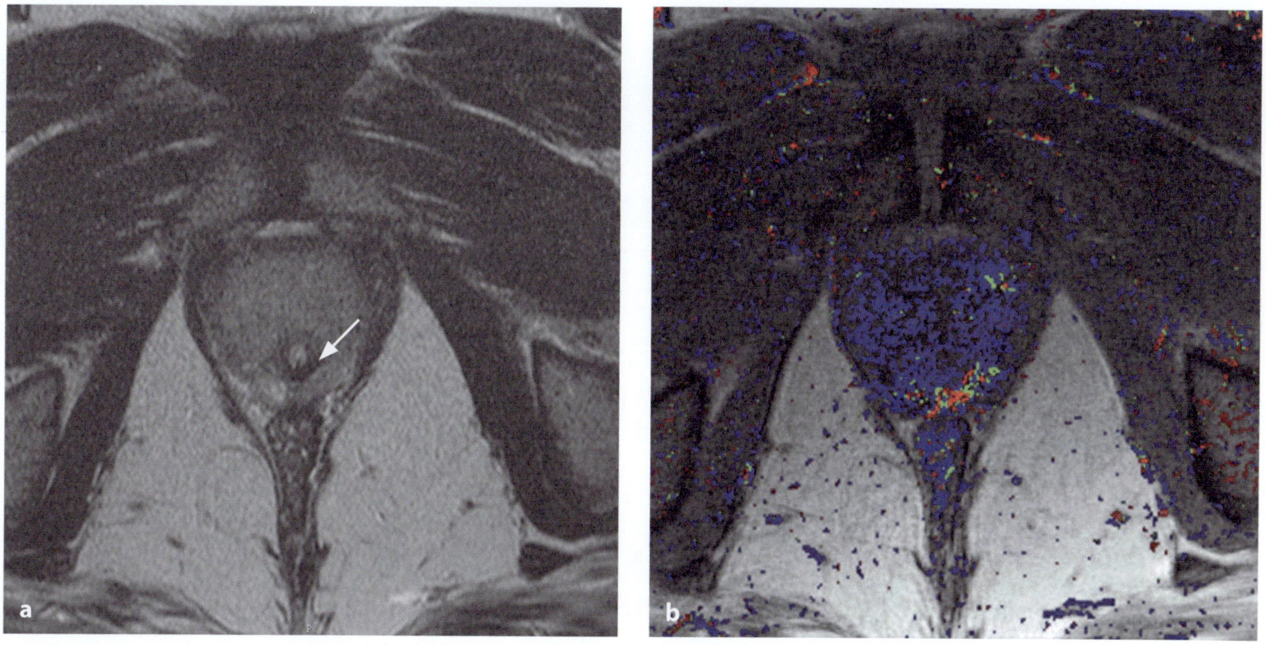

Fig. 2.24 a, b Apical left posterior linear lesion with anterior fibrosis

Fig. 2.25 a, b

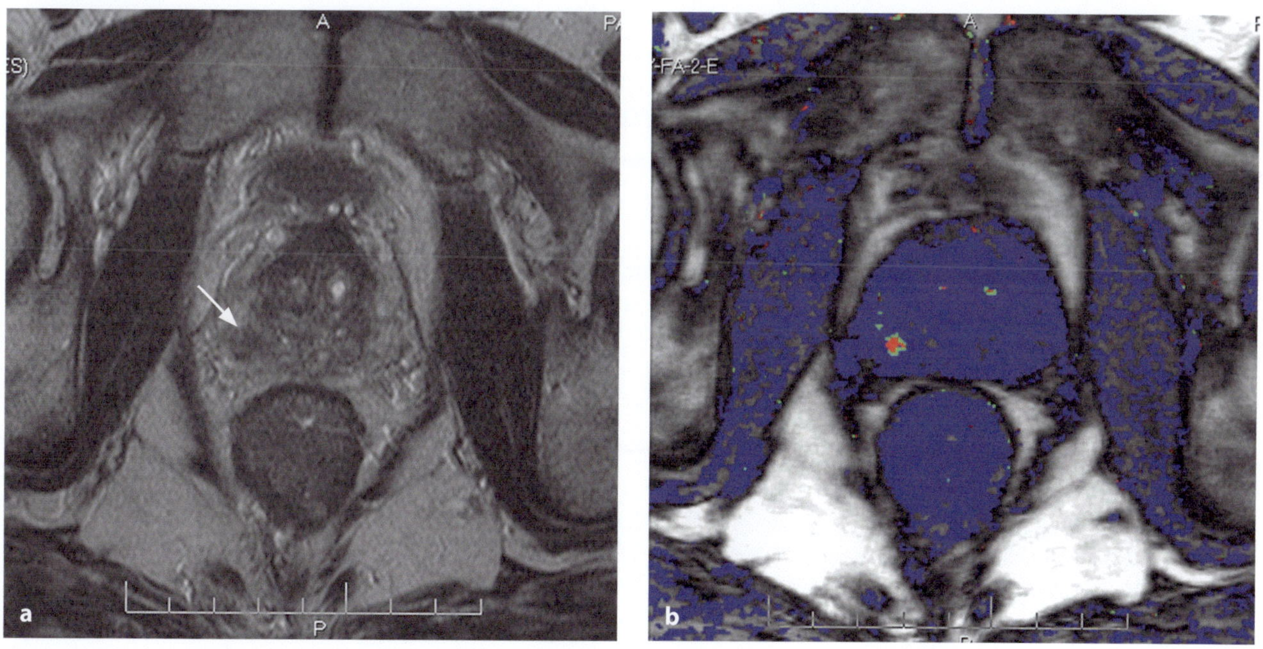

Fig. 2.25 a, b base right posterior focal lesion

Fig. 2.26 a, b

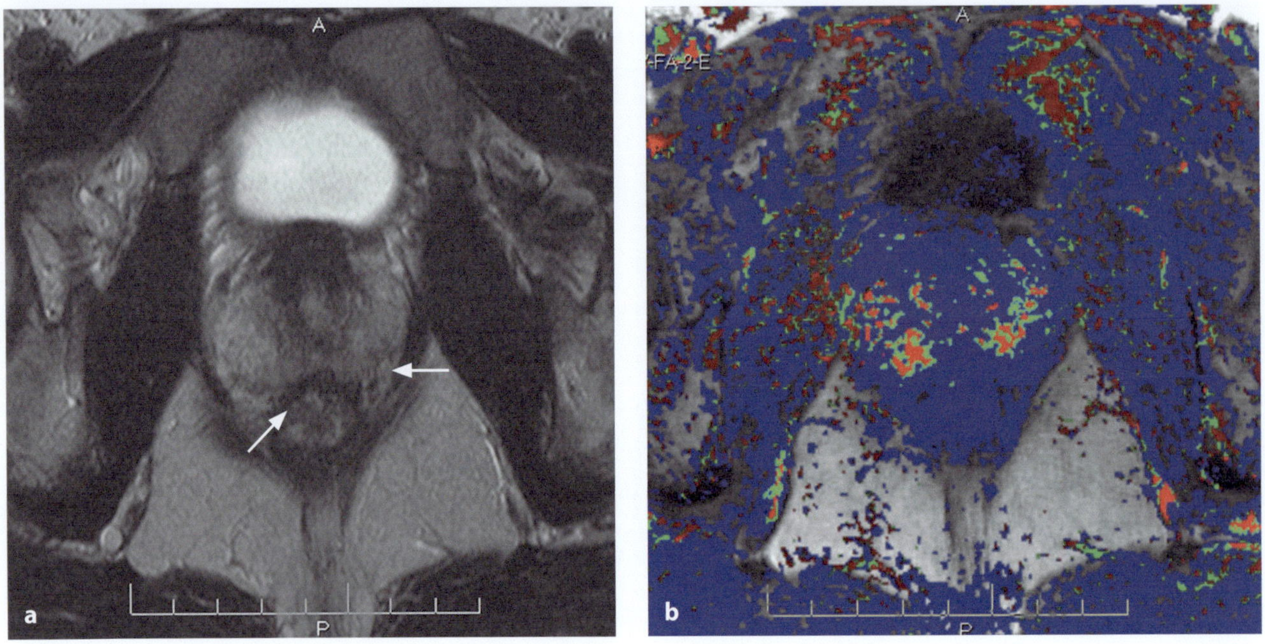

Fig. 2.26 a, b Midgland bilateral posterior focal lesions

Fig. 2.27 a, b

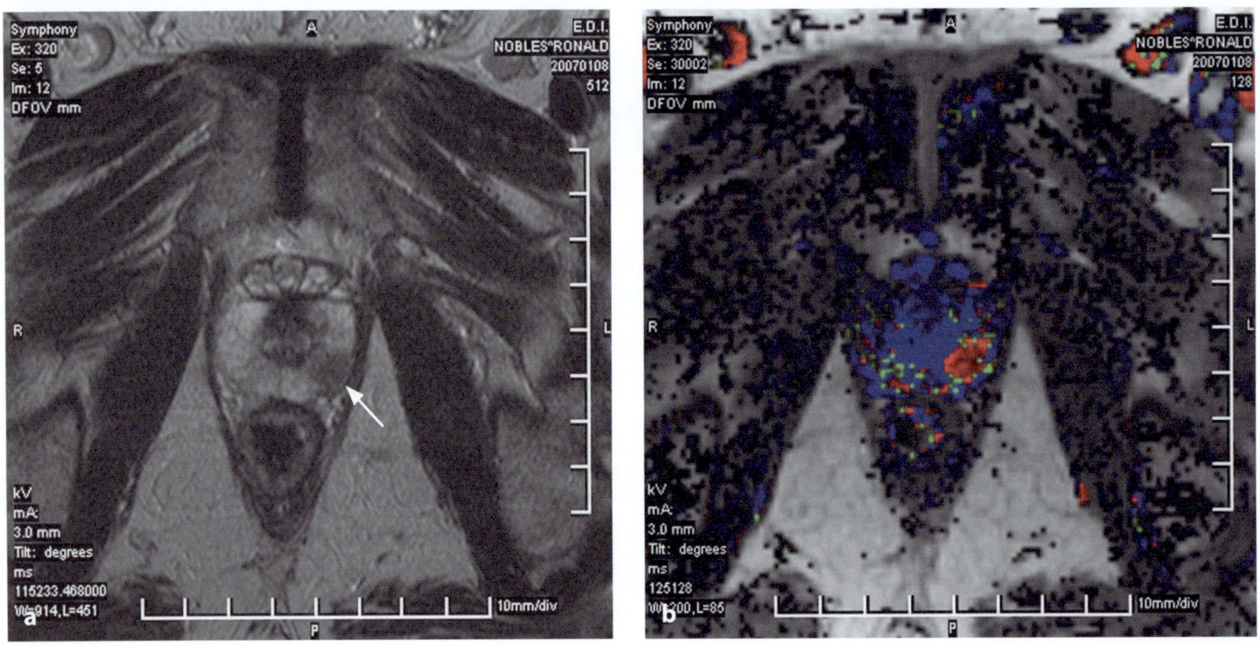

Fig. 2.27 a, b Midgland left posterior lateral focal lesion

Fig. 2.28 a, b

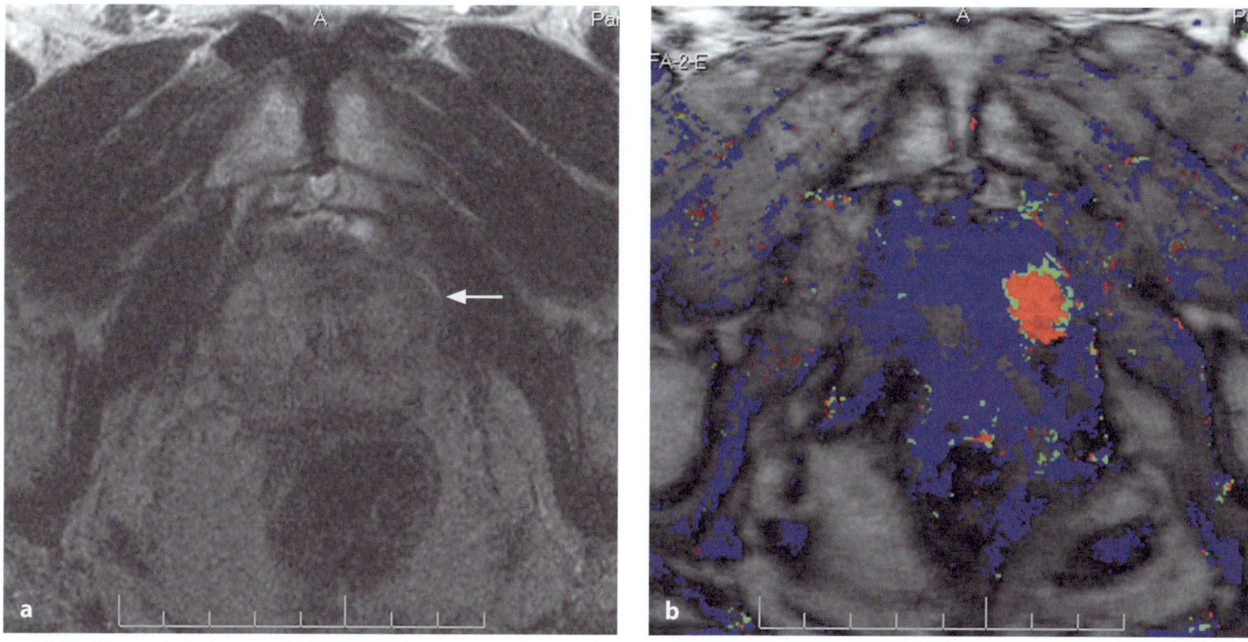

Fig. 2.28 a, b Apical left peripheral lesion eroding into central gland

Fig. 2.29 a, b

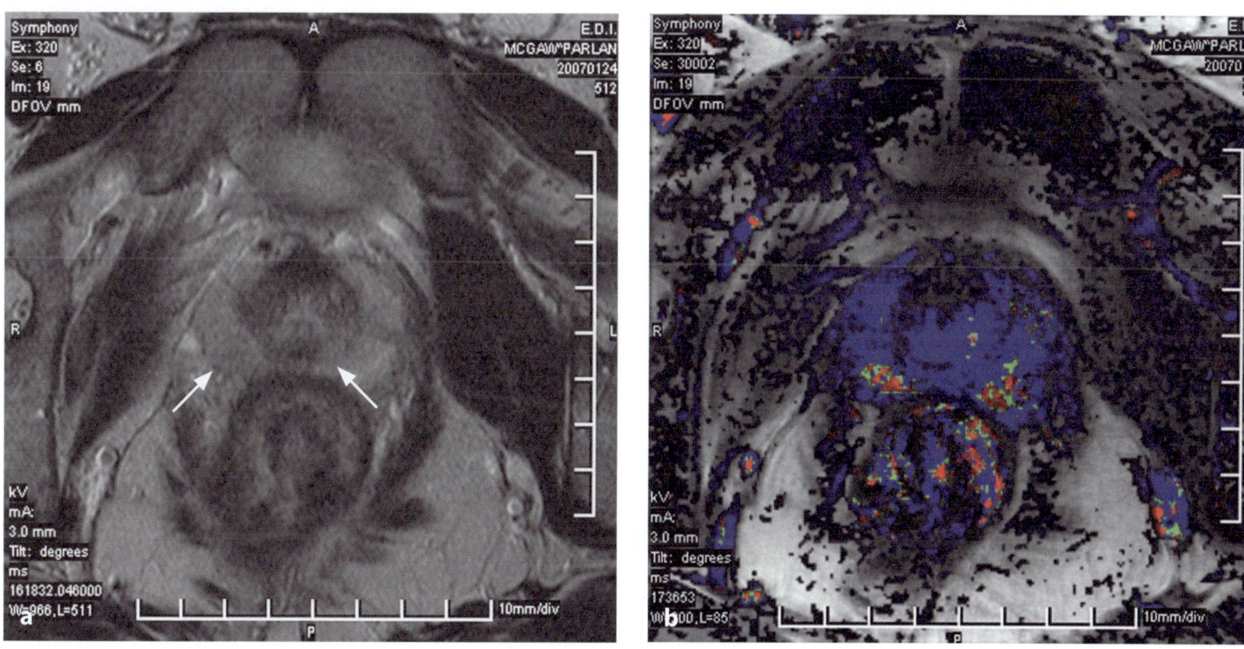

Fig. 2.29 a, b Midgland bilateral posterior lateral focal lesions

Fig. 2.30 a, b

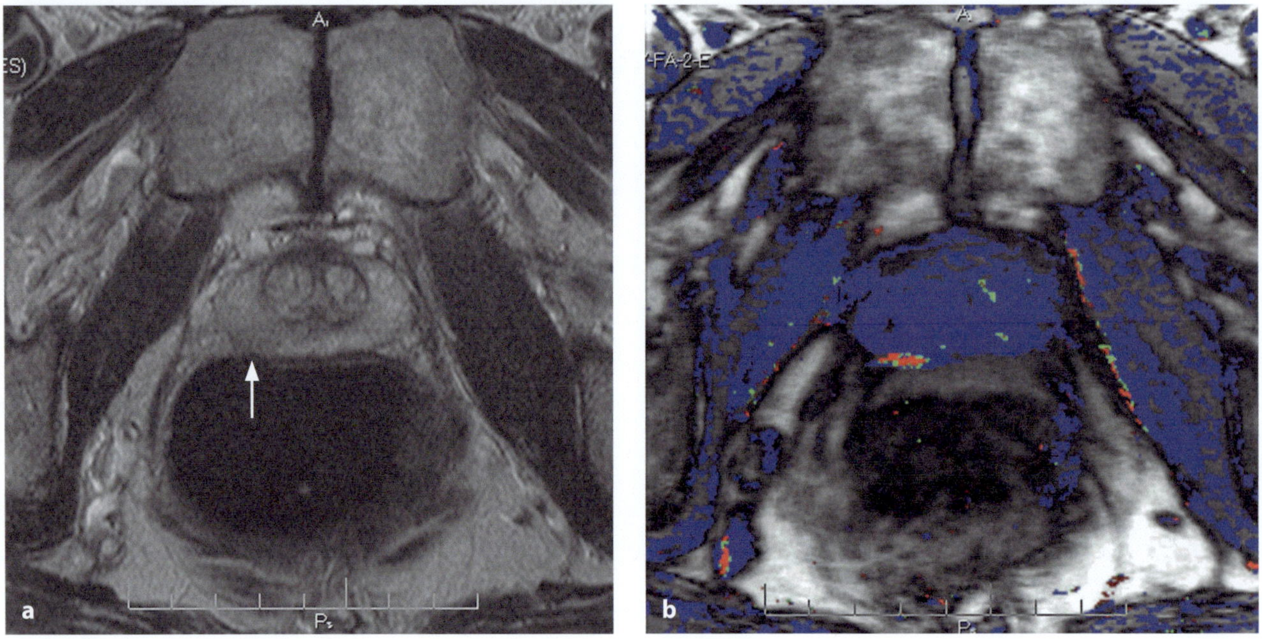

Fig. 2.30 a, b Midgland right posterior linear lesion

Fig. 2.31 a, b

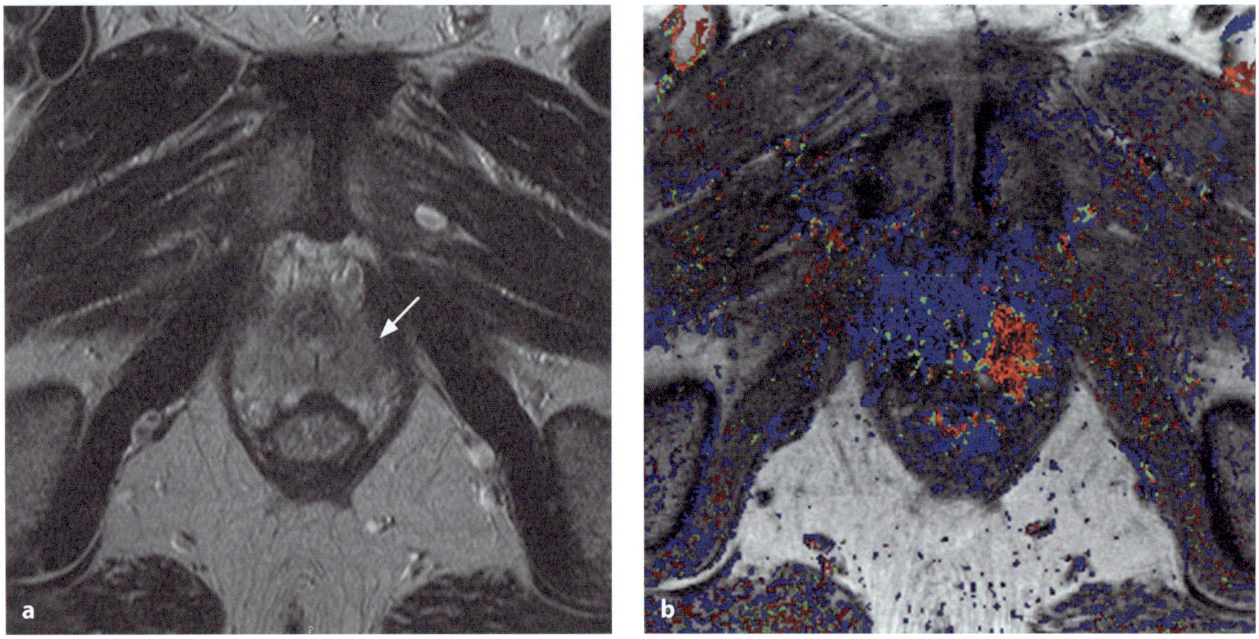

Fig. 2.31 a, b Apical left lateral focal lesion

Fig. 2.32 a, b

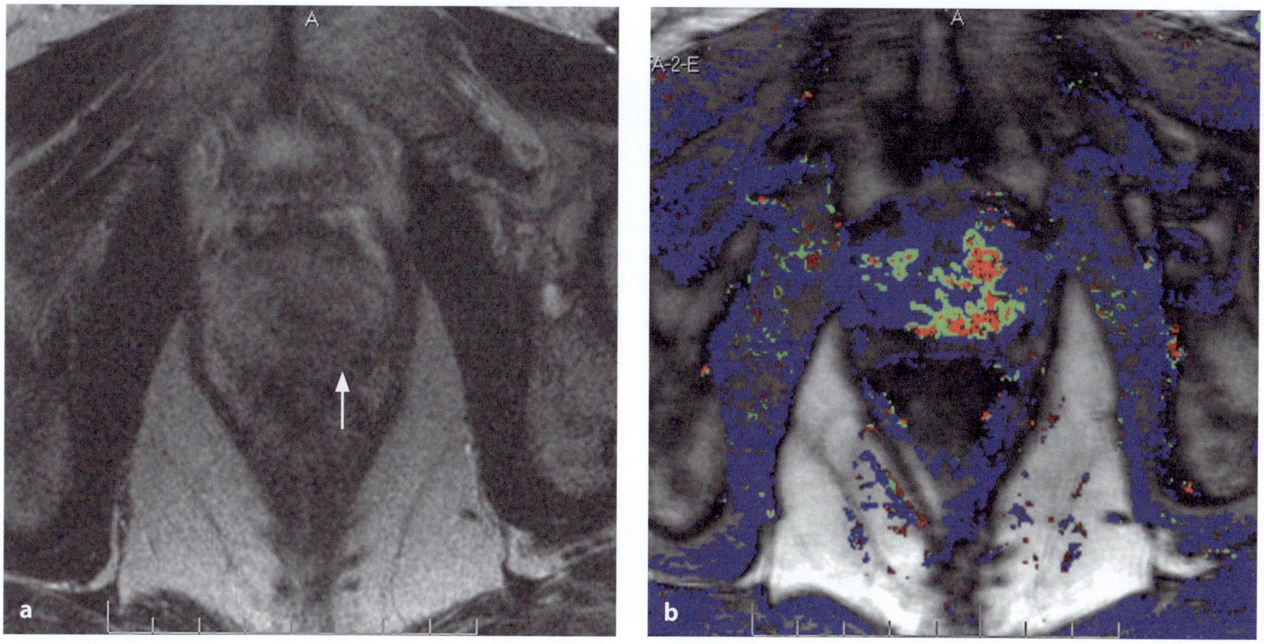

Fig. 2.32 a, b Midgland left posterior tumor crosses midline to right

Fig. 2.33 a, b

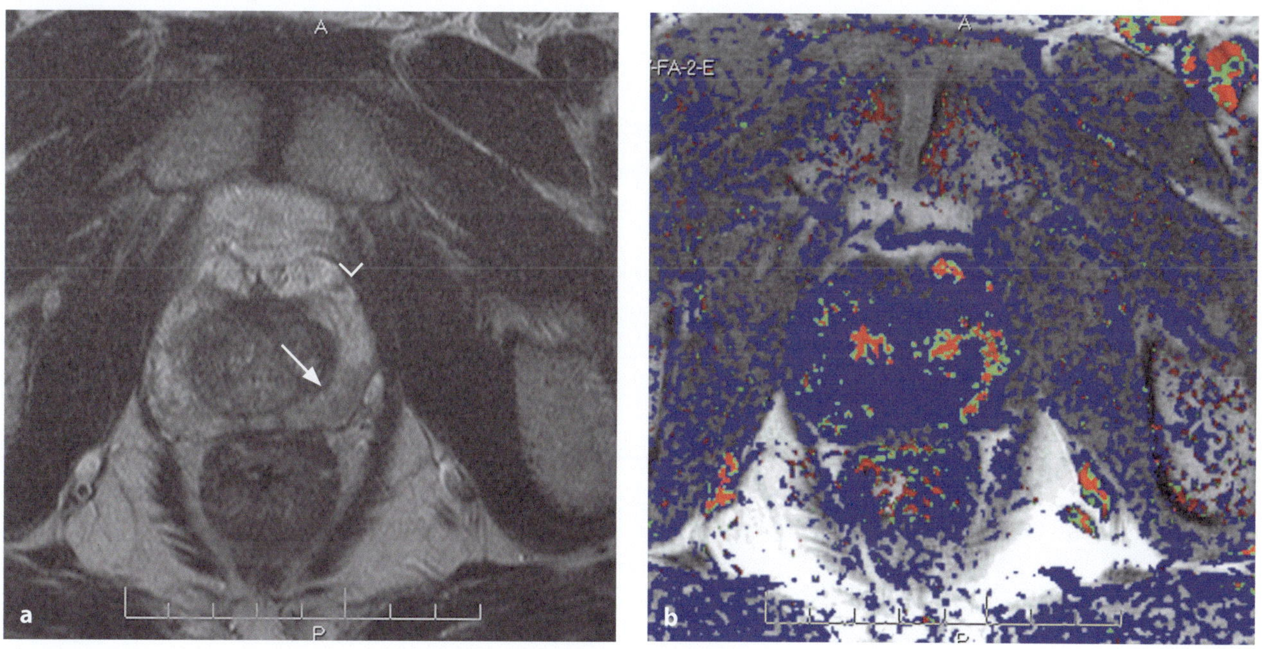

Fig. 2.33 a, b Midgland left lateral linear lesion-note left anterior vein

Fig. 2.34 a, b

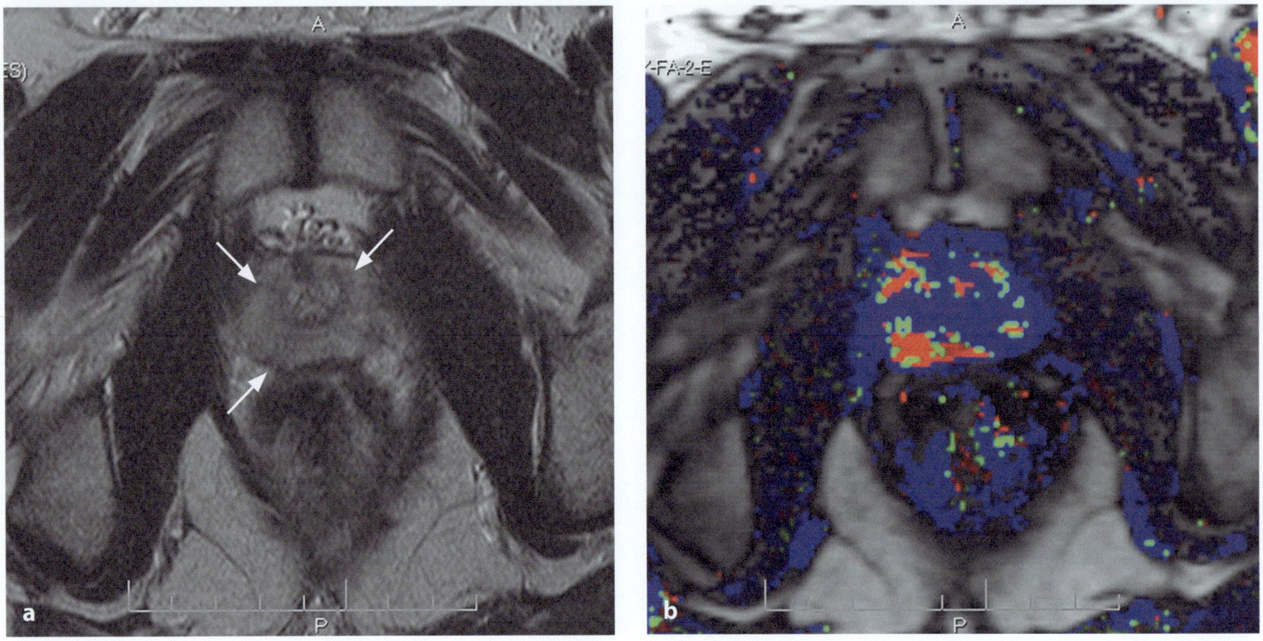

Fig. 2.34 a, b Midgland right posterior/right anterior focal lesions and left anterior linear lesion

Fig. 2.35 a, b

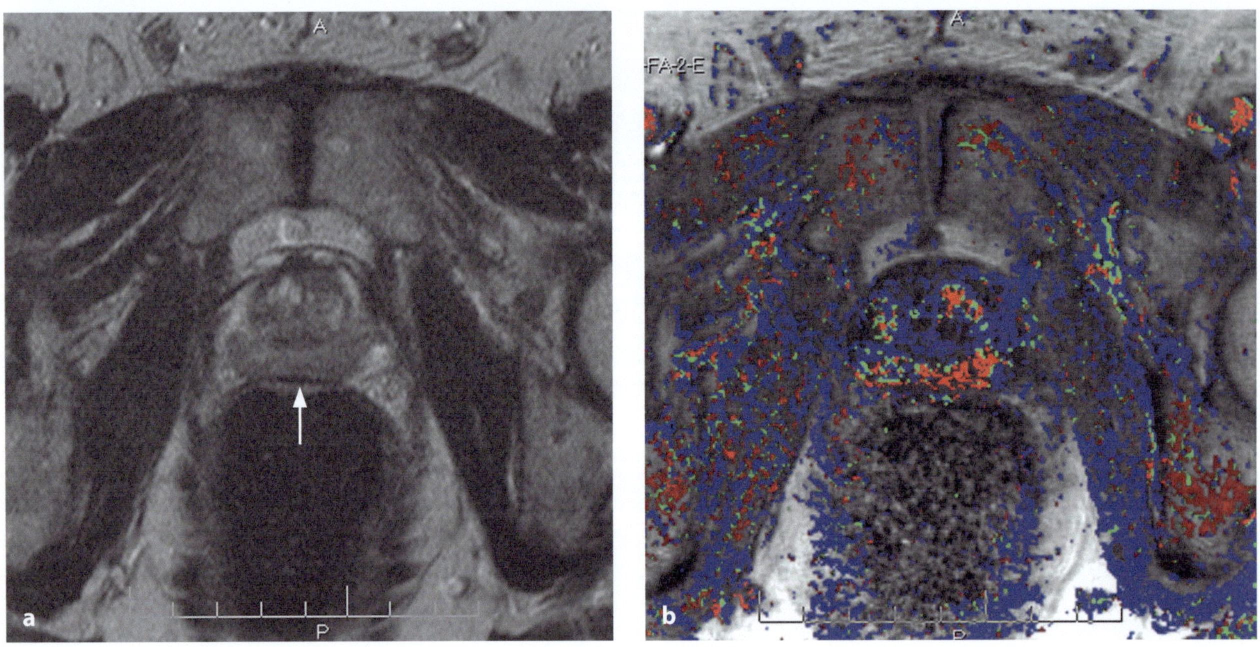

Fig. 2.35 a, b Apical post linear lesion

Fig. 2.36 a, b

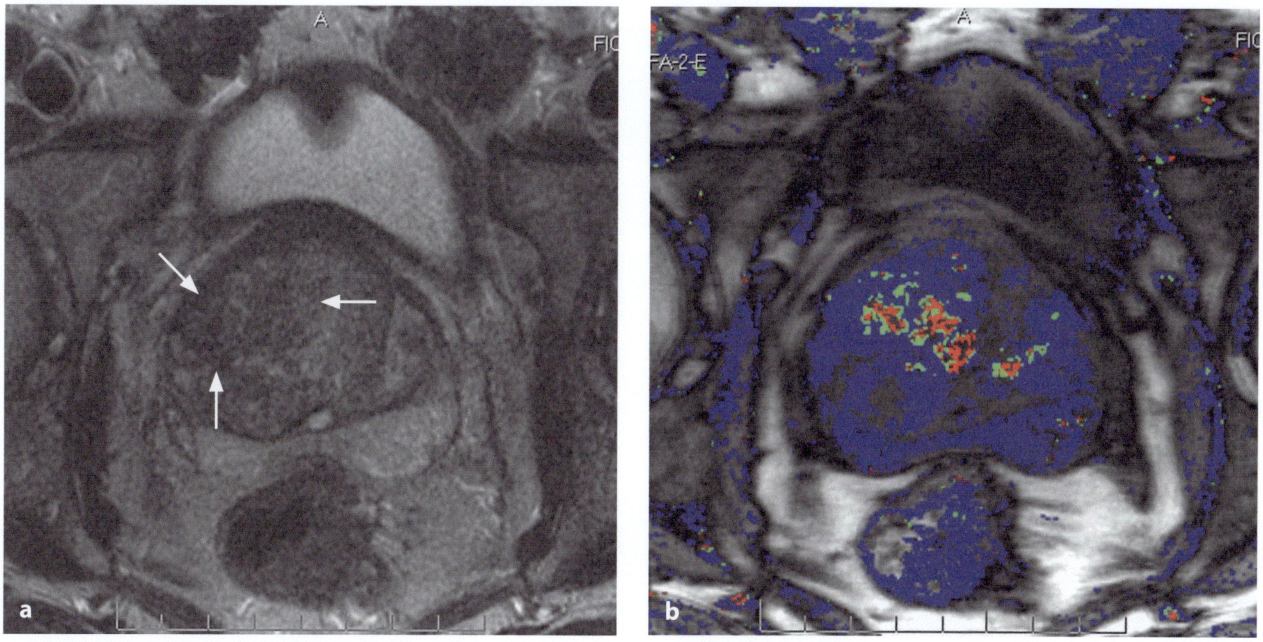

Fig. 2.36 a, b Midgland right central zone lesion-note left anterior BPH has medium T2 weighted signal while right malignant tumor has no T2 weighted signal

Fig. 2.37 a, b

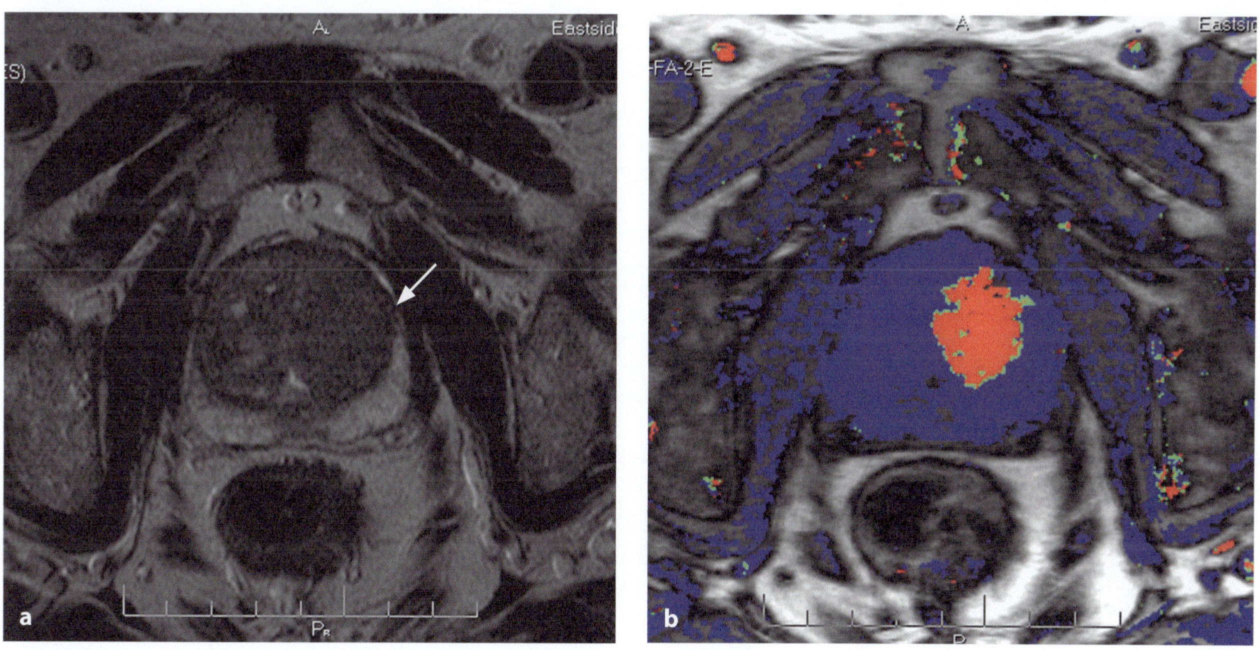

Fig. 2.37 a, b Midgland left central zone lesion

Fig. 2.38 a, b

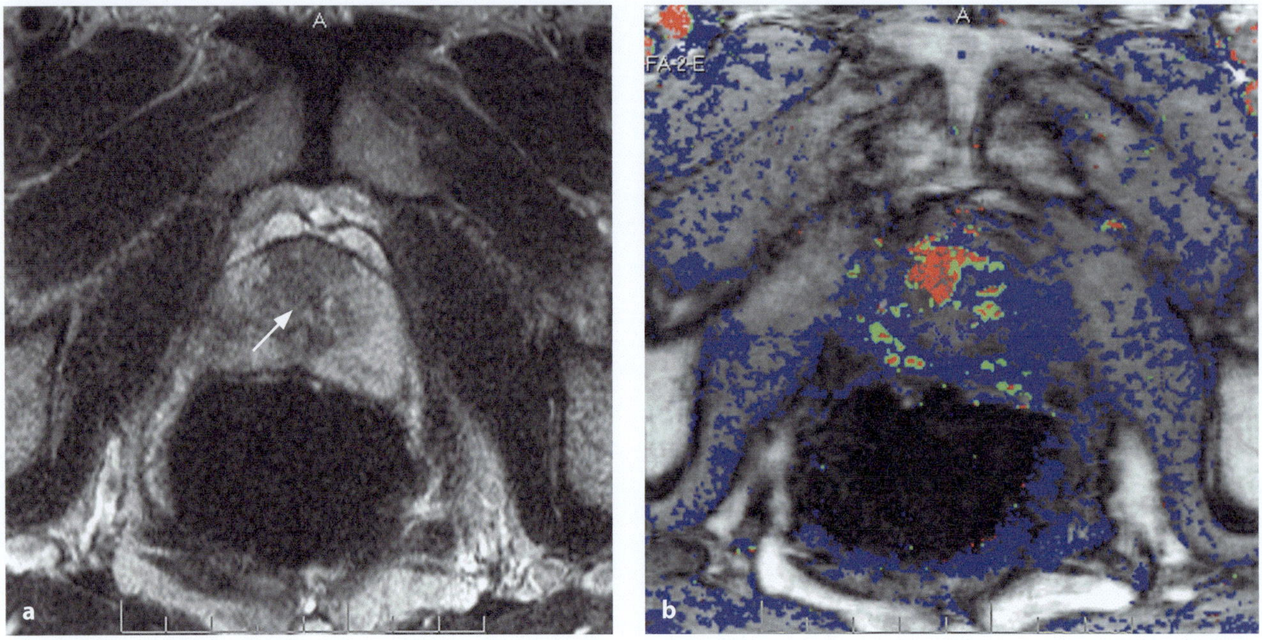

Fig. 2.38 a, b Midgland right anterior focal lesion

Fig. 2.39 a, b

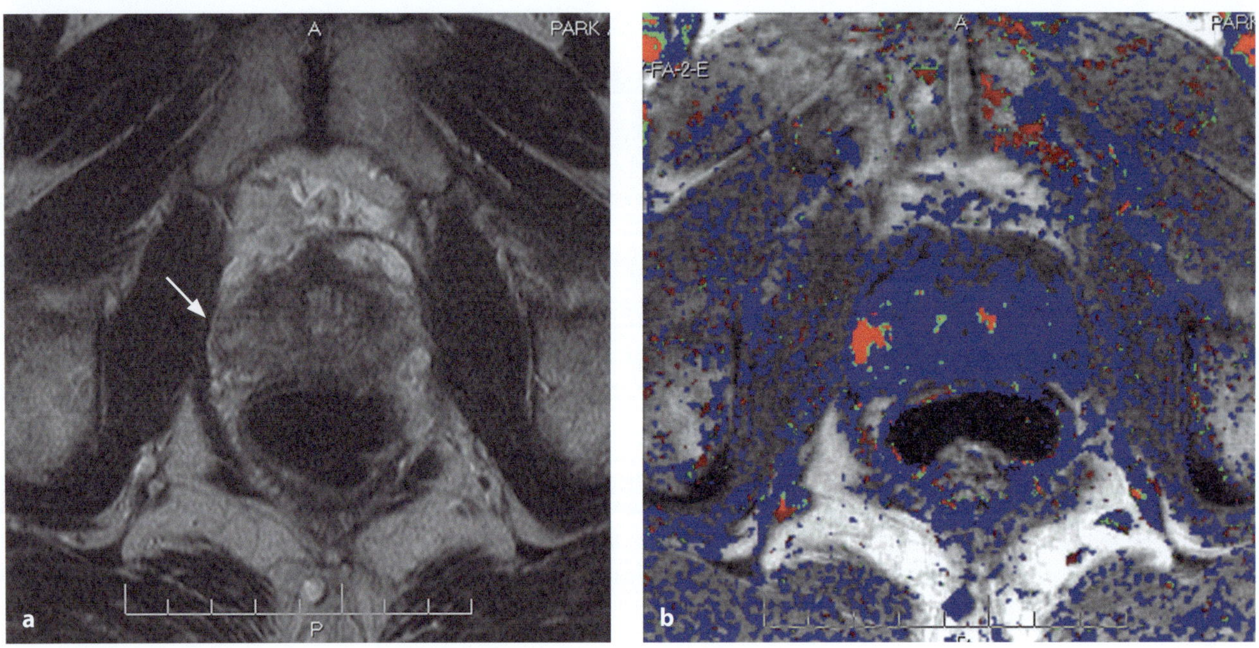

Fig. 2.39 a, b Midgland right anterior focal lesion

Fig. 2.40 a, b

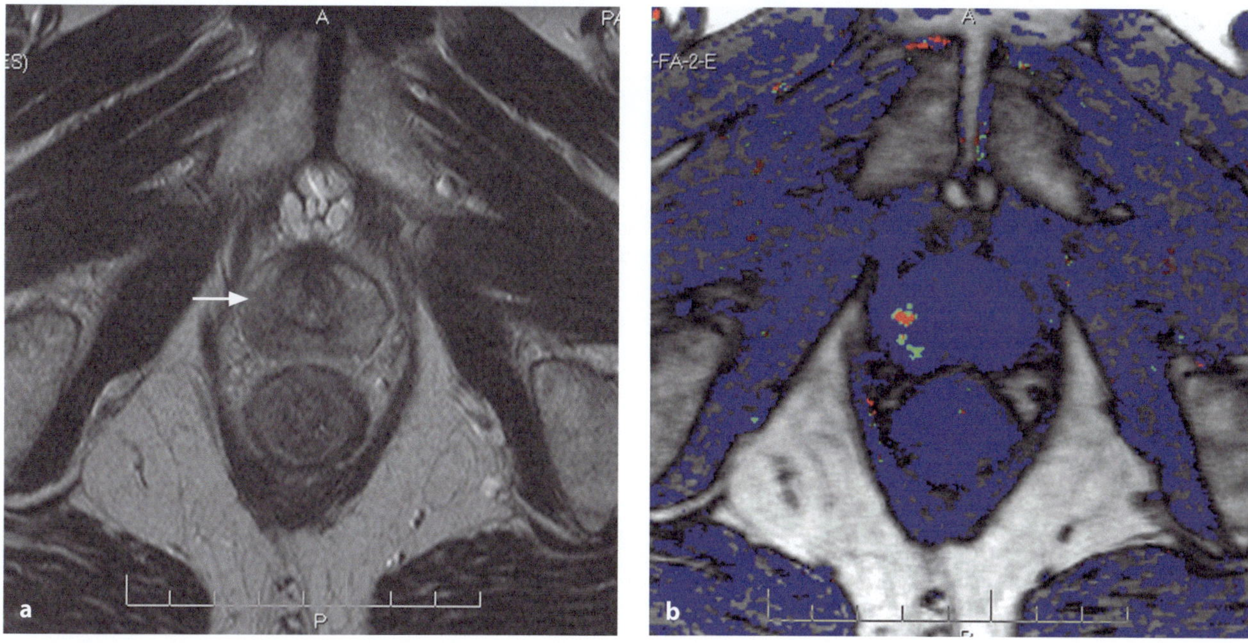

Fig. 2.40 a, b Midgland right anterior focal lesion

Fig. 2.41 a, b

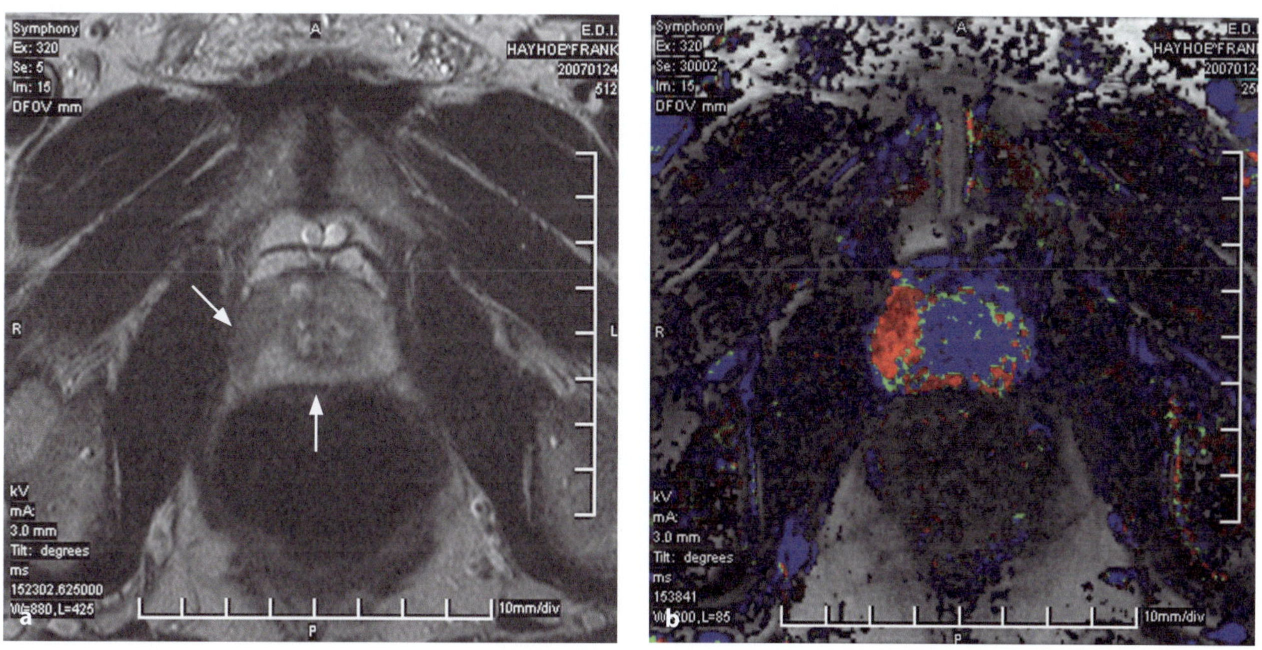

Fig. 2.41 a, b Midgland anterior right focal and posterior linear lesions

Fig. 2.42 a, b

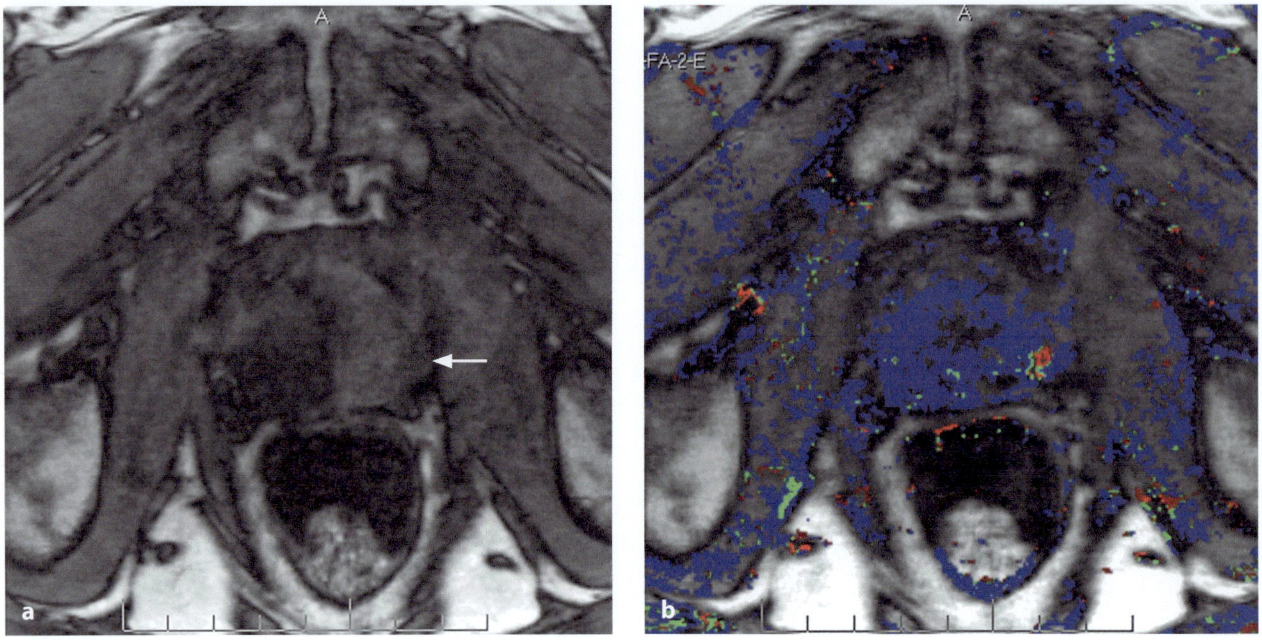

Fig. 2.42 a, b Midgland left anterior focal lesion

Fig. 2.43 a, b

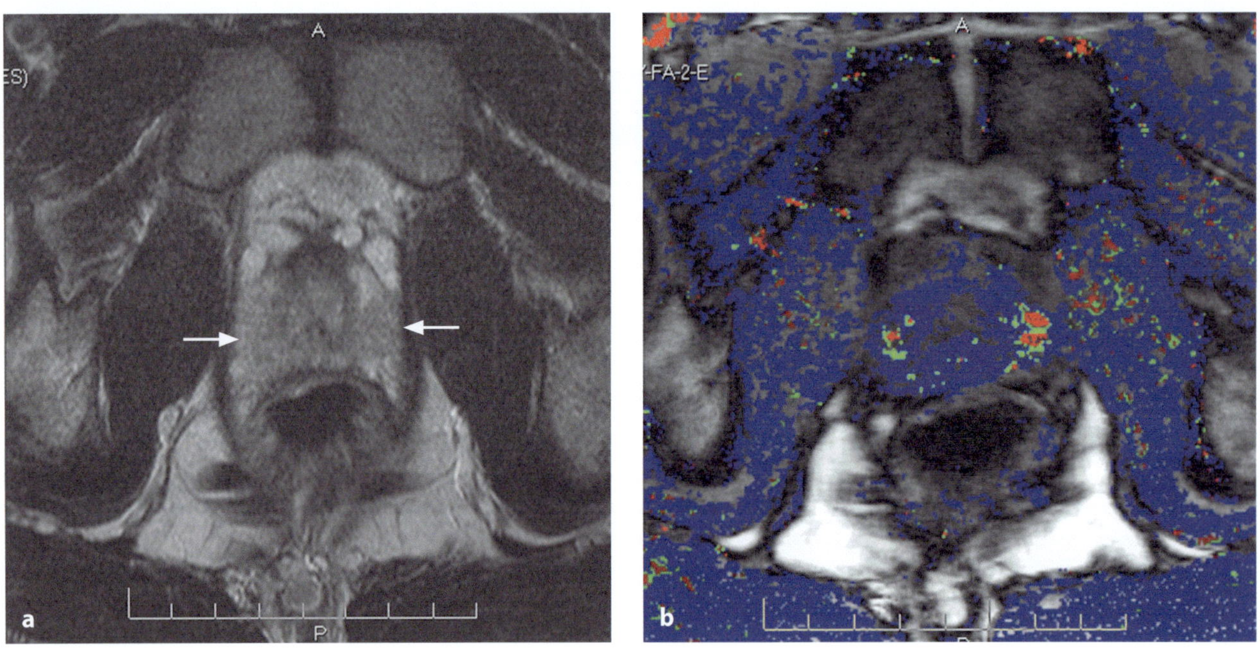

Fig. 2.43 a, b Apical anterior right and left focal lesions

Fig. 2.44 a, b

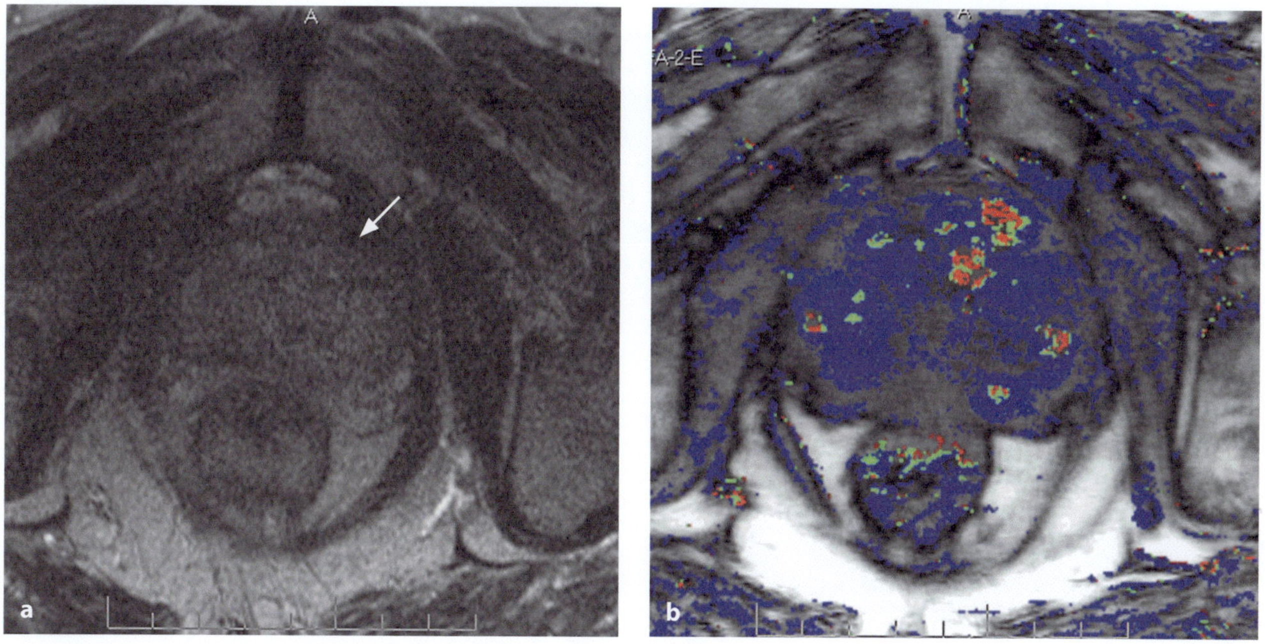

Fig. 2.44 a, b Midgland left anterior lesion-note posterior fibrosis

Fig. 2.45 a, b

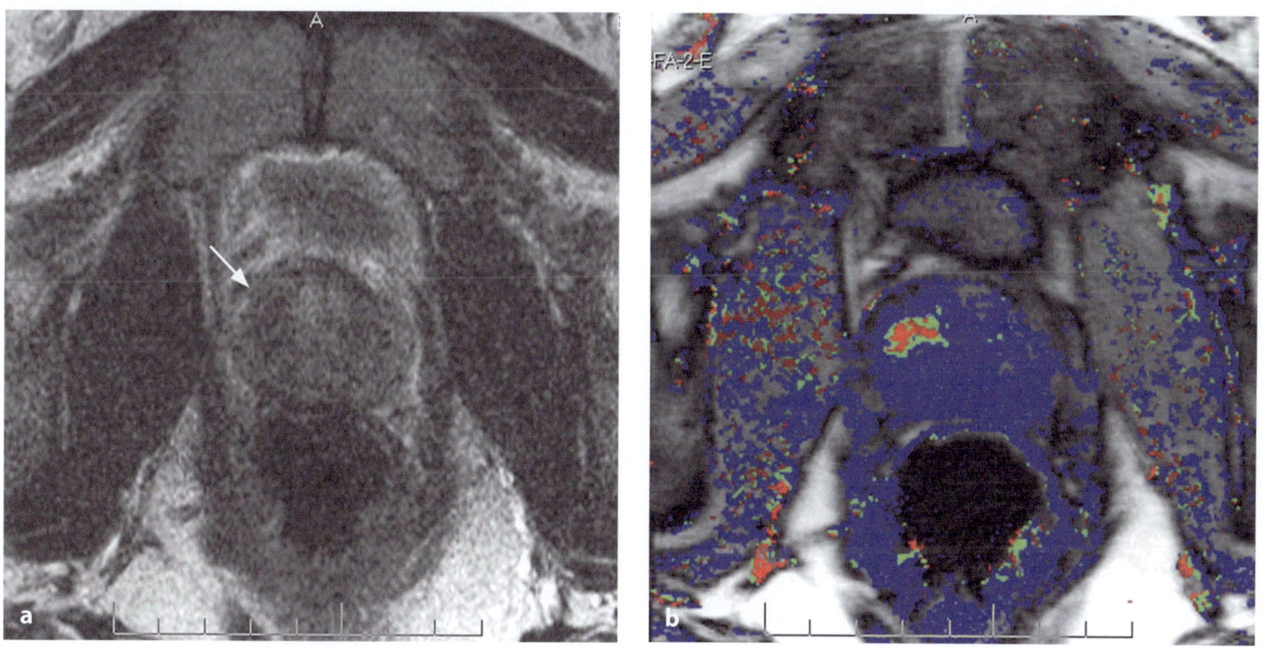

Fig. 2.45 a, b Apical right anterior focal lesion

Fig. 2.46 a, b

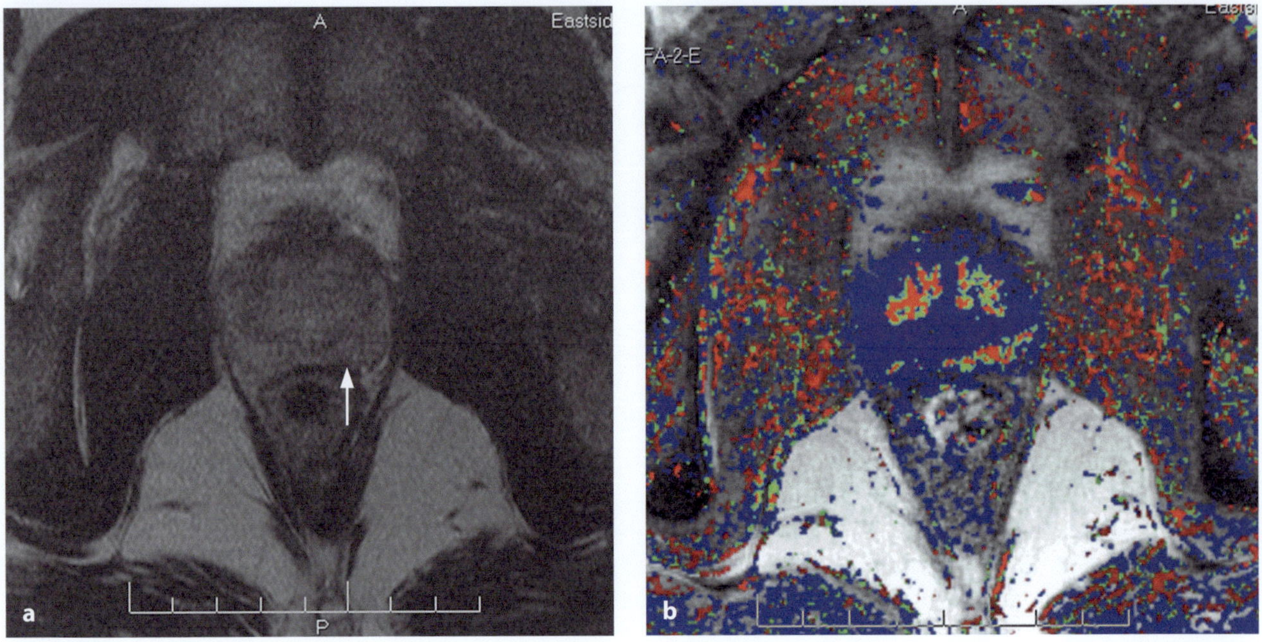

Fig. 2.46 a, b Midgland left posterior linear

Extraprostatic Cancer

3

Tumor extending outside the prostate is malignant.

Benign conditions may bulge the fibrous capsule but do not invade through the prostatic capsule.

Fig. 3.1 a, b

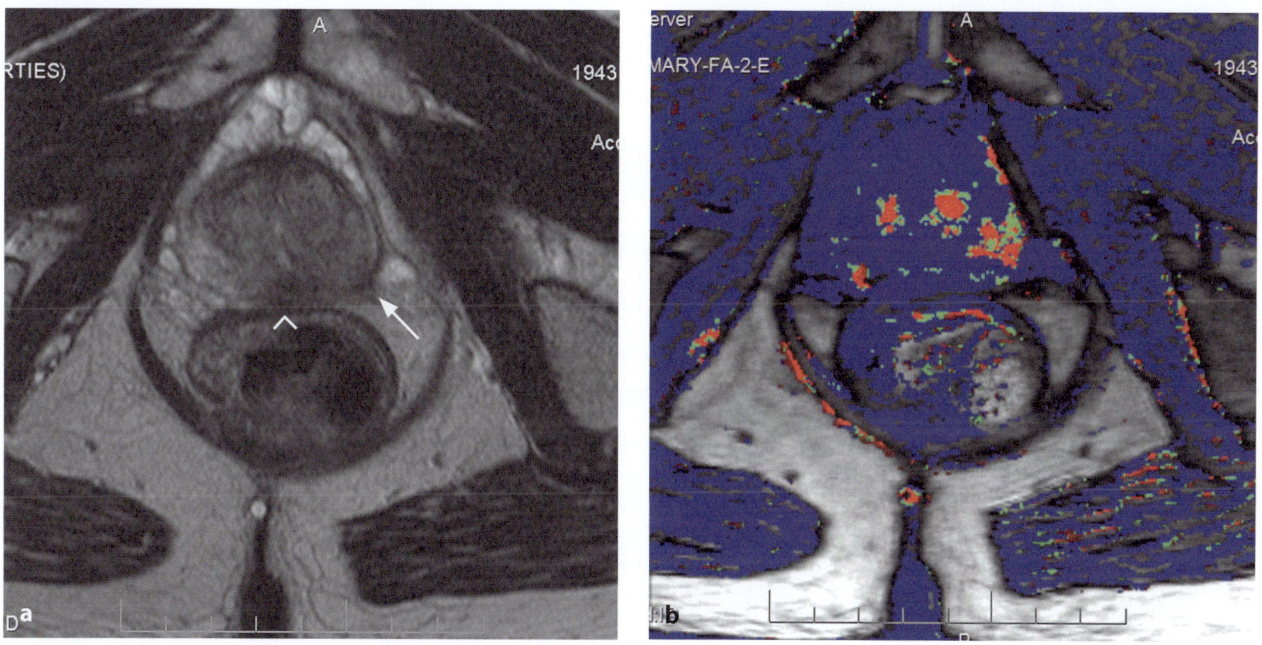

Fig. 3.1 a, b Midgland left lateral capsule erosion-note posterior fibrosis

Fig. 3.2 a, b

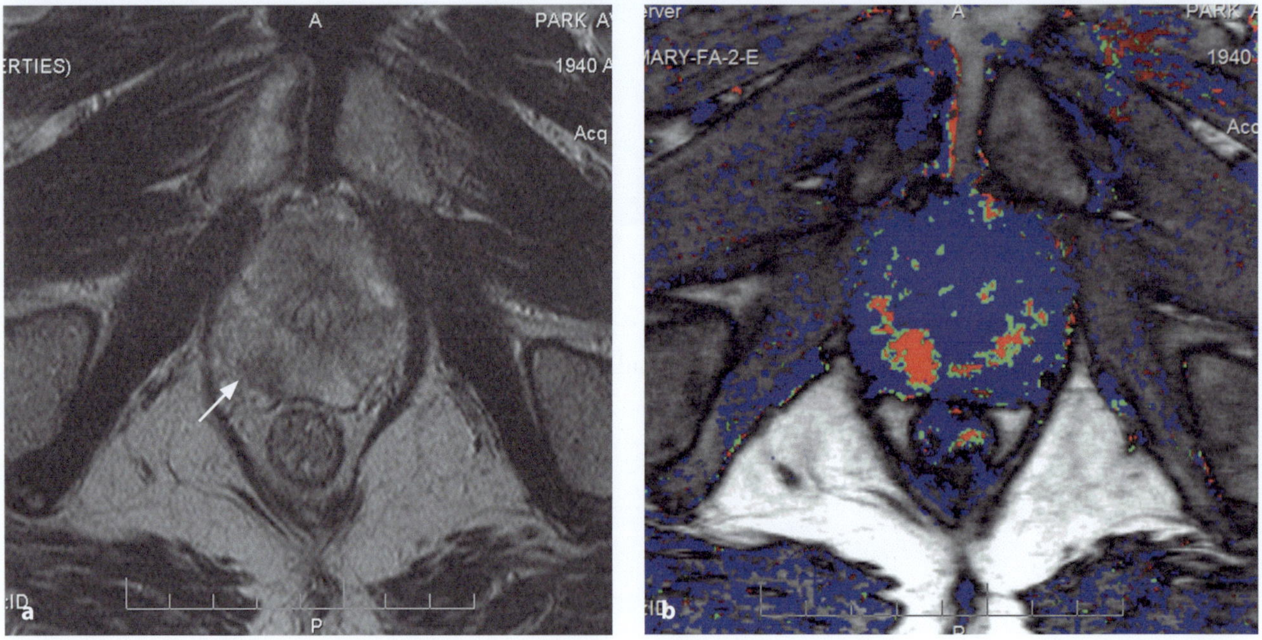

Fig. 3.2 a, b Apical right lateral capsular erosion

Fig. 3.3 a, b

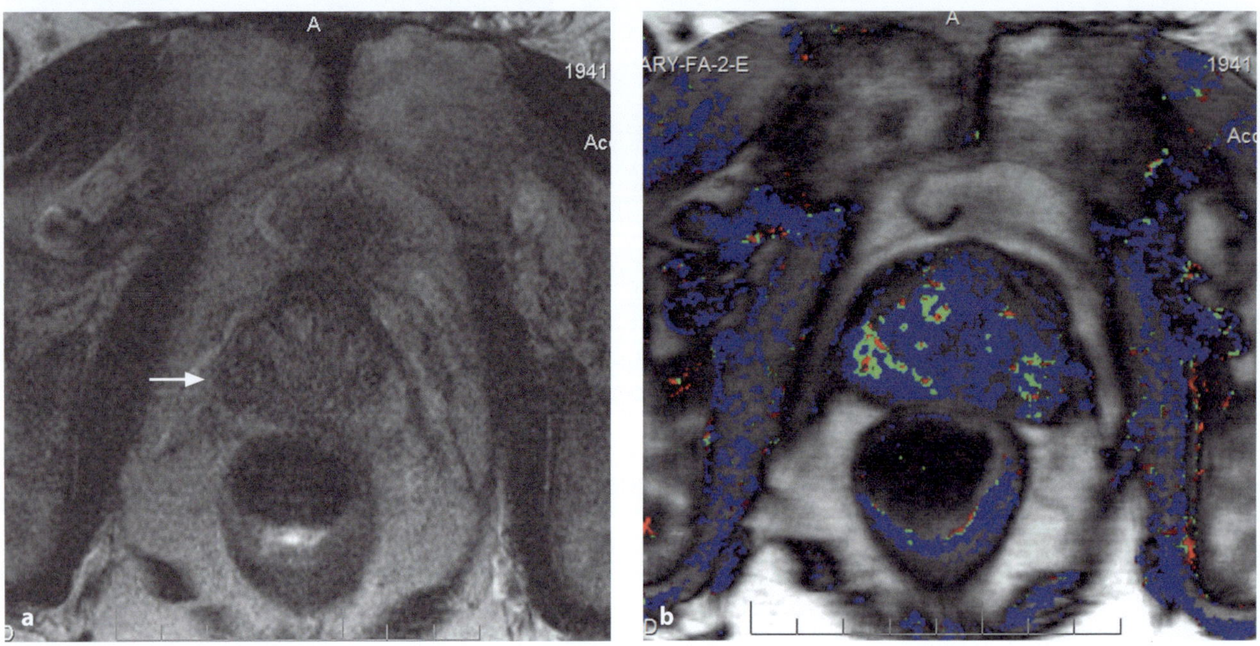

Fig. 3.3 a, b Midgland right capsular erosion

Fig. 3.4 a, b

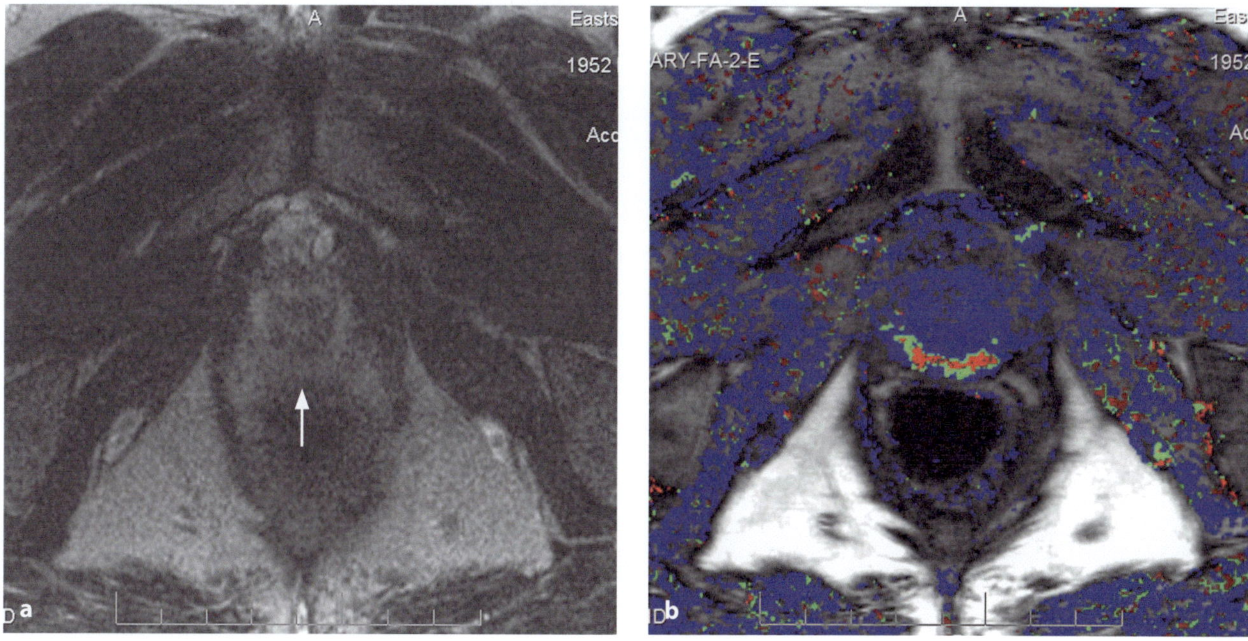

Fig. 3.4 a, b Apical posterior capsular erosion

Fig. 3.5 a, b

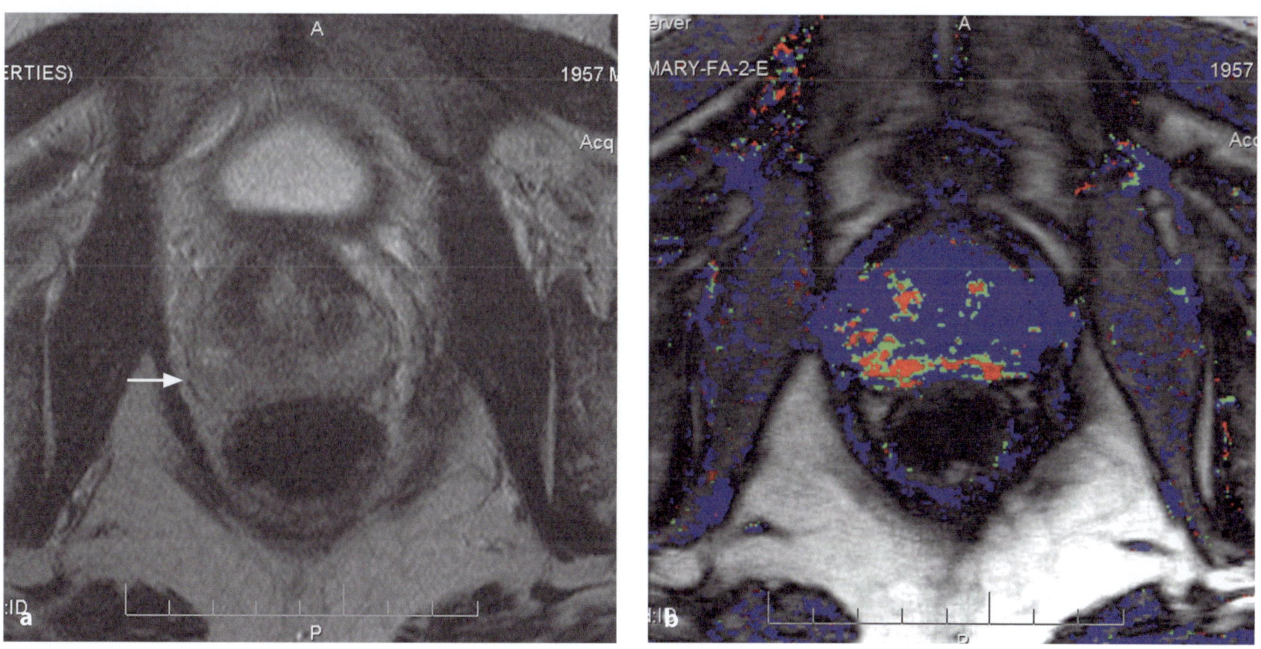

Fig. 3.5 a, b Midgland right lateral posterior capsular erosion

Fig. 3.6 a, b

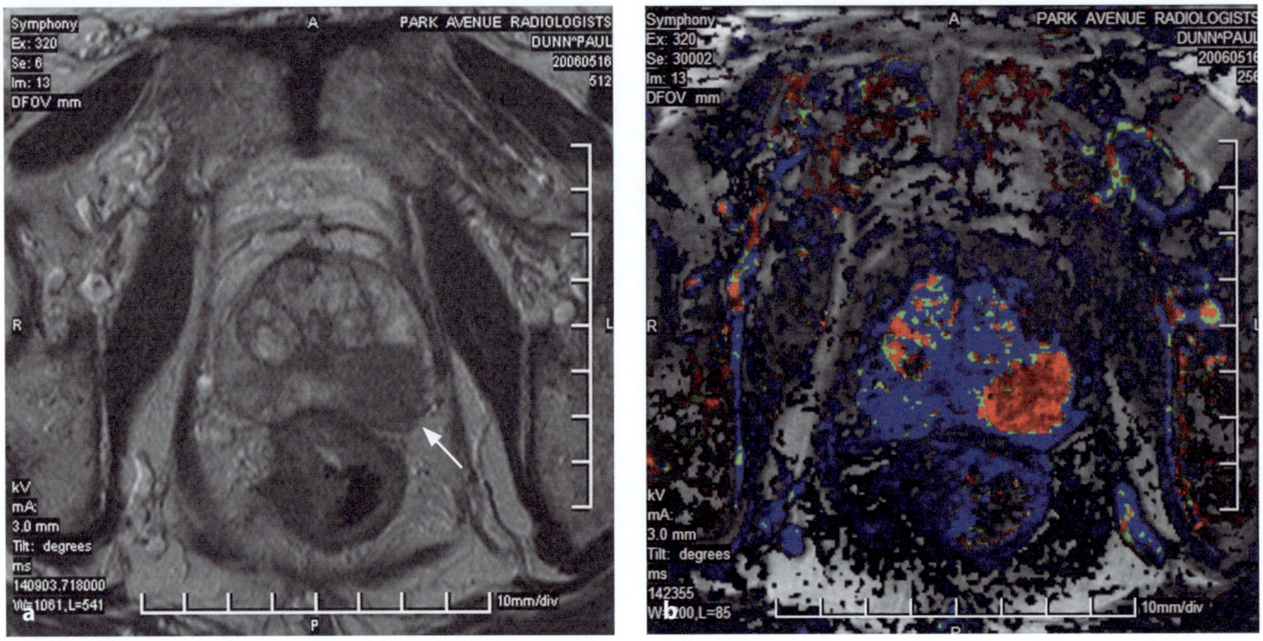

Fig. 3.6 a, b Midgland left lateral capsular erosion

Fig. 3.7 a, b

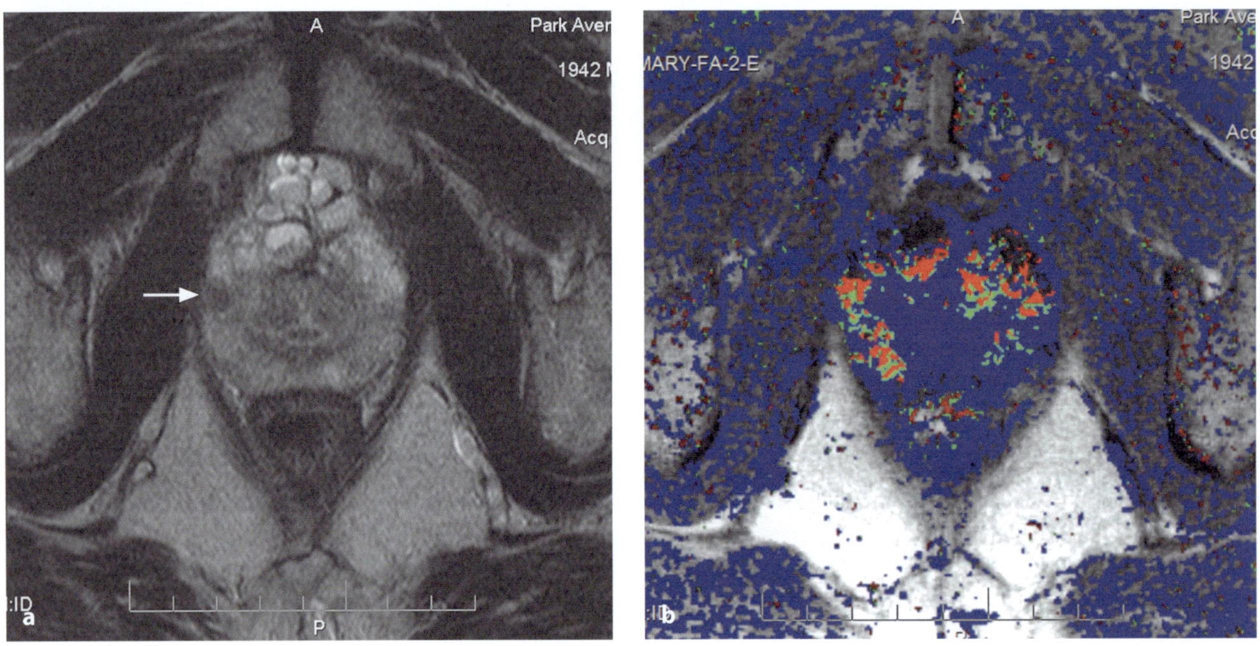

Fig. 3.7 a, b Midgland right anterolateral capsular erosion

Fig. 3.8 a, b

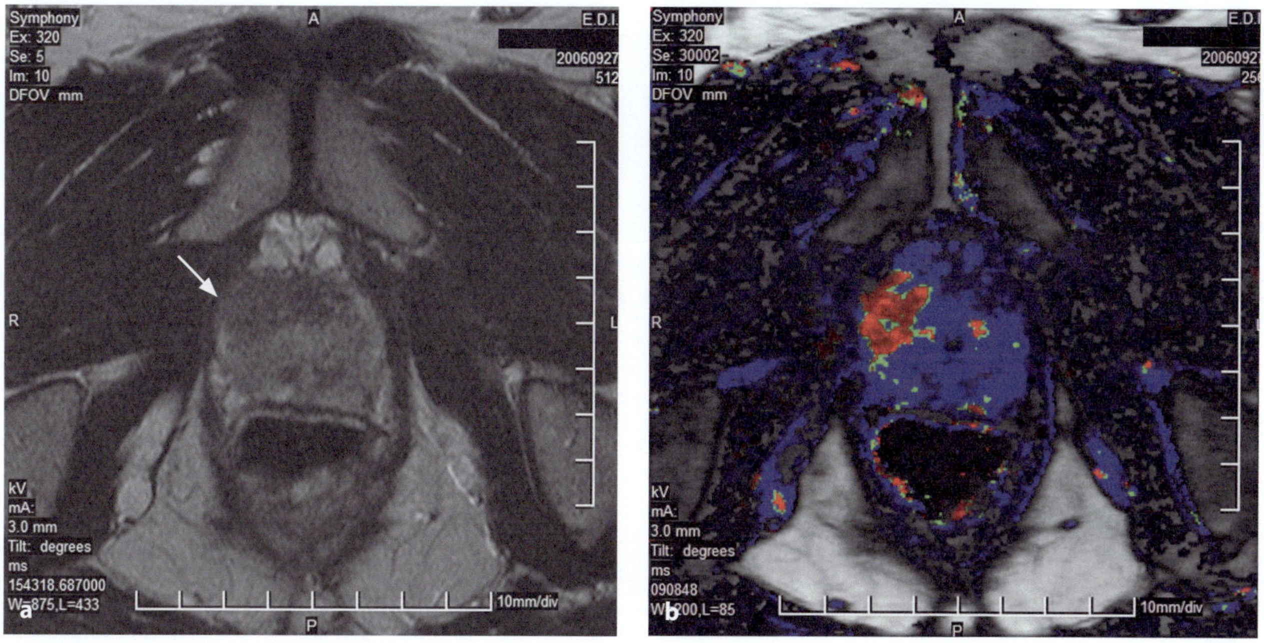

Fig. 3.8 a, b Midgland right anterior capsular erosion

Fig. 3.9 a, b

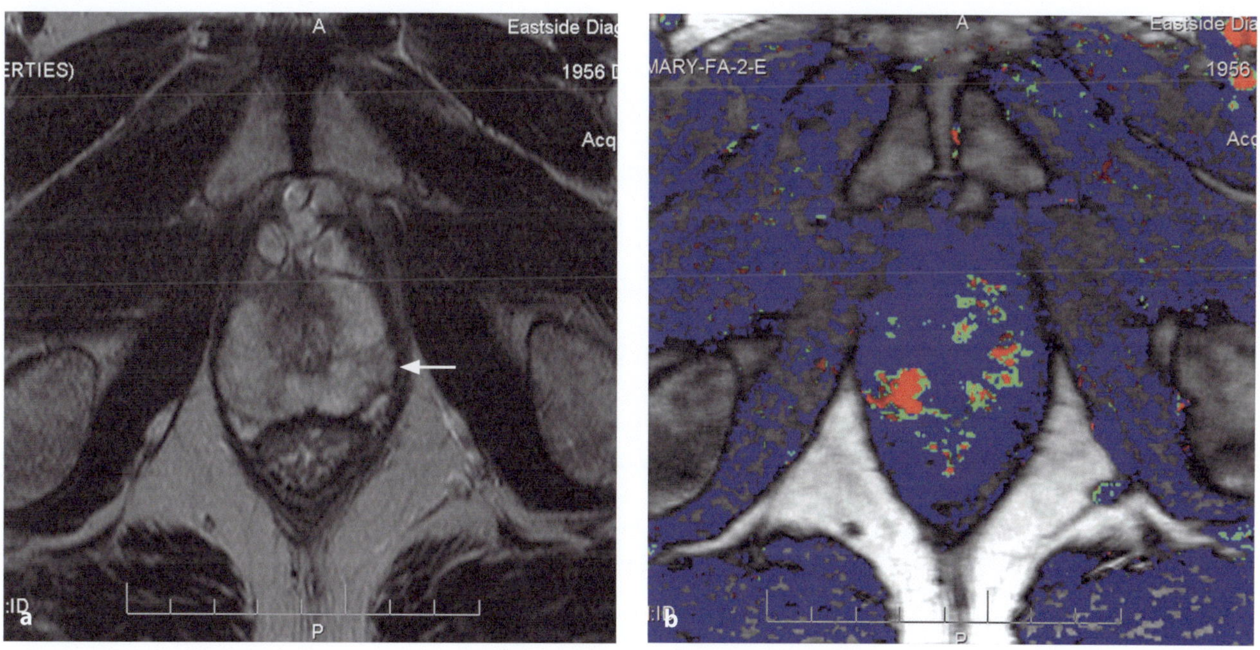

Fig. 3.9 a, b Midgland right and left anterior lesions with left lateral capsular erosion

Fig. 3.10 a, b

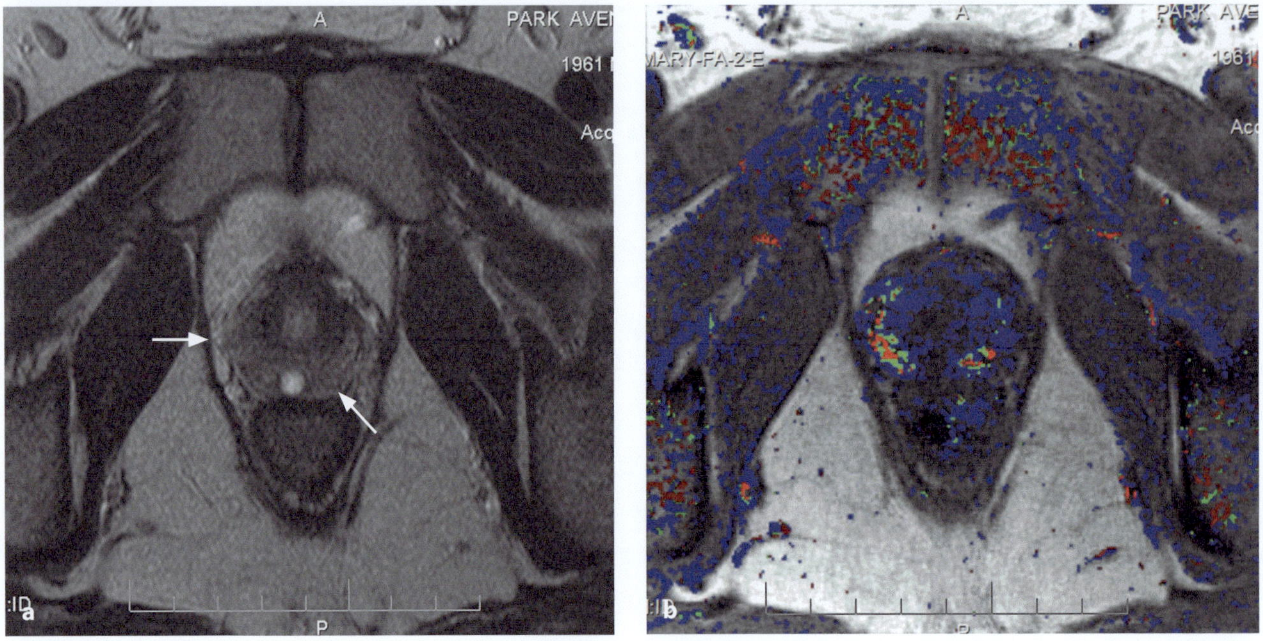

Fig. 3.10 a, b Apical left focal lesion and right anterolateral focal lesion with capsular erosion

Fig. 3.11 a, b

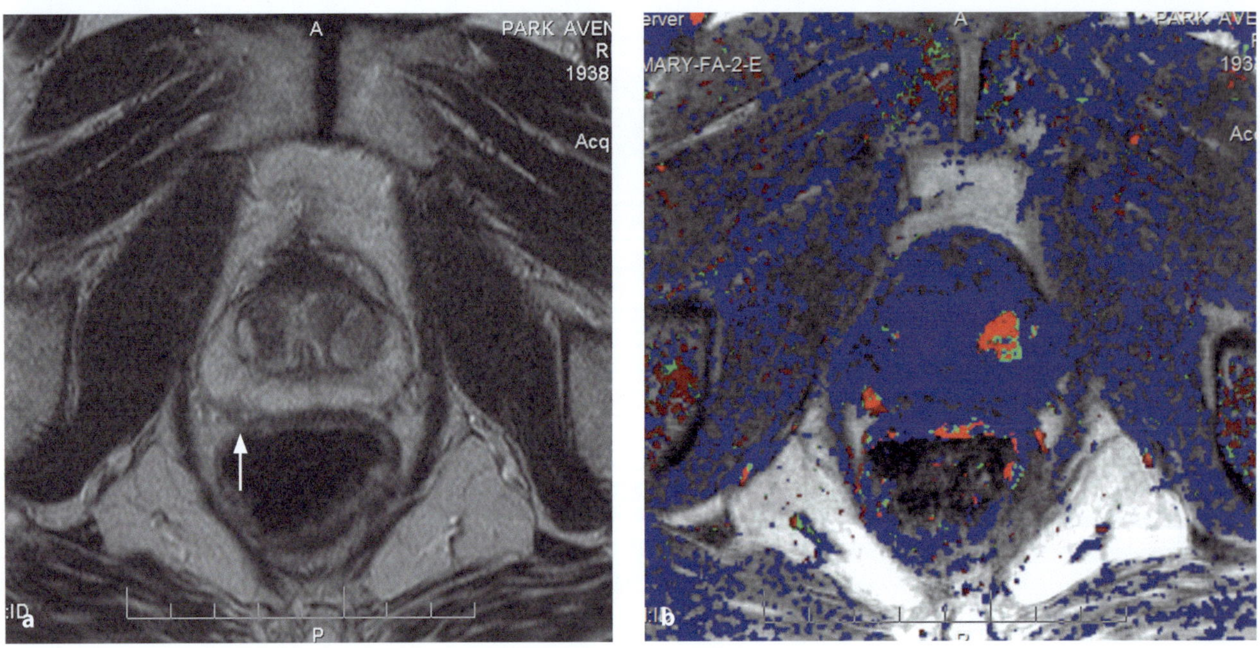

Fig. 3.11 a, b Midgland right lateral posterior 4 mm lesion with capsular erosion

Fig. 3.12 a, b

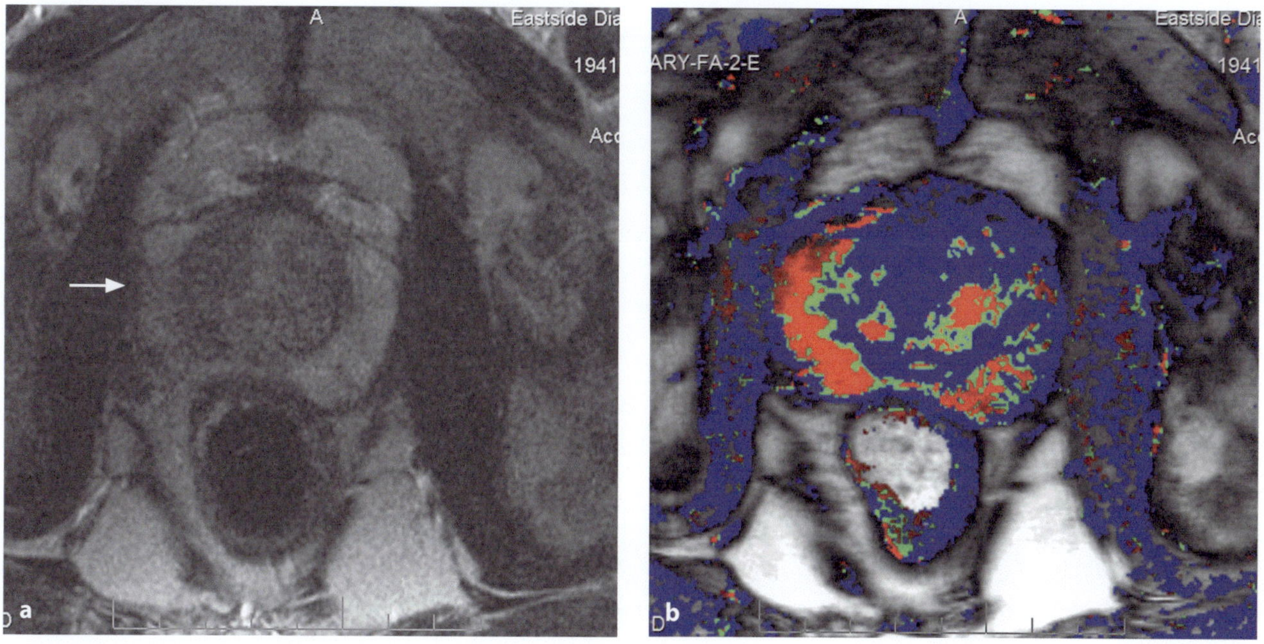

Fig. 3.12 a, b Midgland right lateral capsular erosion

Fig. 3.13 a, b

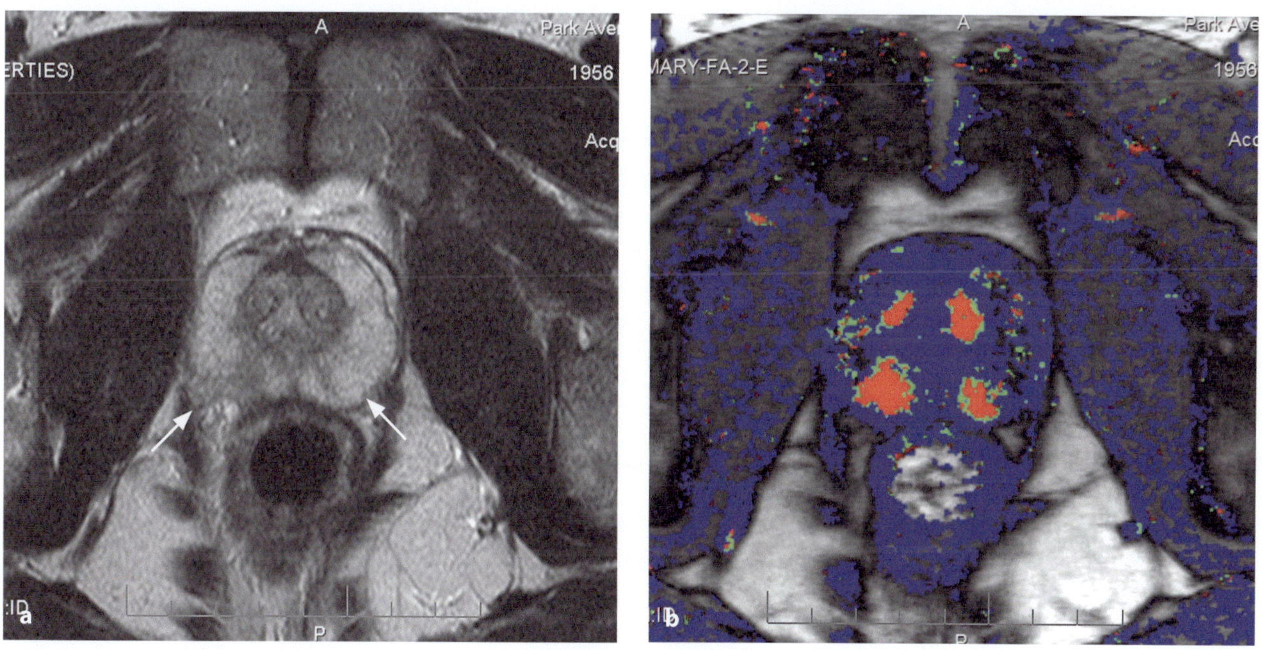

Fig. 3.13 a, b Midgland right lateral capsular erosion with left focal posterior prostatitis

Fig. 3.14 a, b

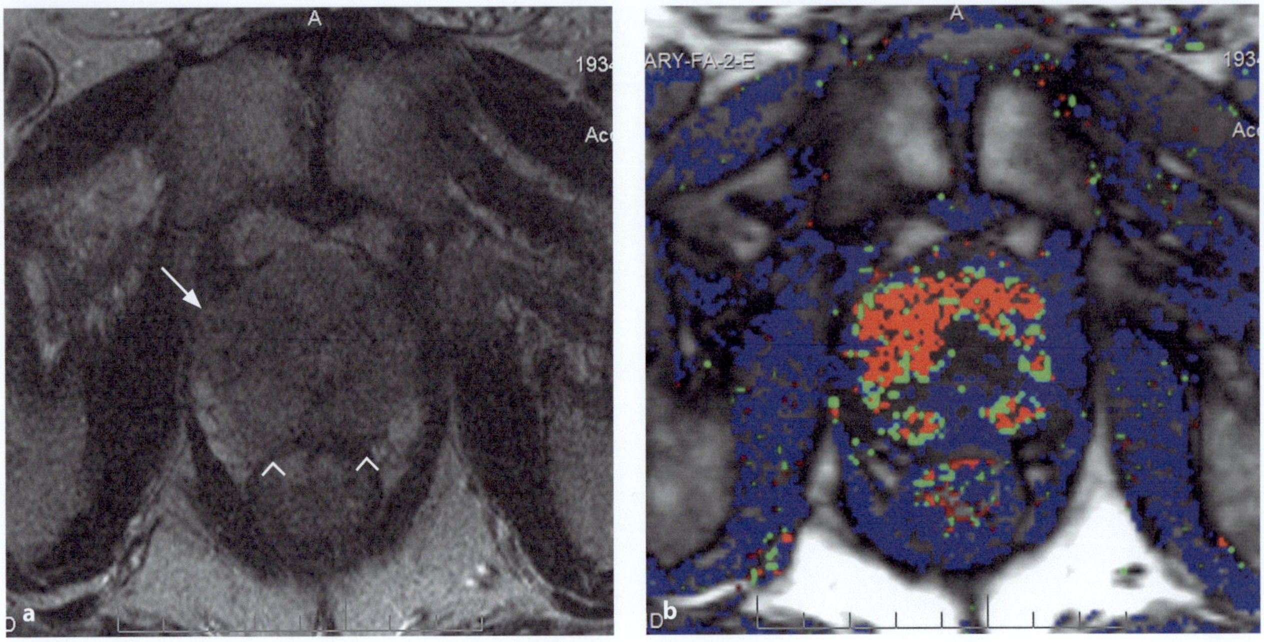

Fig. 3.14 a, b Midgland right anterior lesion with capsular erosion and bilateral posterior lesions

Chapter

Seminal Vesicle Cancer Invasion

4

Tumor extending into the seminal vesicles often do not produce hyperemia. Tumor may invade from central prostatic cancer of the base into the seminal vesicles or engulf the seminal vesicles from lateral large midgland tumors.

Fig. 4.1 a, b

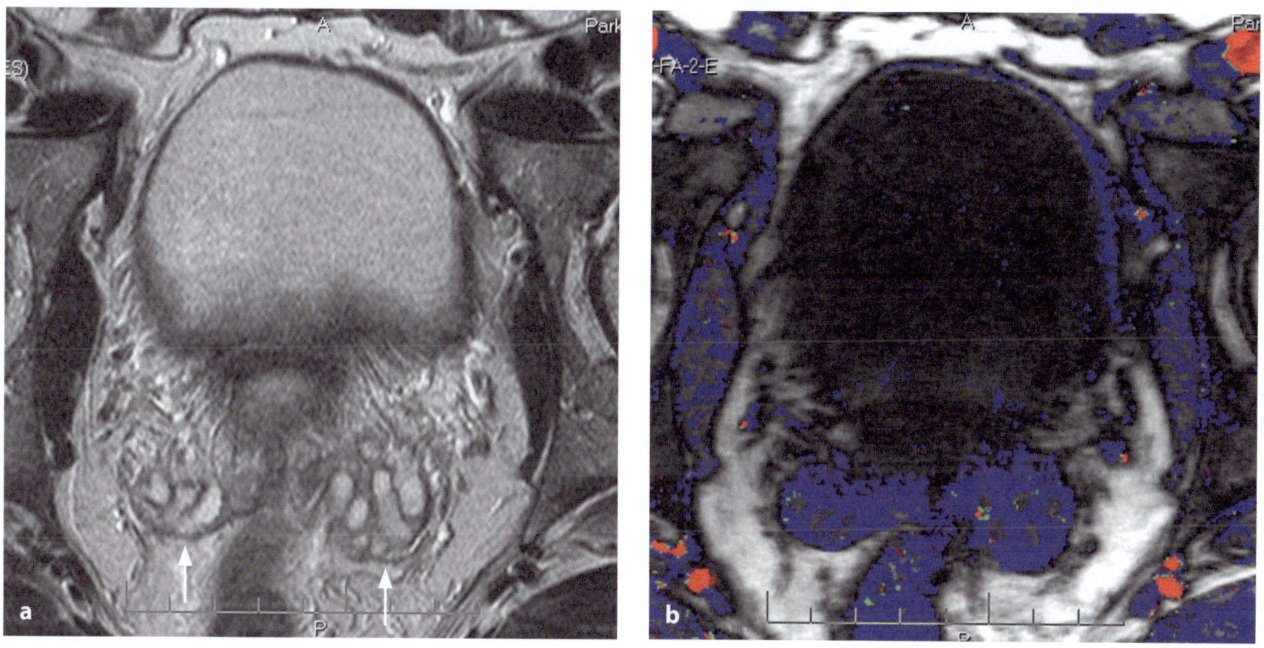

Fig. 4.1 a, b Normal seminal vesicles-note normal vascularity adjacent to semen containing regions with honeycomb appearance

Fig. 4.2 a, b

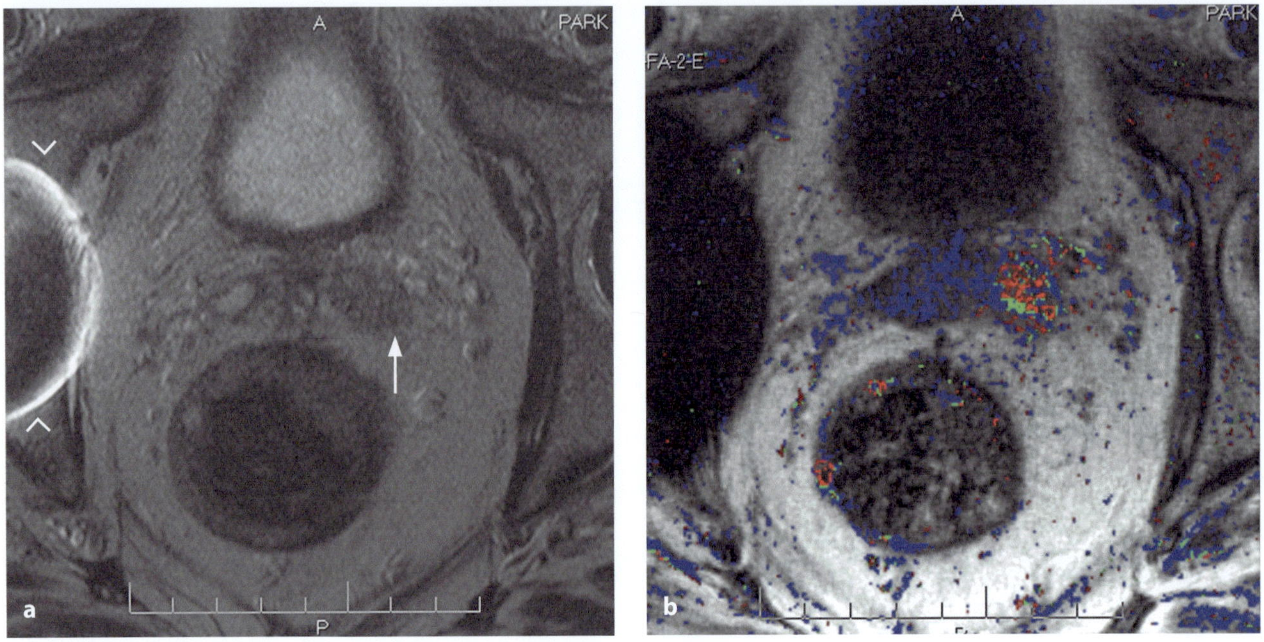

Fig. 4.2 a, b Left seminal vesicle invasion-note right hip metal artifact

Fig. 4.3 a, b

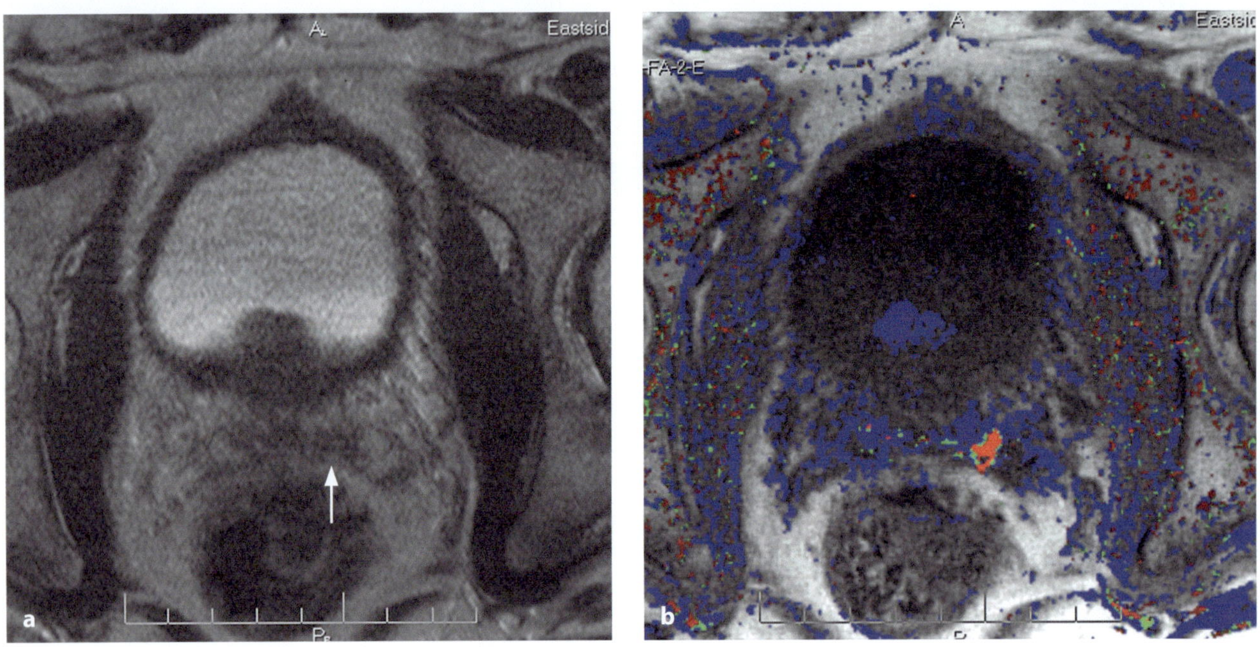

Fig. 4.3 a, b Left medial seminal vesicle invasion

Fig. 4.4 a, b

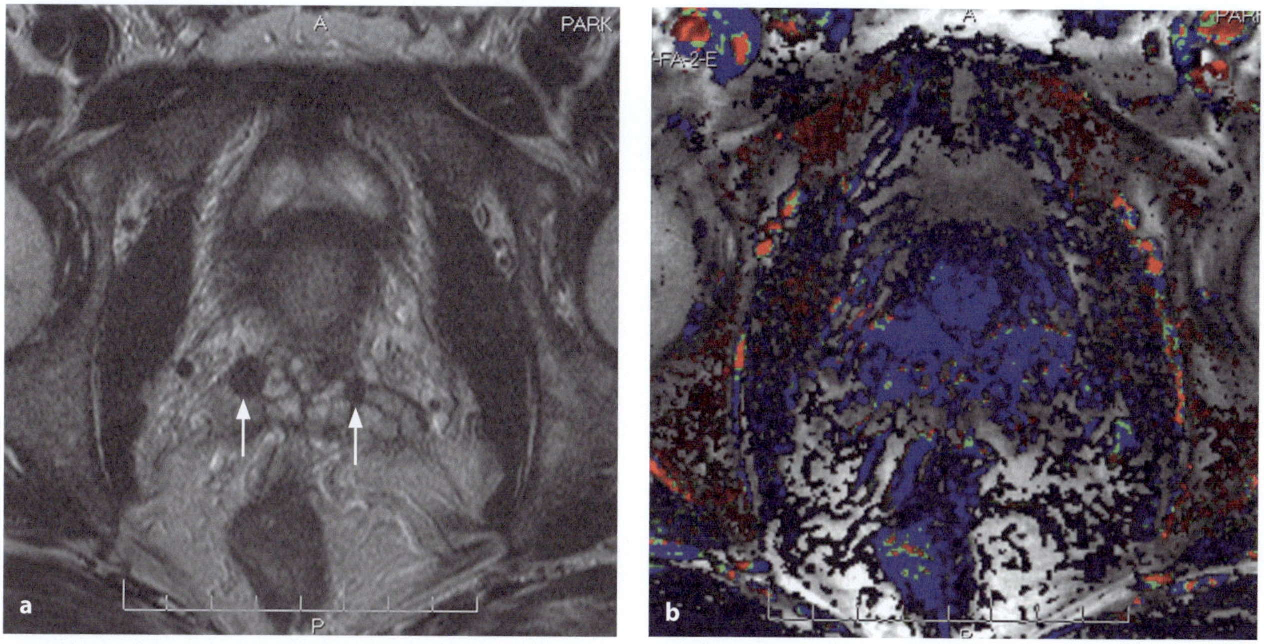

Fig. 4.4 a, b Bilateral seminal vesical invasion

Fig. 4.5 a, b

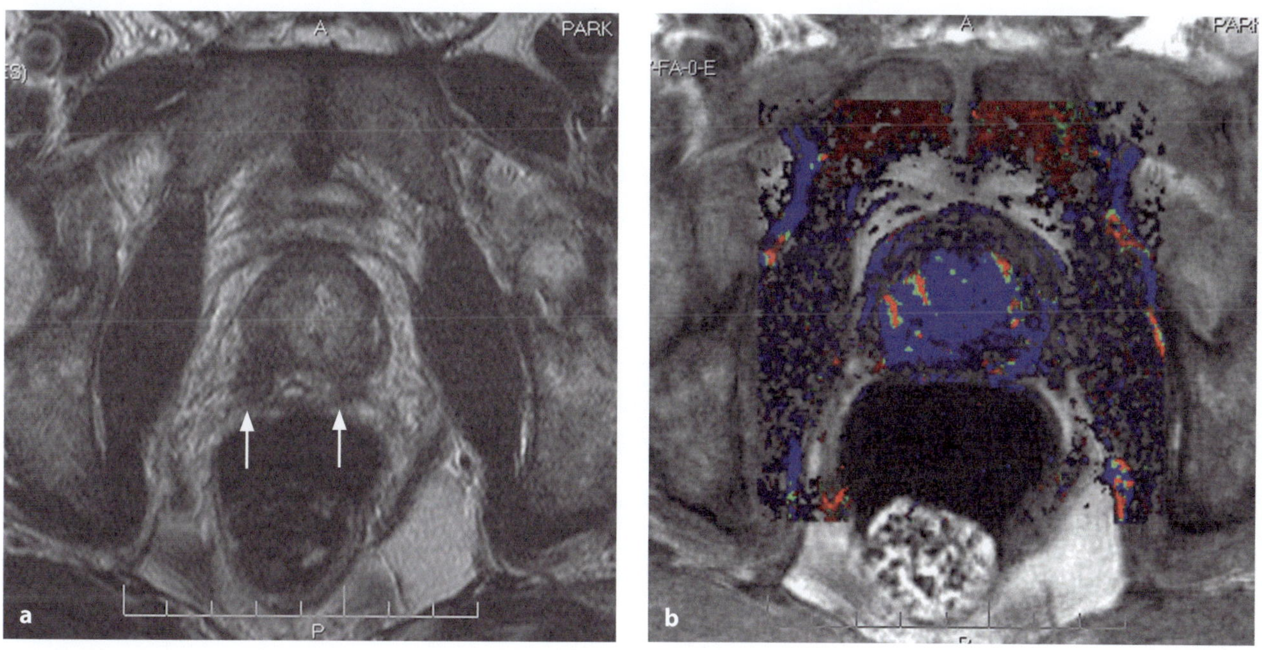

Fig. 4.5 a, b Bilateral seminal vesical invasion

Chapter 5

Nodal Cancer-Perirectal and Pelvic Adenopathy

Perirectal adenopathy 4mm or greater has strong correlation with metastatic disease since prostate metastases are usually subcentimeter in size. Findings must confirmed by lymph node MRI or biopsy.

Vascularized lymph nodes best correlate with active malignancy, however, normal lymph nodes have expected hilar vascularity that may produce hyperemia during the DCE exam.

Fig. 5.1 a–d

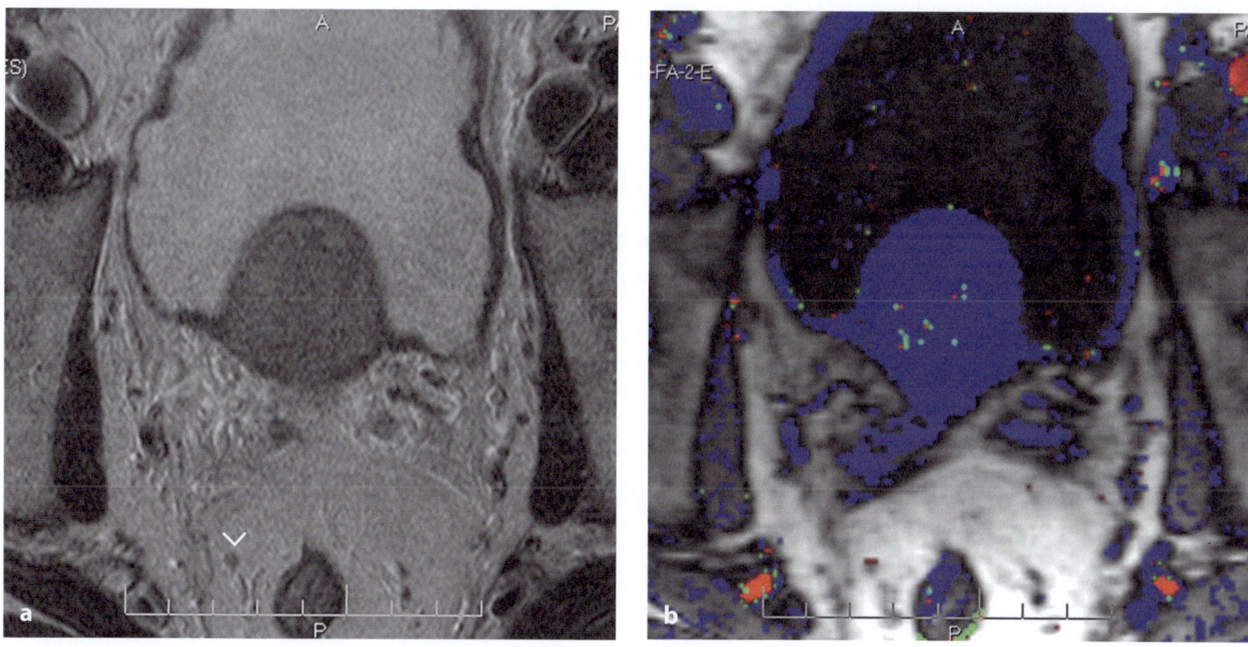

Fig. 5.1 a, b Right perirectal node 3 mm with homogeneous signal

Fig. 5.1 c,d

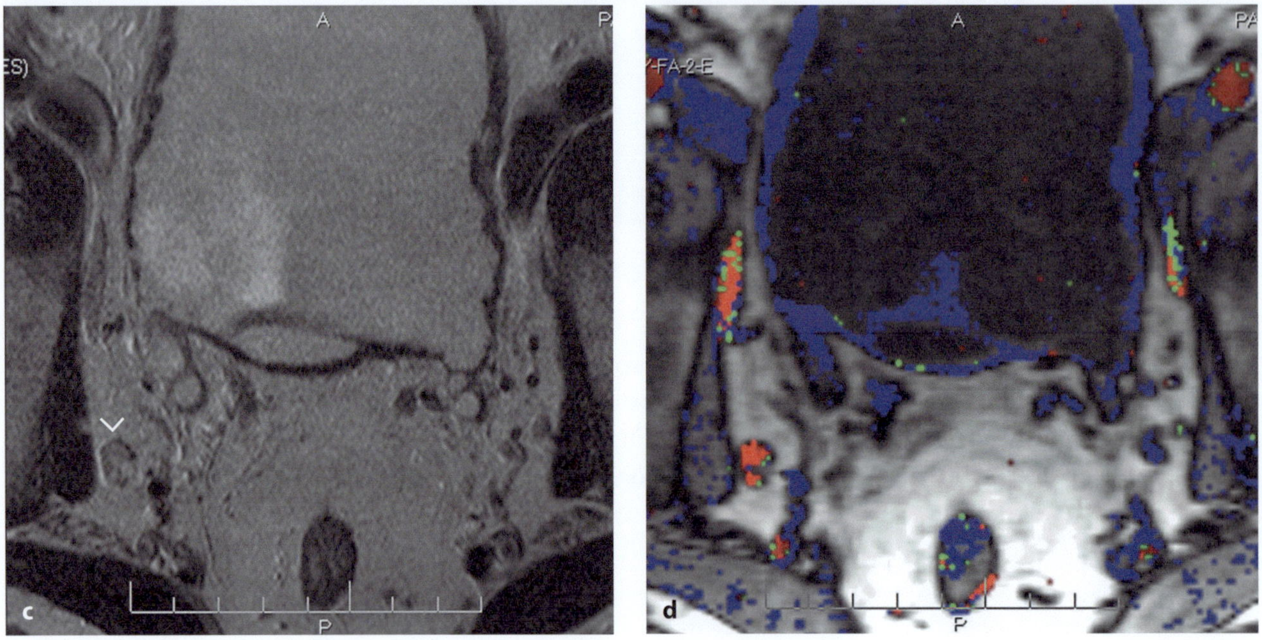

Fig. 5.1 c, d Right obturator node 9 mm with inhomogeneous signal

Fig. 5.2 a–l

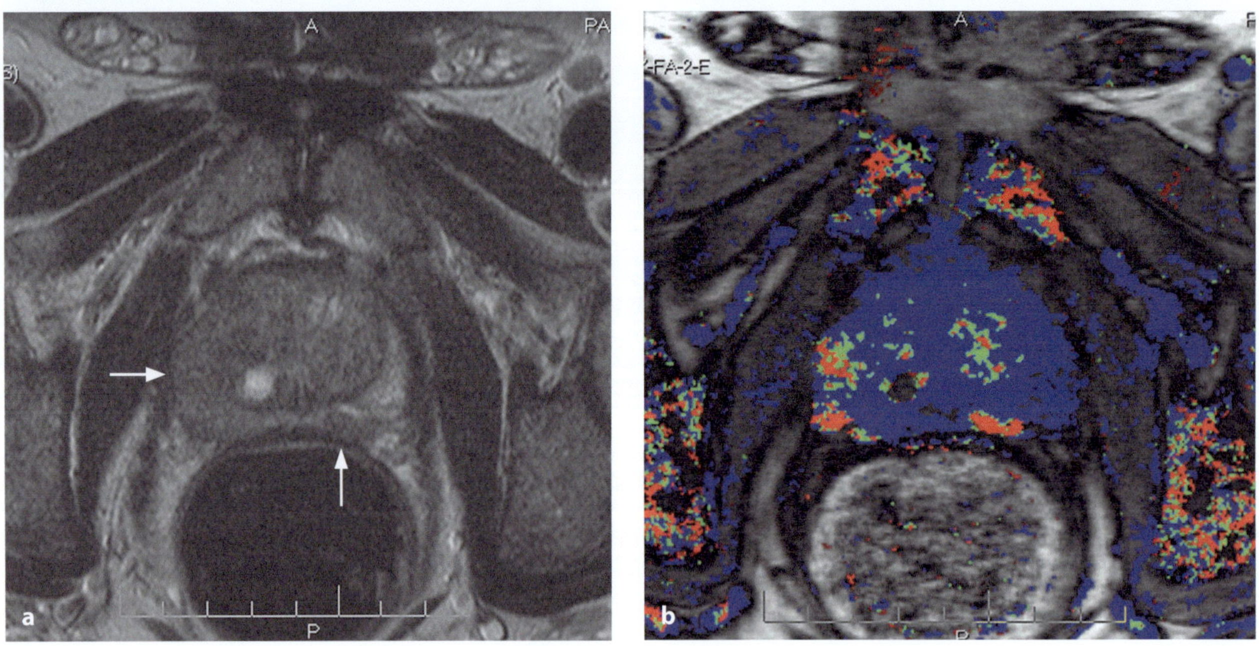

Fig. 5.2 a, b Gleason 4 left base and Gleason 5 right base

Fig. 5.2 c, d

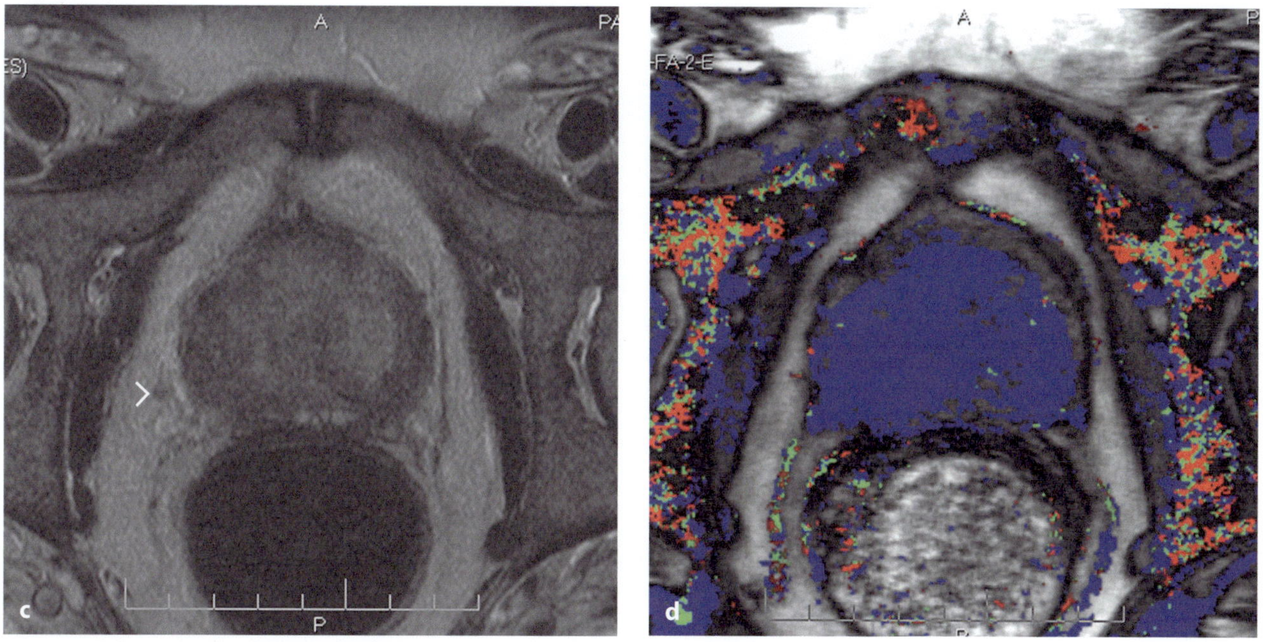

Fig. 5.2 c, d Right periprostatic 3 mm node

Fig. 5.2 e, f

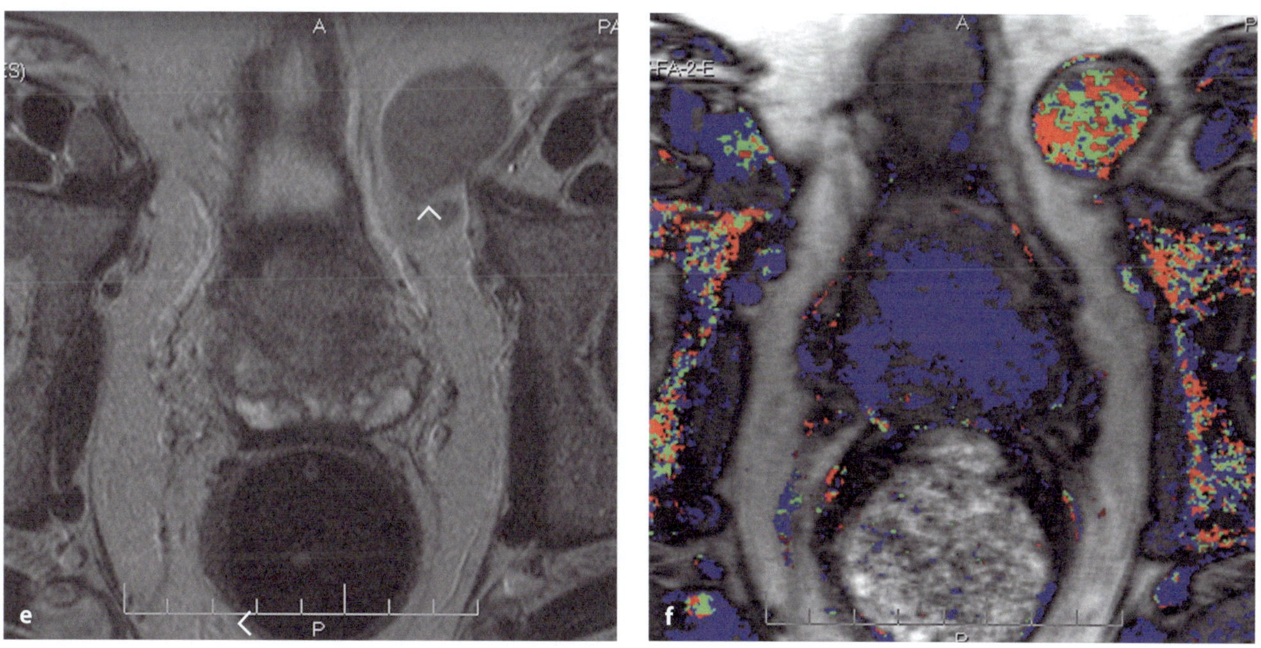

Fig.5.2 e, f Right perirectal node and left obturator nodes

Fig. 5.2 g, h

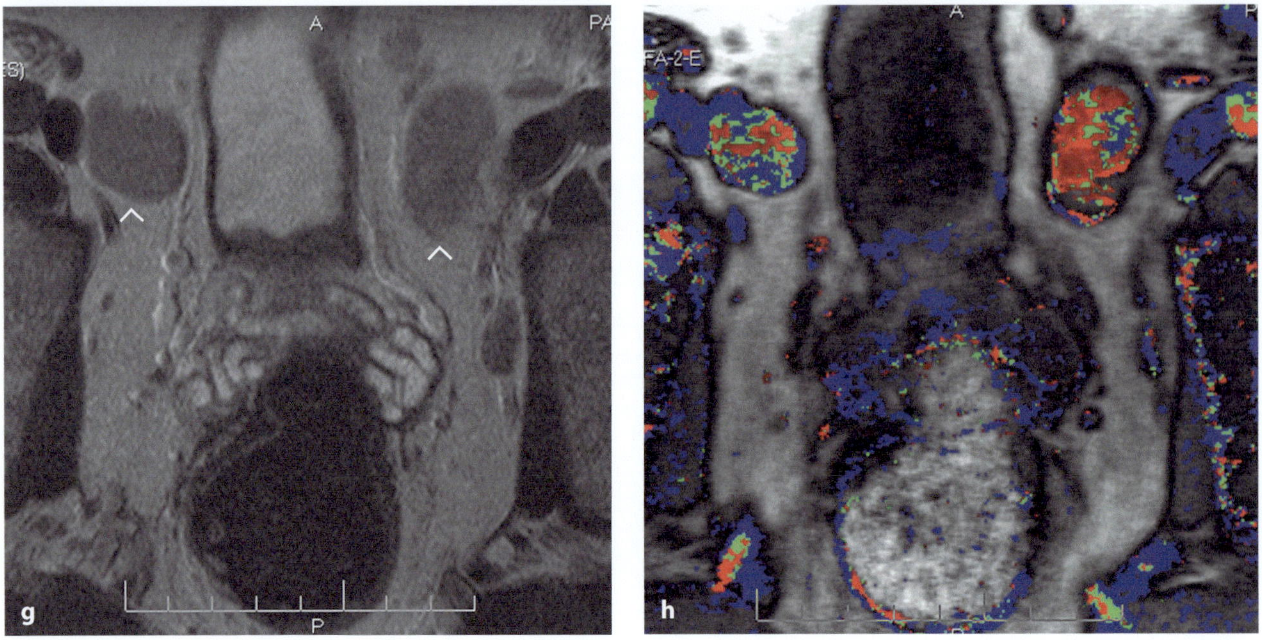

Fig. 5.2 g, h Bilateral vascular obturator nodes and bone metastases

Fig. 5.2 i, j

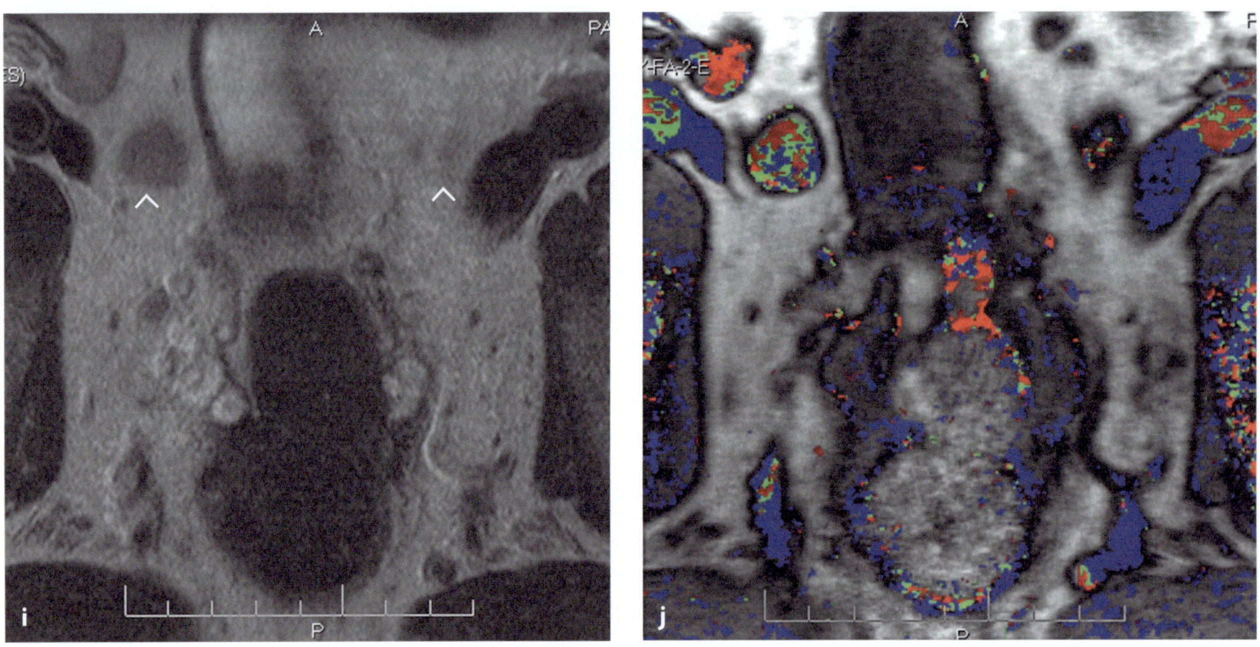

Fig. 5.2 i, j Bilateral vascular internal iliac nodes and bone metastases

Fig. 5.2 k, l

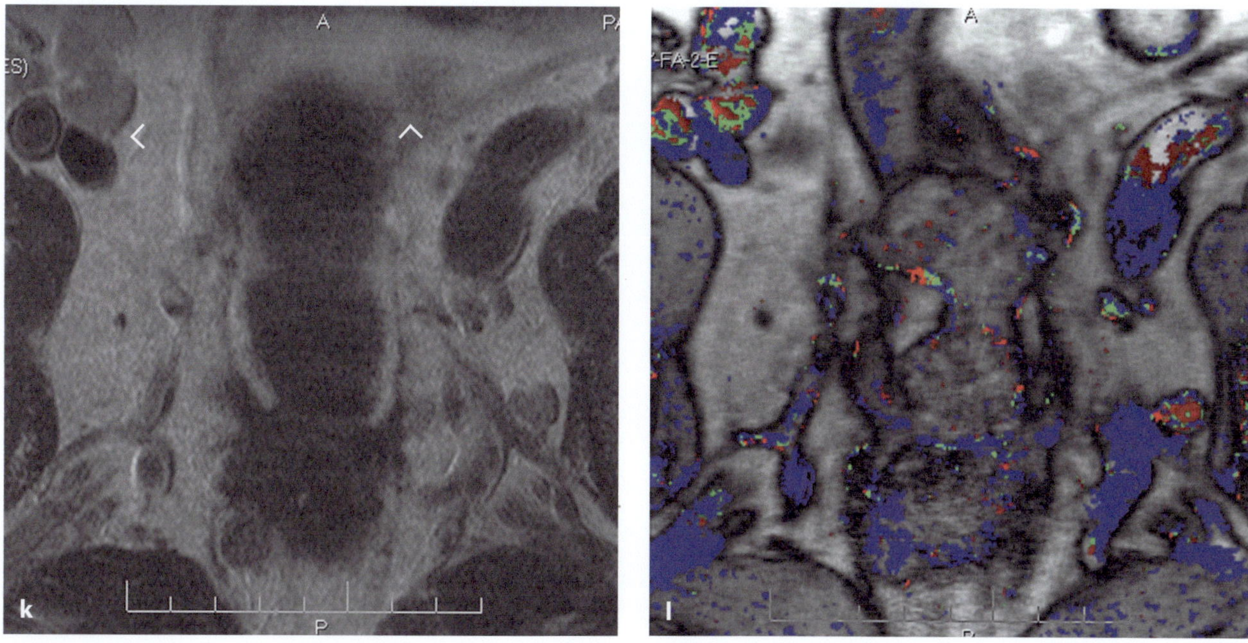

Fig. 5.2 k, l Bilateral vascular external iliac nodes and bone metastases

Fig. 5.3 a–d

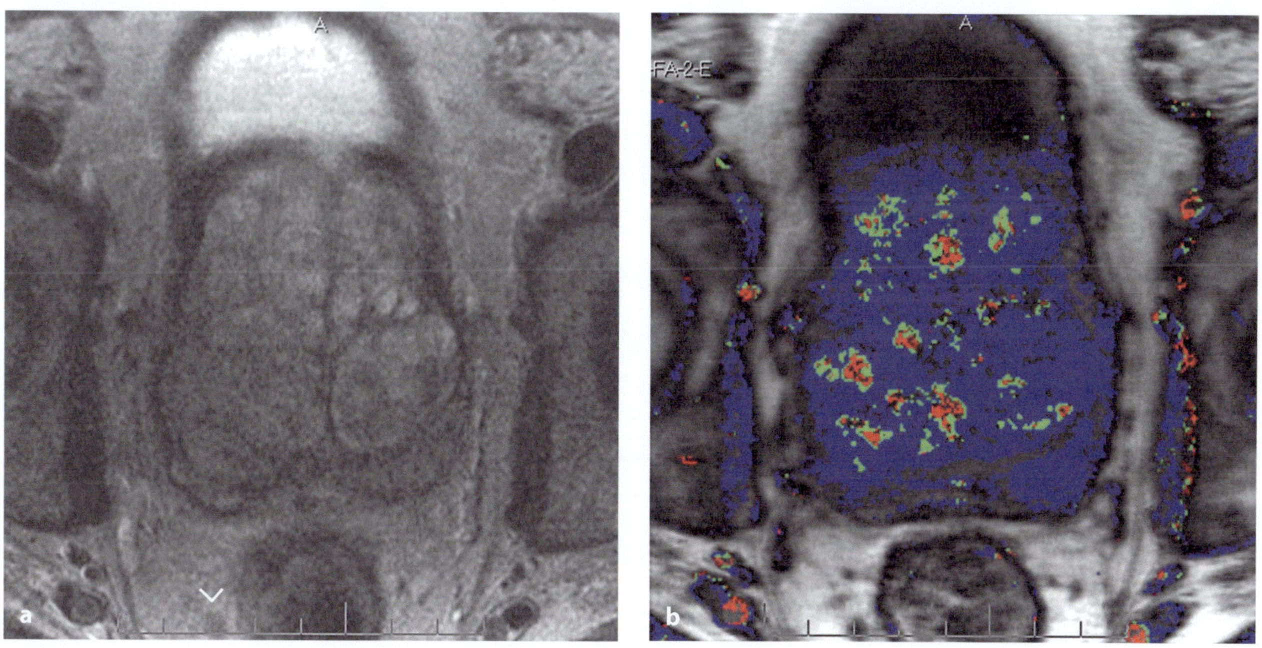

Fig. 5.3 a, b Right perirectal node 6 mm with homogeneous signal

Fig. 5.3 c,d

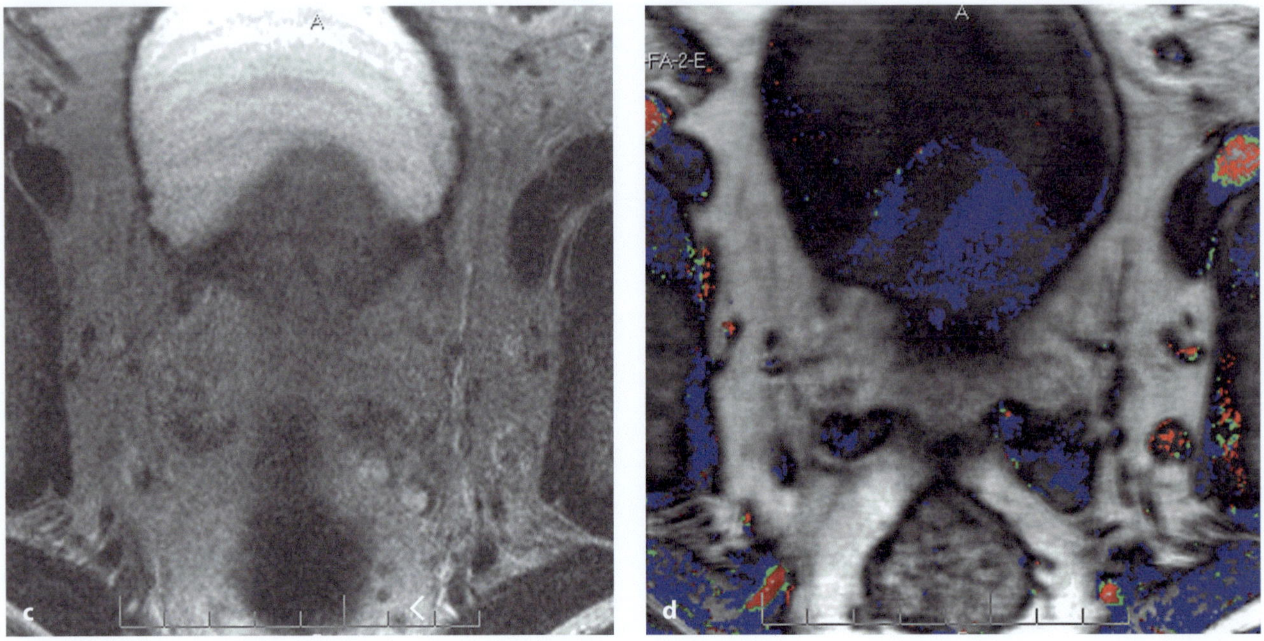

Fig. 5.3 c, d Left perirectal node 3mm-note 2 anterior vessels

Fig. 5.4 a, b

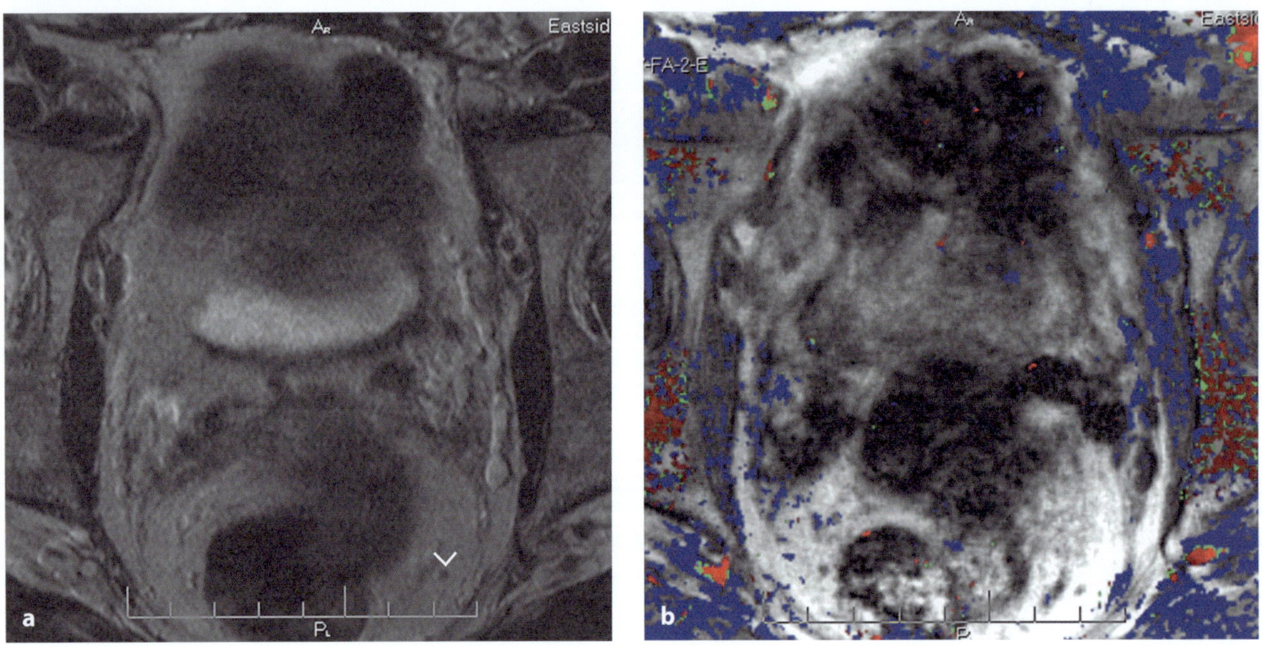

Fig. 5.4 a, b Left 3mm perirectal node-avascular

Fig. 5.5 a, b

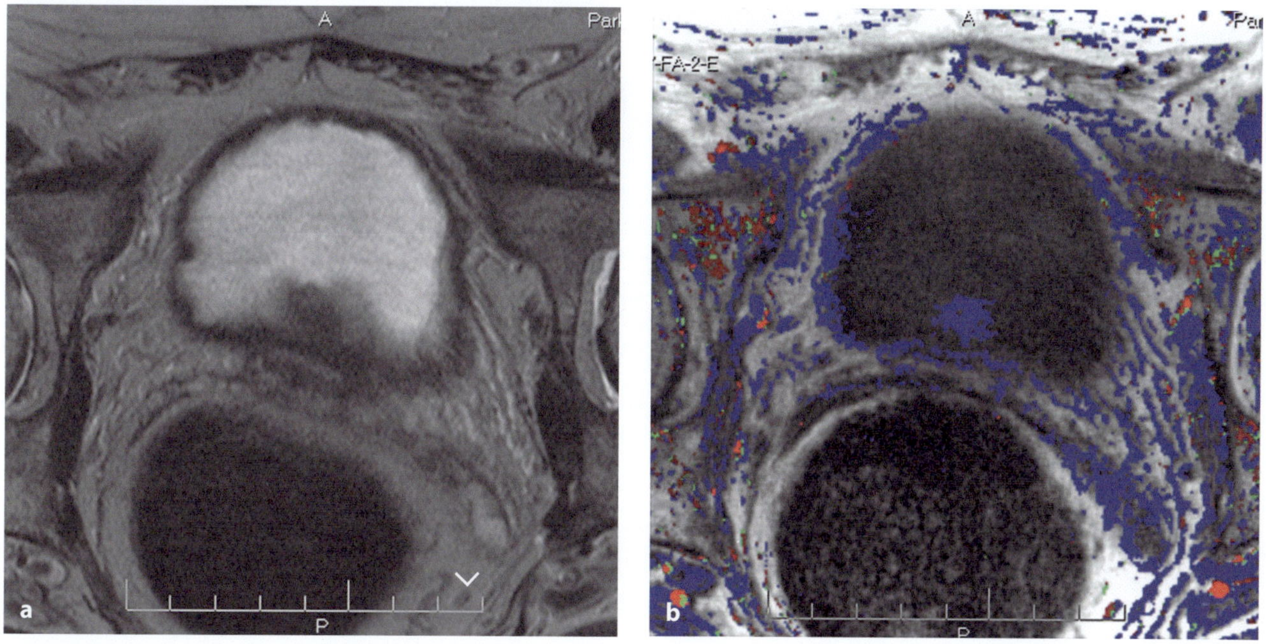

Fig. 5.5 a, b Left 3x5 mm perirectal node-vascular

Fig. 5.6 a, b

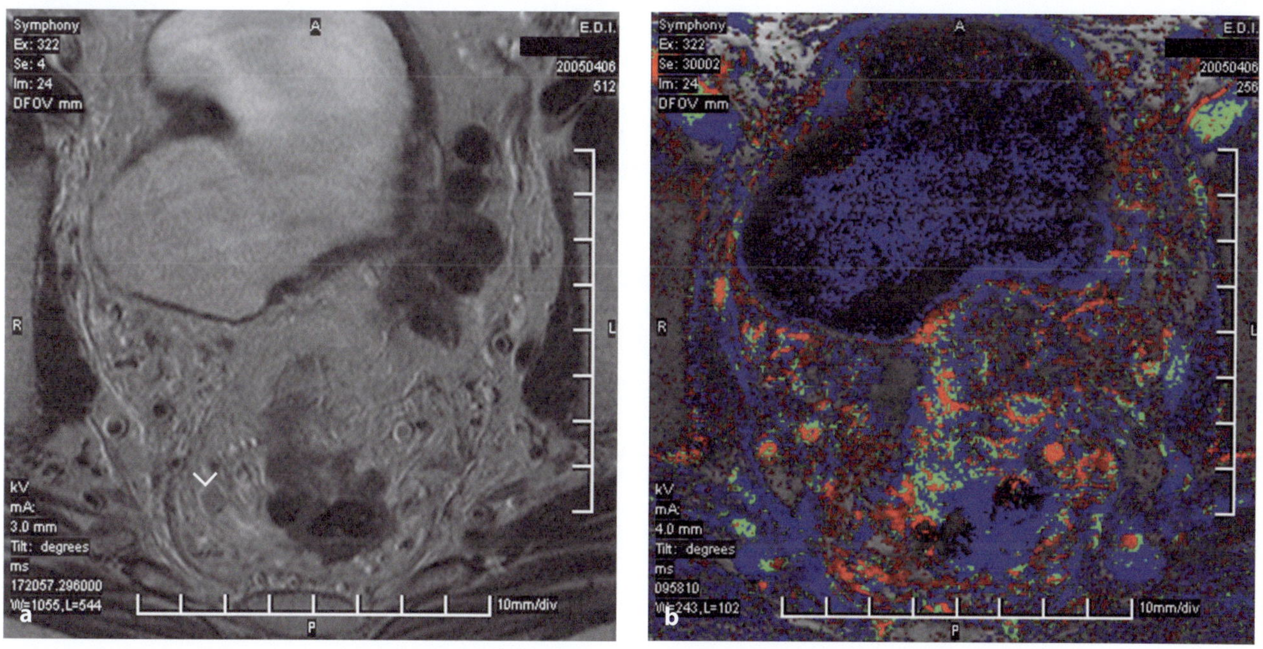

Fig. 5.6 a, b Right perirectal vascular node from squamous cell carcinoma-note massive rectal invasion

Bone Metastases

6

Metastatic foci are generally sclerotic and focal although diffuse widespread boney disease may occur. Abnormal bone findings must be correlated clinically and with other studies such as plain radiograph, CT scan and bone scan. T2 weighted lesions appear as signal loss. DCE images show color based on current degree of tumor vascularization.

Fig. 6.1 a–h

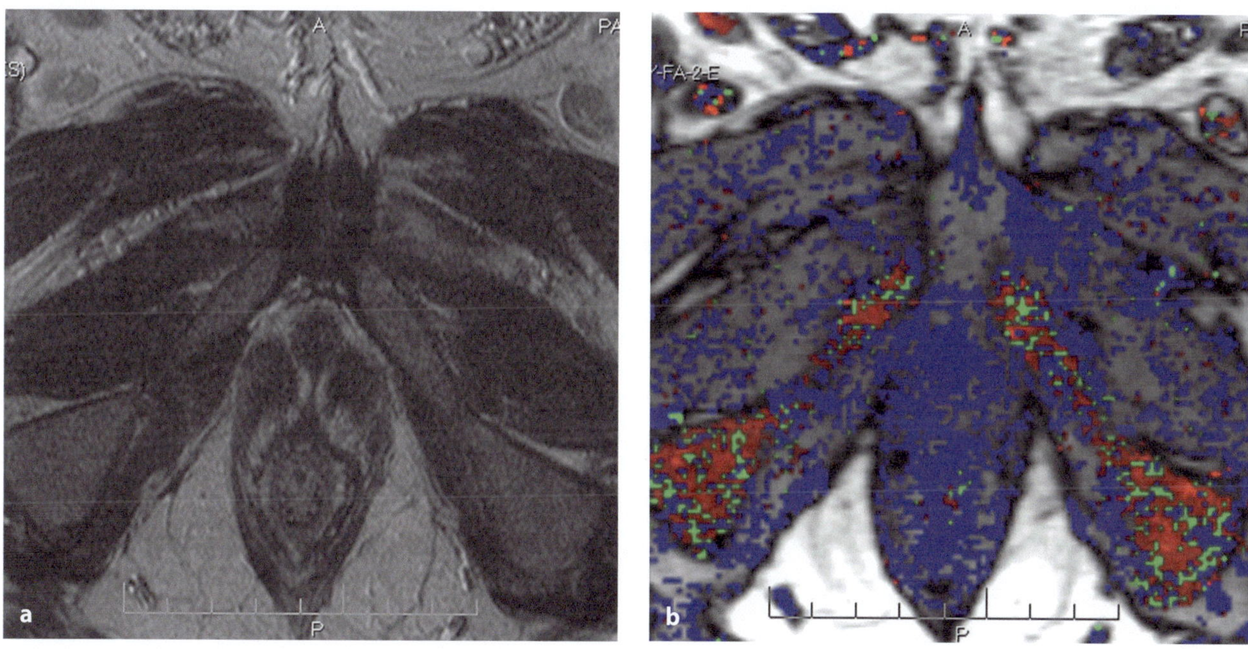

Fig. 6.1 a, b Bilateral inferior pubic rami disease

Fig. 6.1 c,d

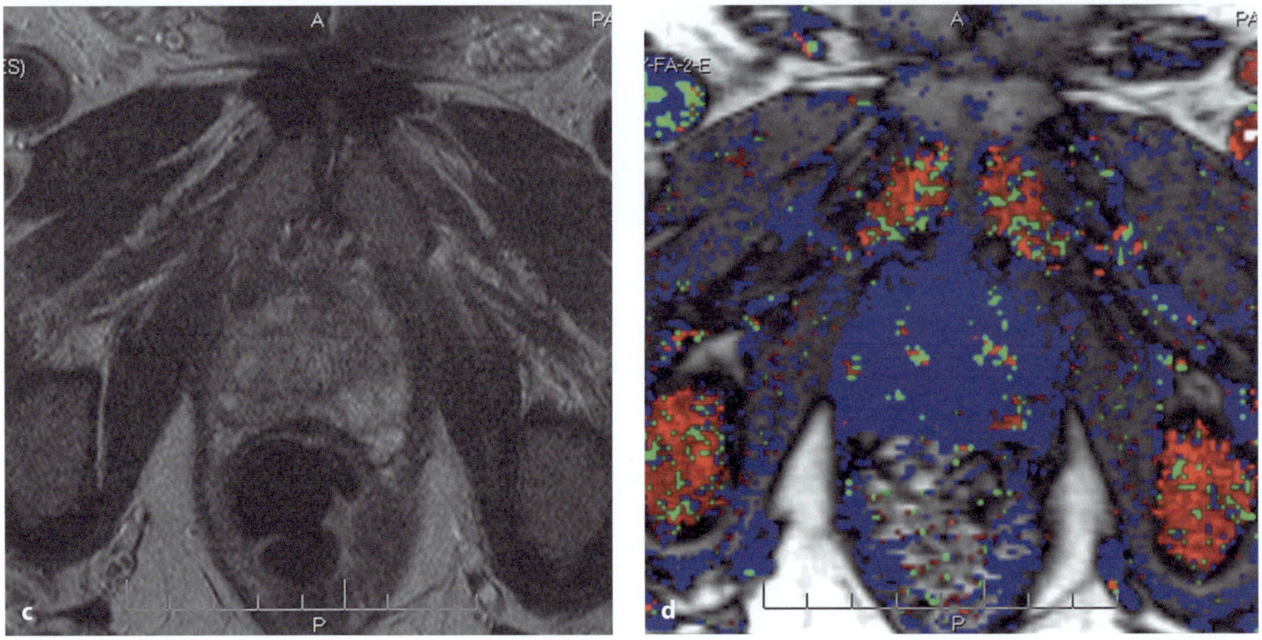

Fig. 6.1 c, d Bilateral ischial tuberosity disease

Fig. 6.1 e, f

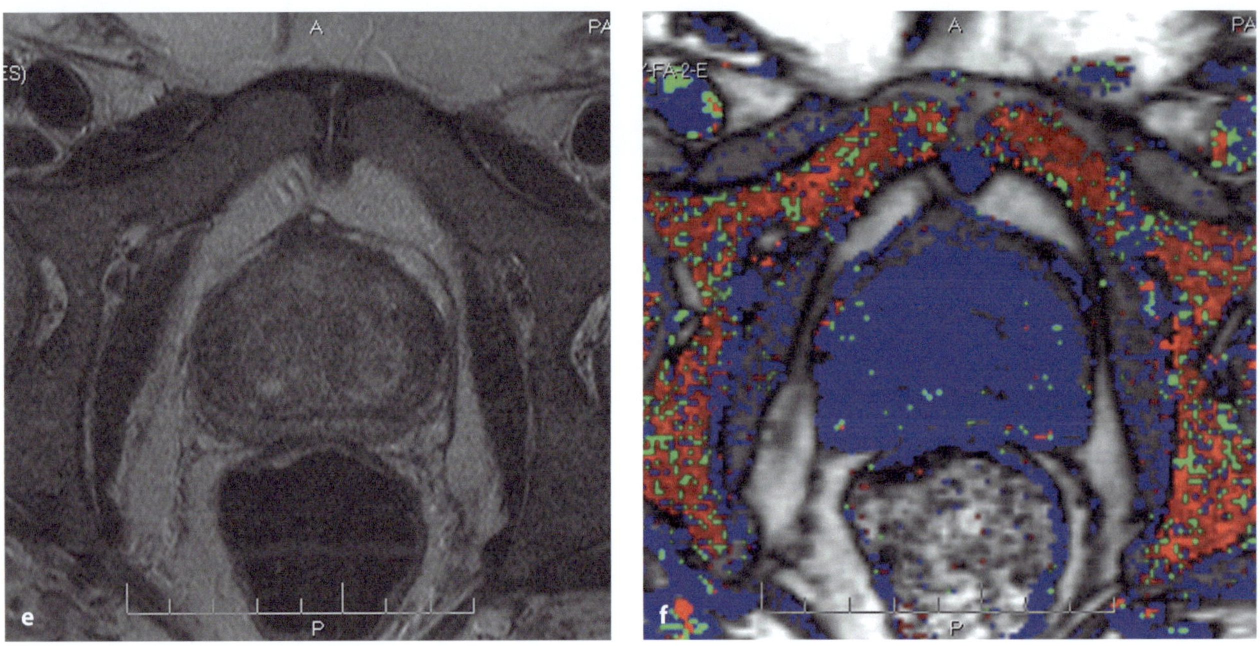

Fig. 6.1 e, f Bilateral acetabular disease

Fig. 6.1 g, h

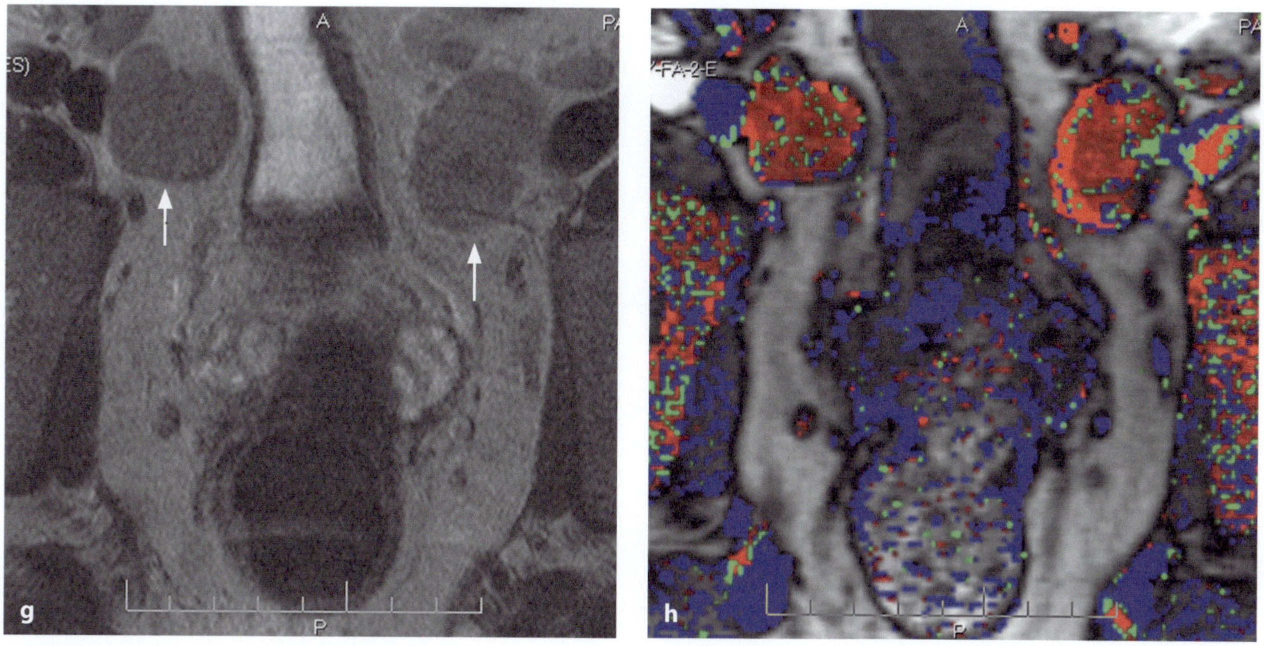

Fig. 6.1 g, h Bilateral superior pubic ramus and iliac disease-note adenopathy producing hour-glass bladder deformity

Fig. 6.2 a–h

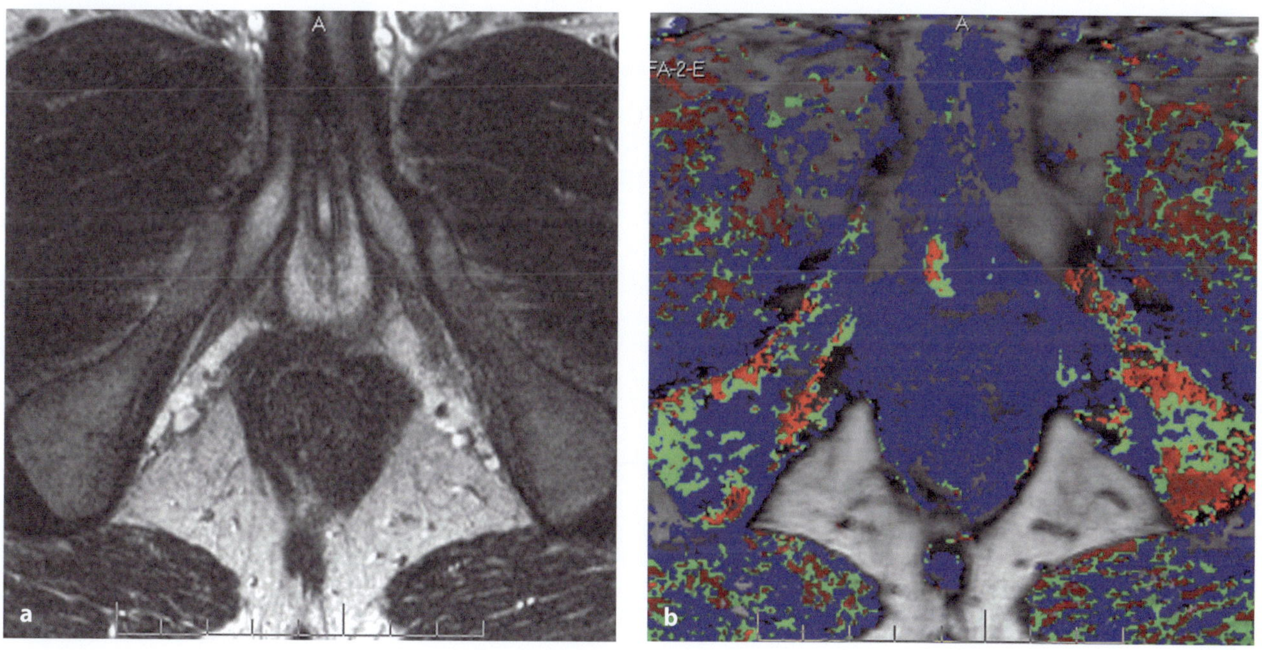

Fig. 6.2 a, b Bilateral ischial tuberosity and inferior pubic ramus disease

Fig. 6.2 c, d

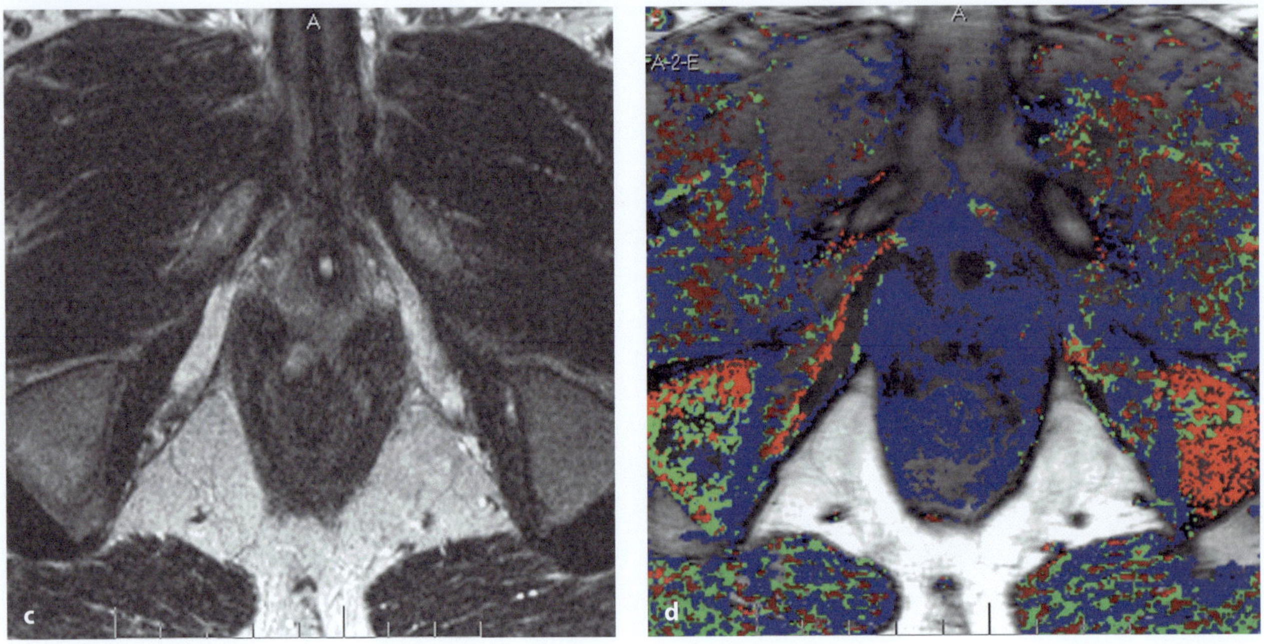

Fig. 6.2 c, d Bilateral ischial tuberosity disease

Fig. 6.2 e, f

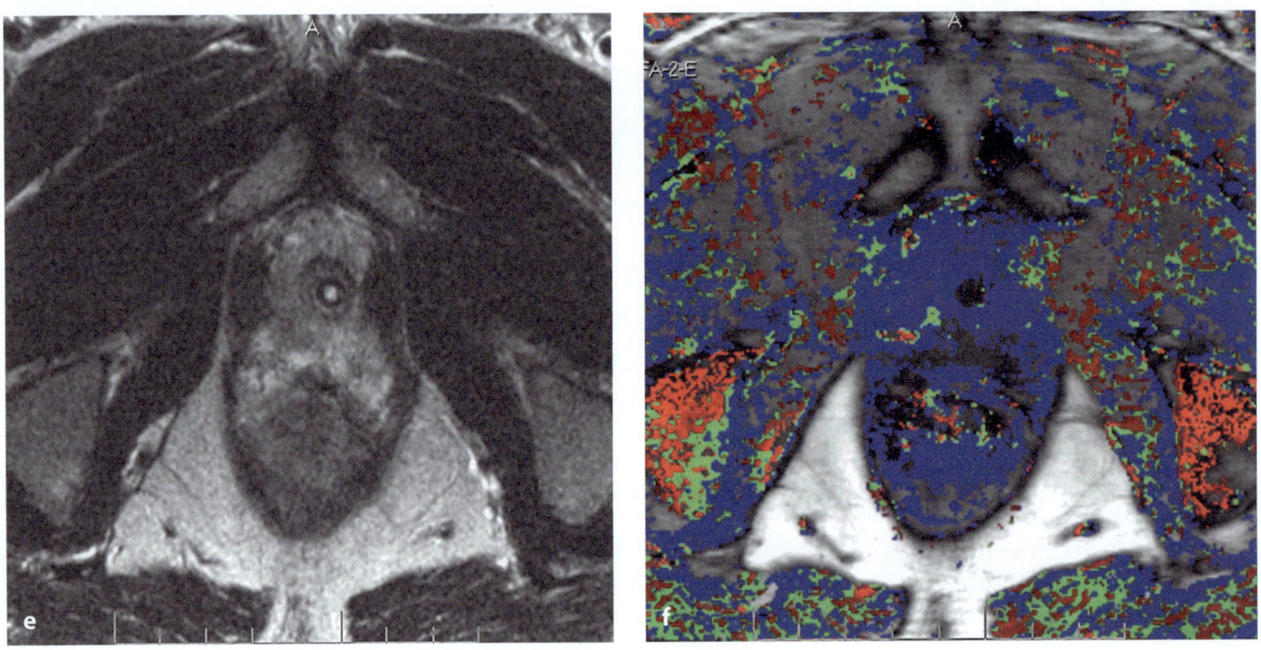

Fig. 6.2 e, f Bilateral ischial disease-note postoperative prostate

Fig. 6.2 g, h

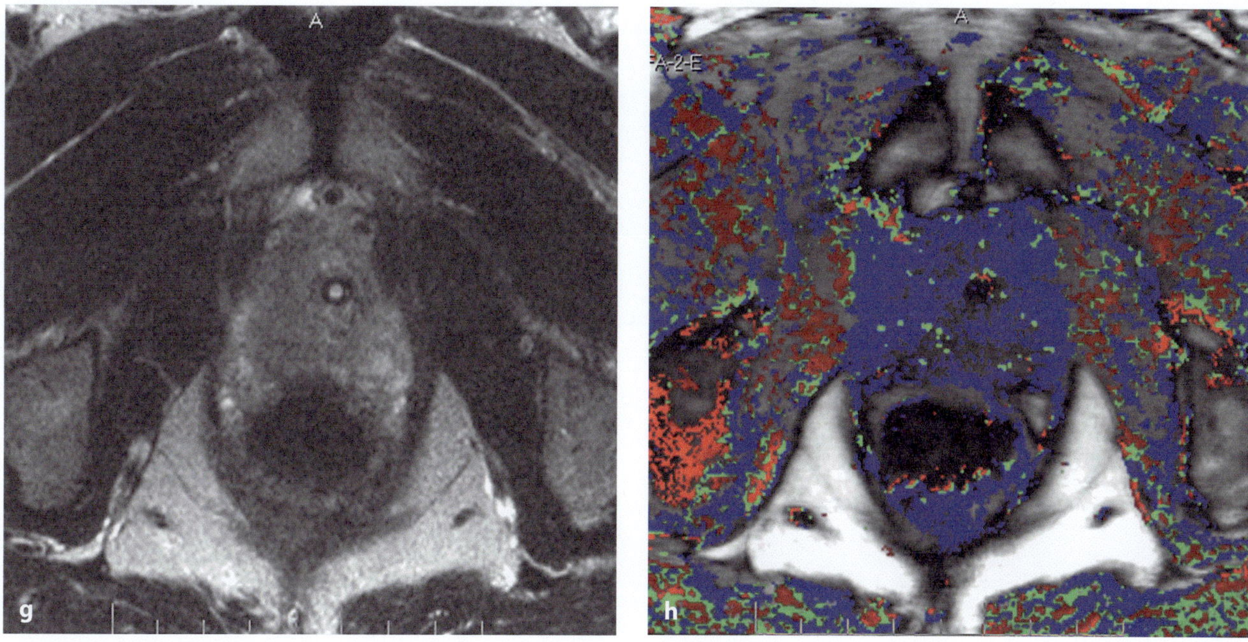

Fig. 6.2 g, h Right ischial disease

Fig. 6.3 a–l

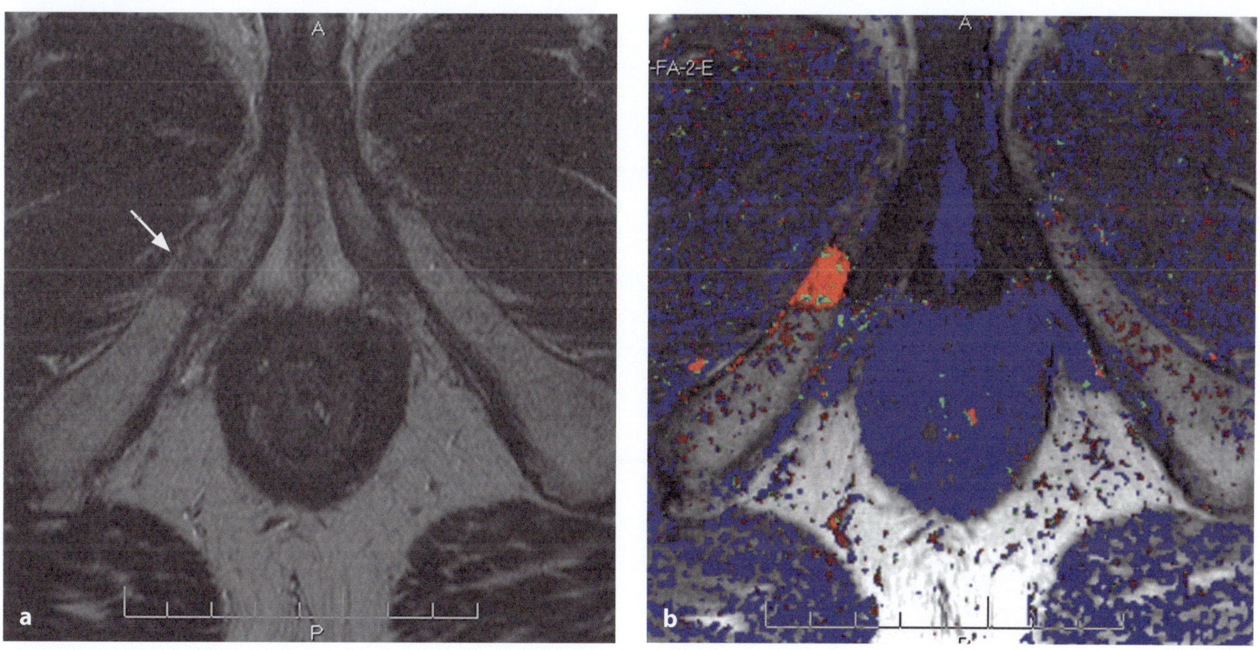

Fig. 6.3 a, b Focal right anterior inferior pubic ramus disease

Fig. 6.3 c, d

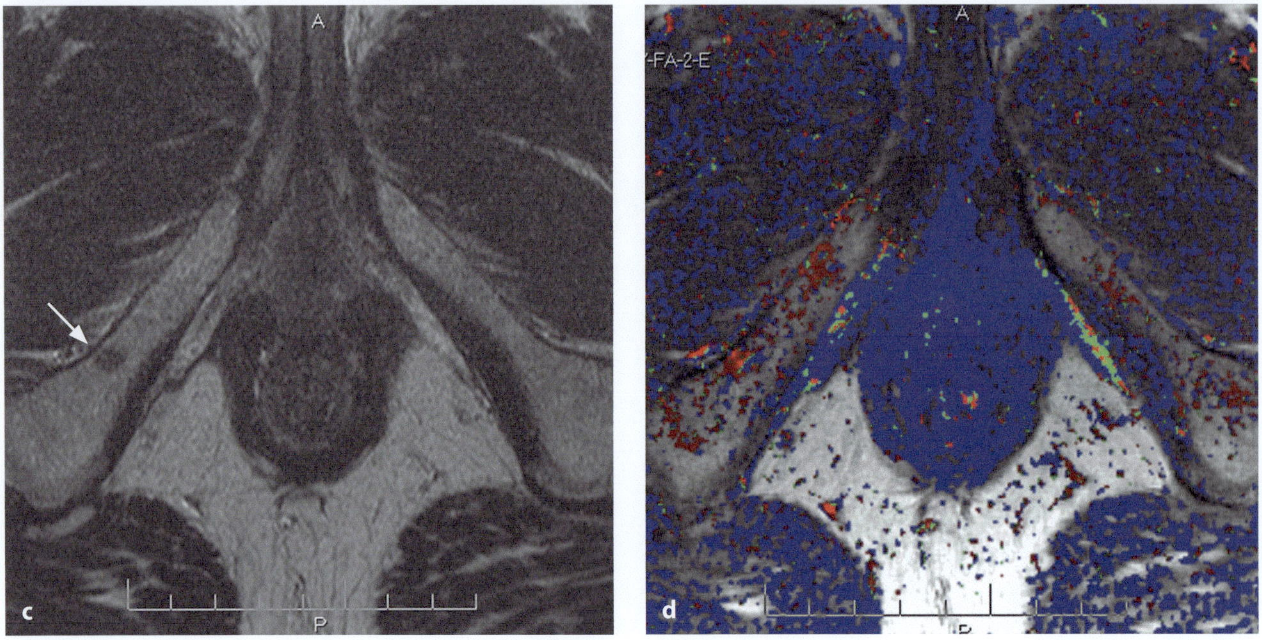

Fig. 6.3 c, d Focal right posterior inferior pubic ramus disease

Fig. 6.3 e, f

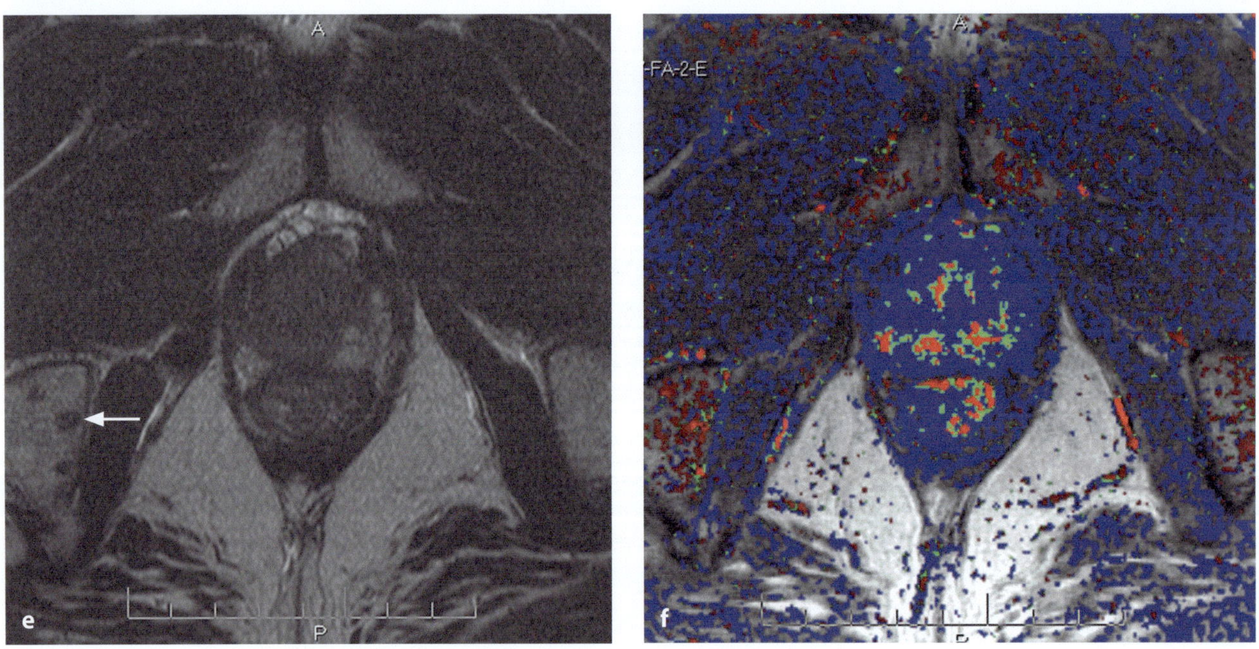

Fig. 6.3 e, f Focal right ischial tuberosity disease

Fig. 6.3 g, h

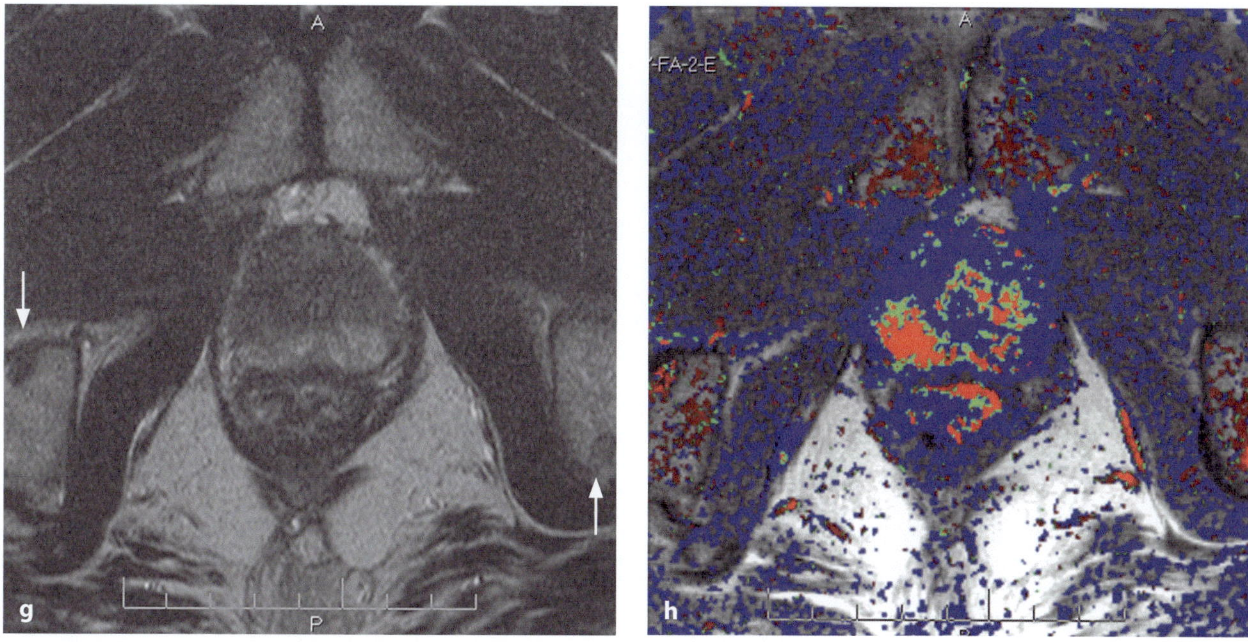

Fig. 6.3 g, h Bilateral right ischial tuberosity disease

Fig. 6.3 i, j

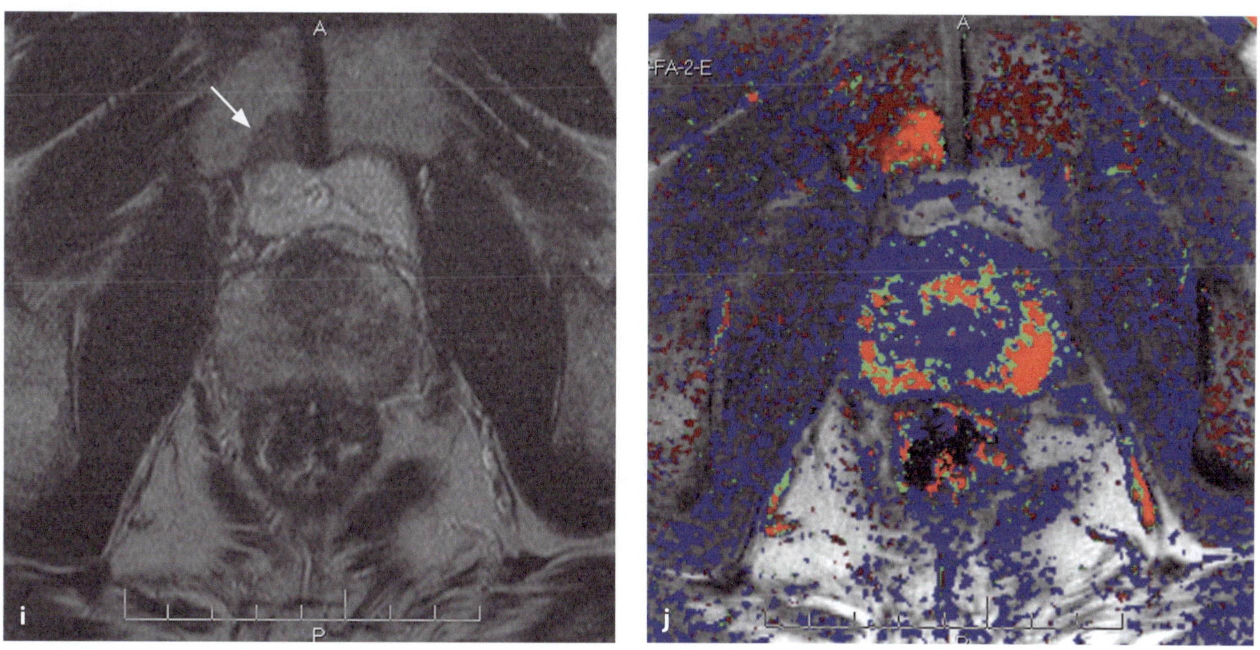

Fig. 6.3 i, j Focal right pubic symphysis disease

Fig. 6.3 k, l

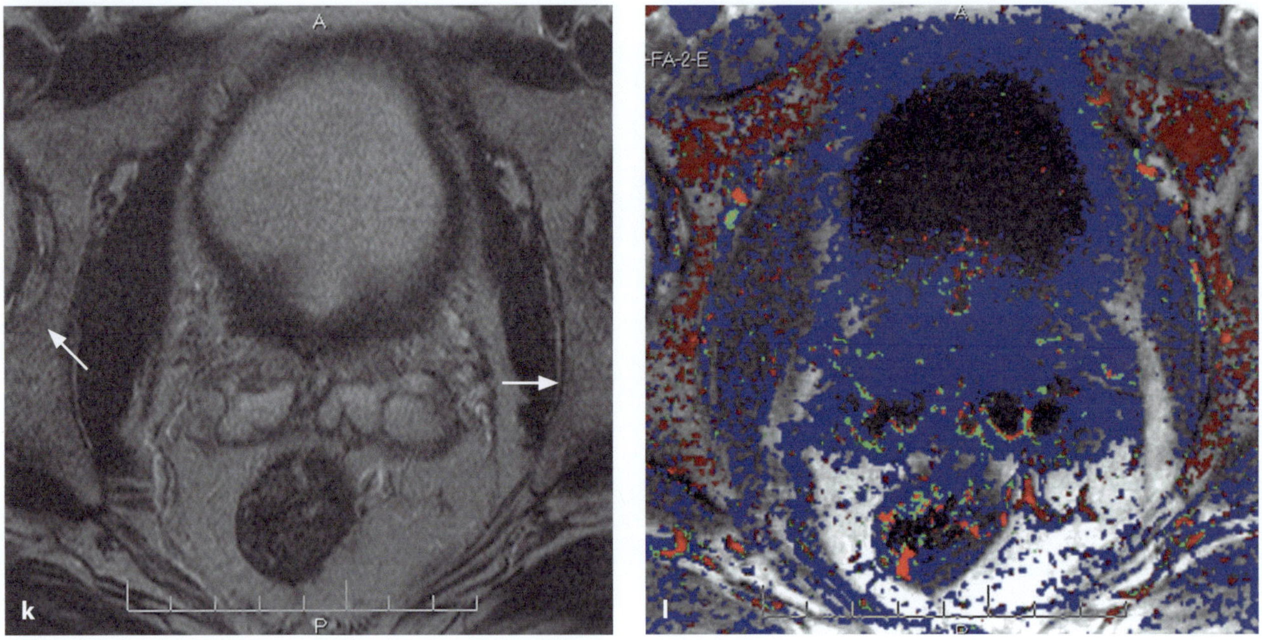

Fig. 6.3 k, l Focal right and left anterior acetabular disease

Fig. 6.4 a–f

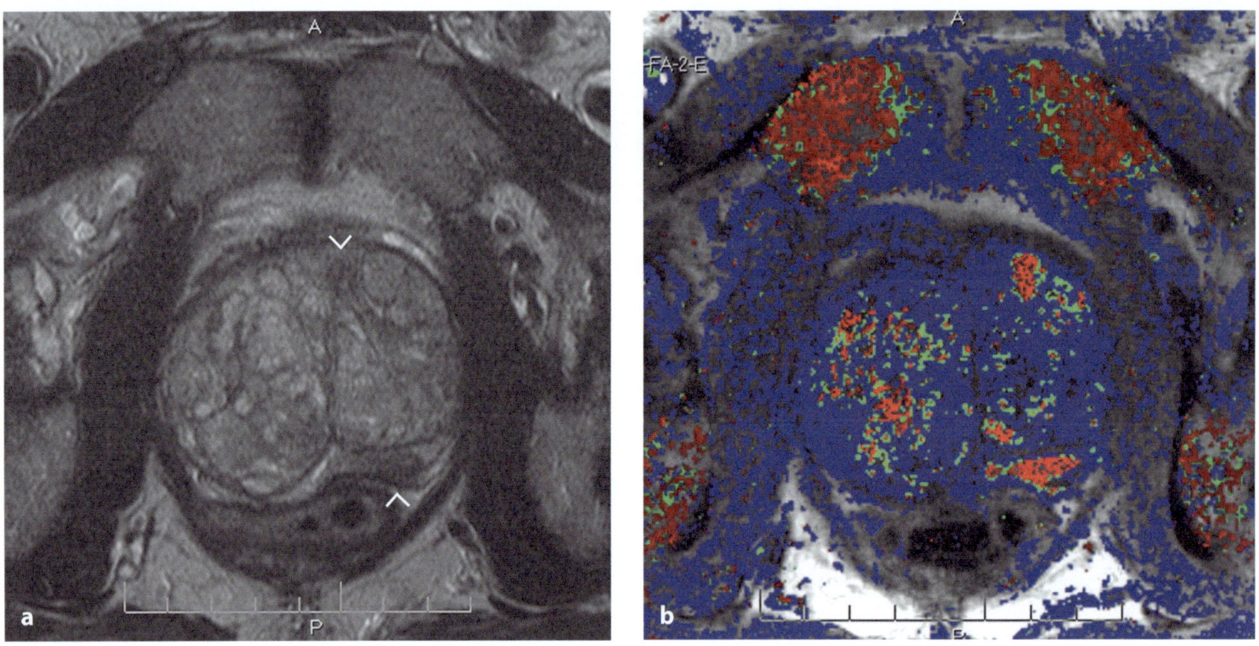

Fig. 6.4 a, b Focal right and left pubic symphysis disease-note left anterior and posterior tumors

Fig. 6.4 c, d

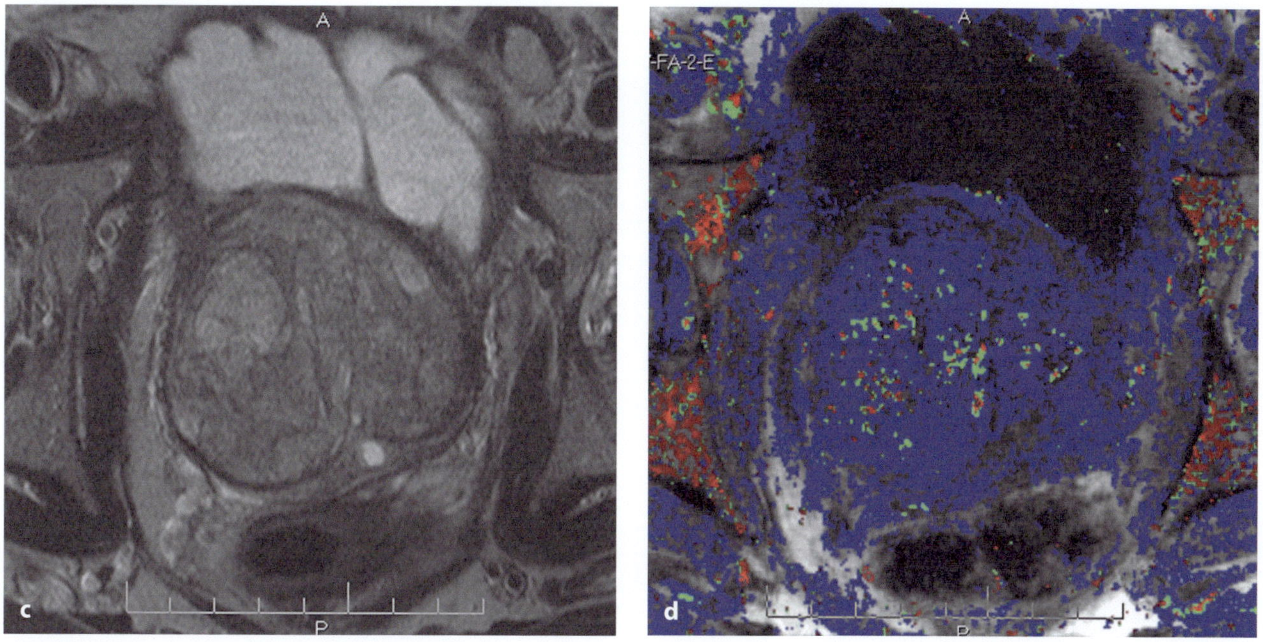

Fig. 6.4 c, d Right and left acetabular disease

Fig. 6.4 e, f

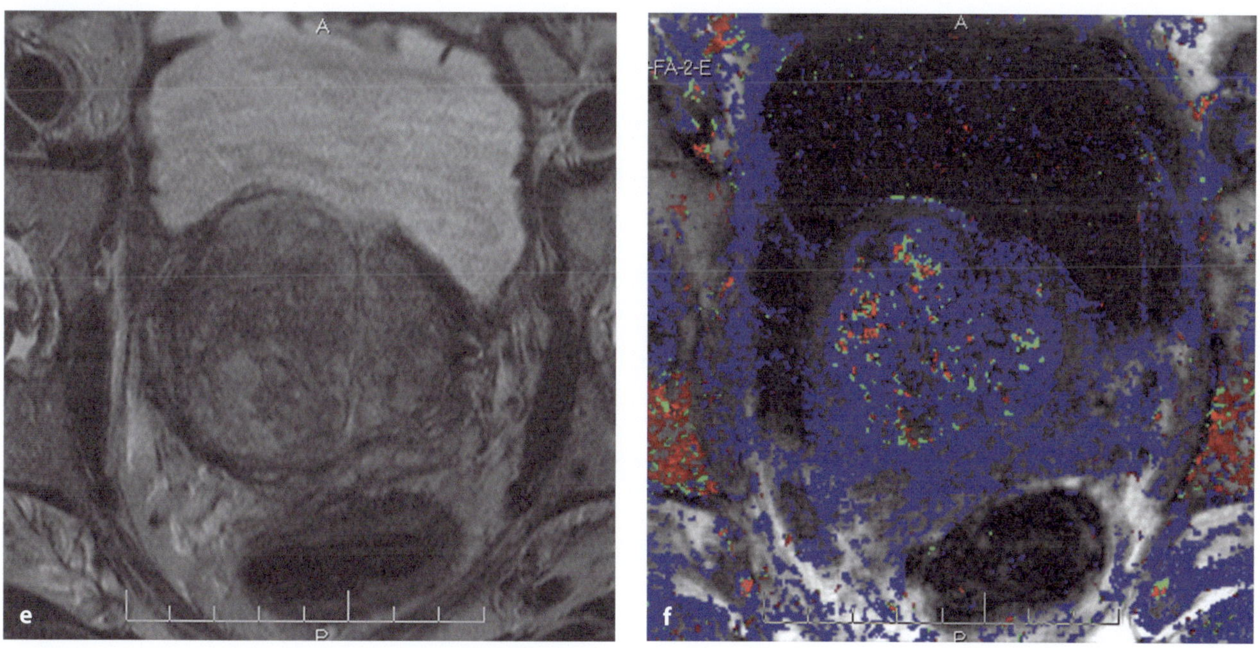

Fig. 6.4 e, f Right and left posterior acetabular disease

Chapter

Treatment: Improvement

7

Improvement is first detected by decreased or absent vascularity in previously vascular region. This may occur within minutes from thermal therapies to months following hormonal treatments. A lack of vascular change in 2 months signals the treatment is not working. Size changes are indeterminate since internal necrosis with fluid retention may enlarge the size and fibrosis may decrease tumor volume.

Fig. 7.1 a, b

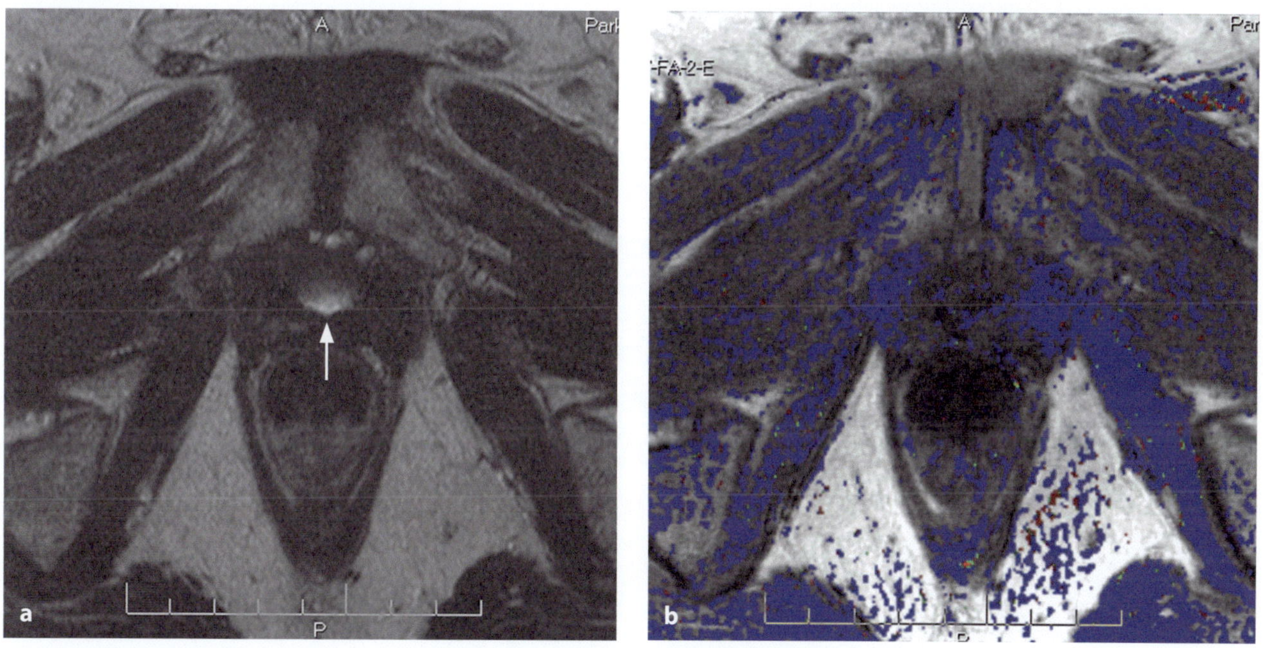

Fig. 7.1 a, b Normal postoperative gland-no tissue and no flow present-note dilated urethra

Fig. 7.2 a–d

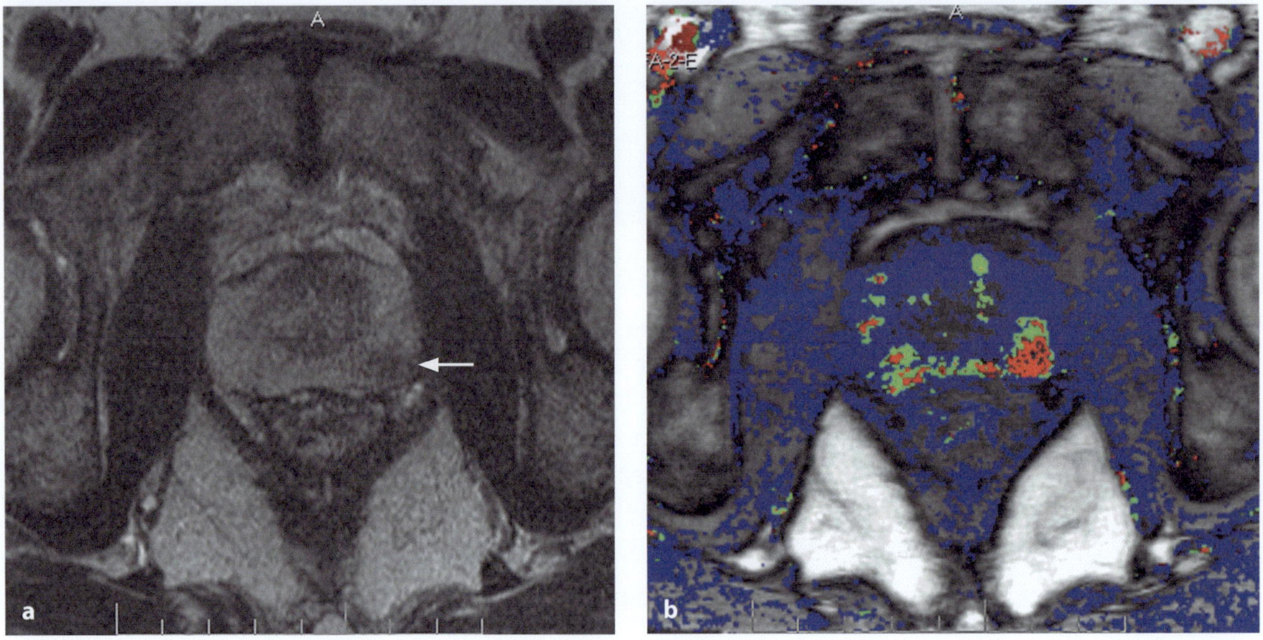

Fig. 7.2 a, b Left lateral and posterior lesion-Gleason 4

Fig. 7.2 c, d

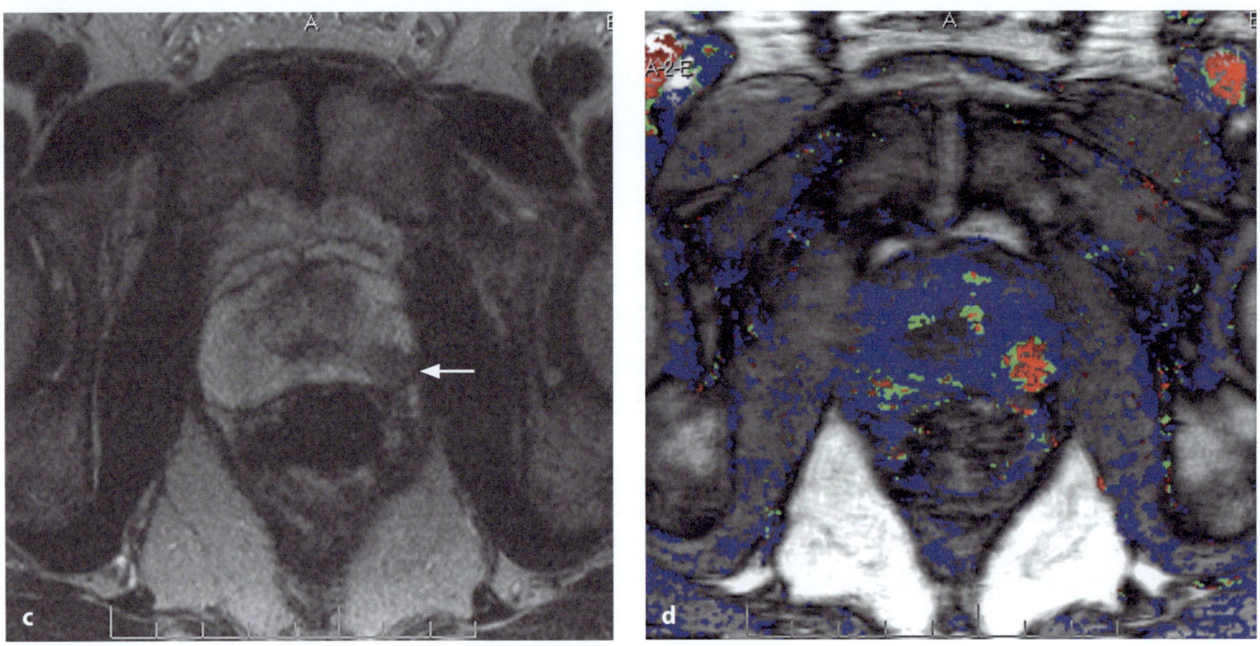

Fig. 7.2 c, d 6 months post antioxidant therapy decreased vascularity

Fig. 7.3 a–h

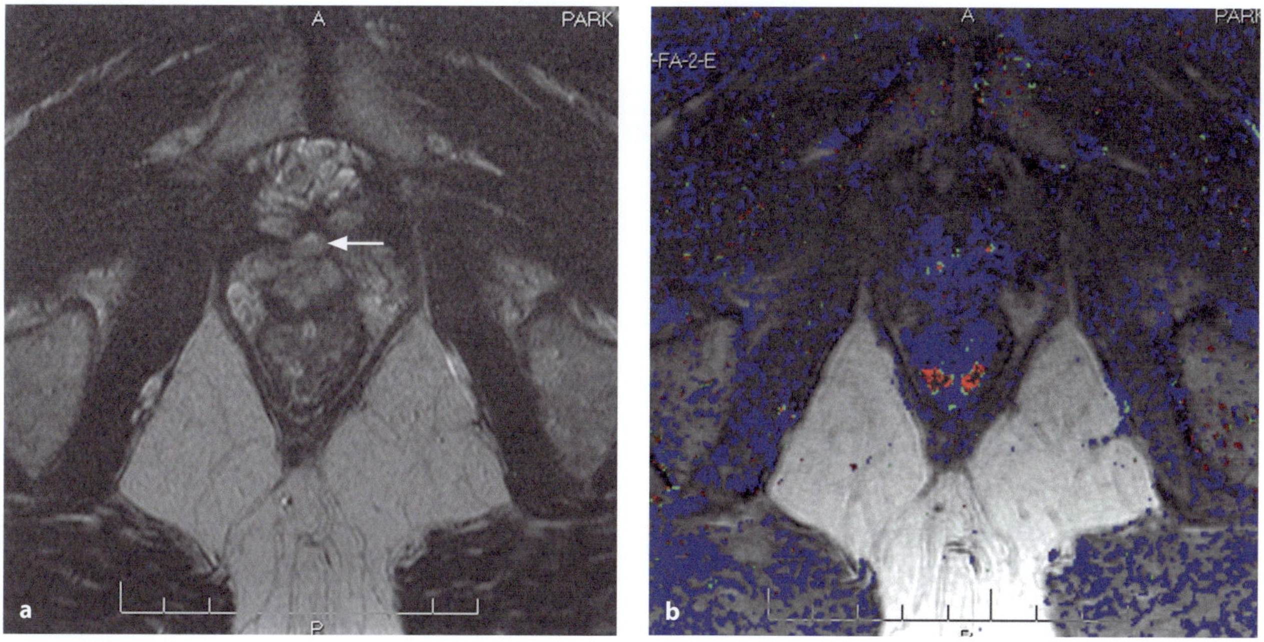

Fig. 7.3 a, b Post HIFU irregular prostate bed

Fig. 7.3 c, d

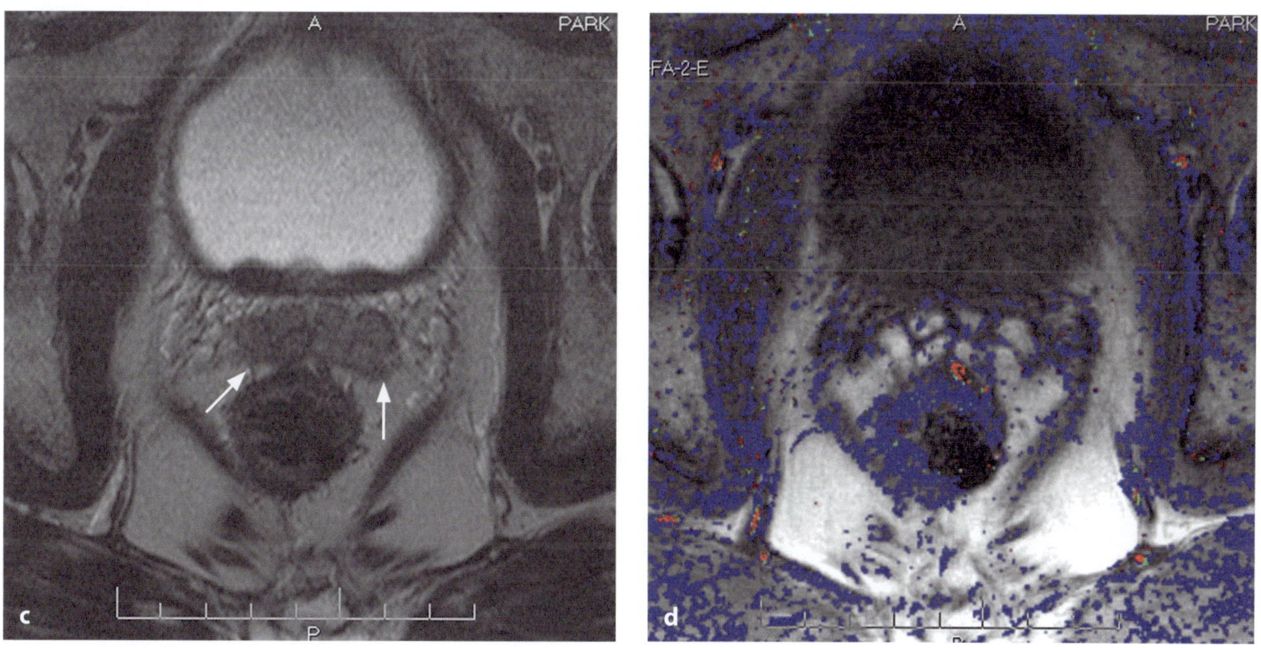

Fig. 7.3 c, d Post HIFU seminal vesicles are avascular

Fig. 7.3 e, f

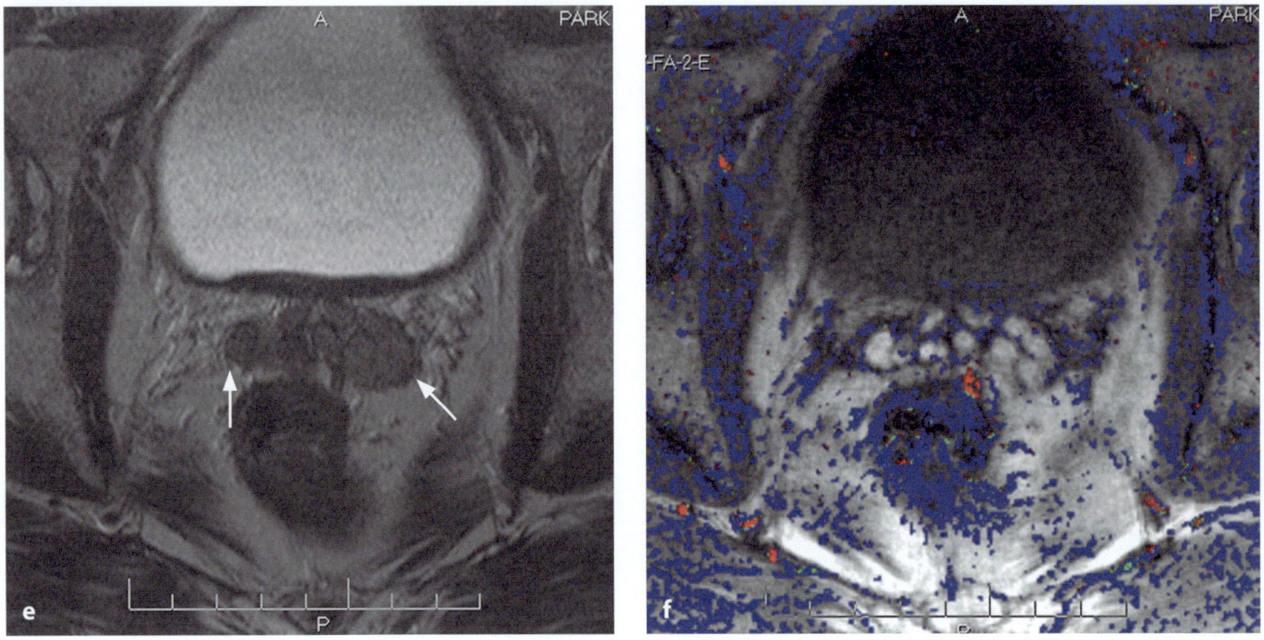

Fig. 7.3 e, f Post HIFU seminal vesicles are avascular

Fig. 7.3 g, h

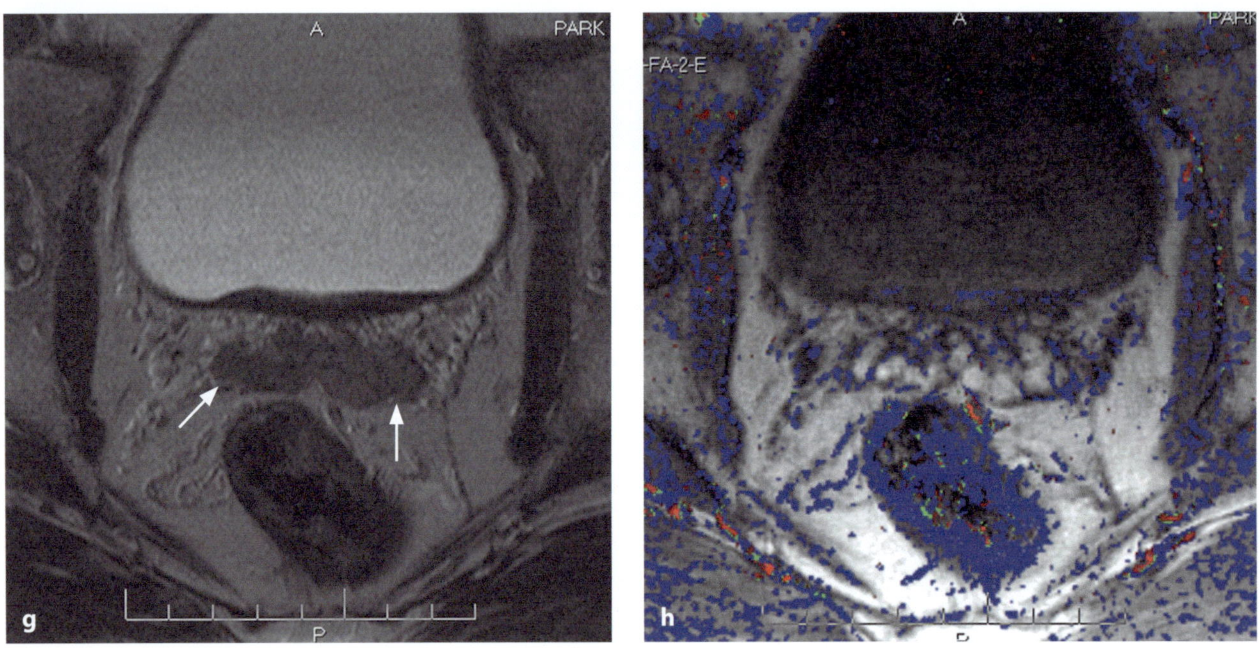

Fig. 7.3 g, h Post HIFU seminal vesicles are avascular

Fig. 7.4 a–h

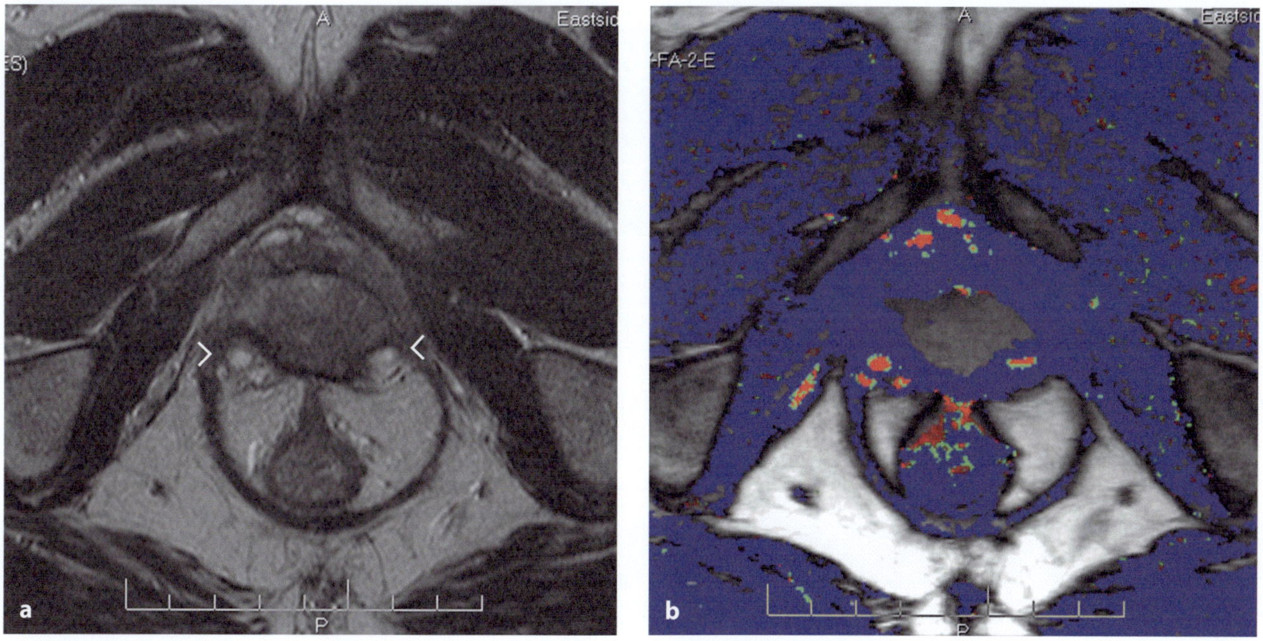

Fig. 7.4 a, b Post HIFU apex-note adjacent neurovascular bundles are well imaged due to volume loss

Fig. 7.4 c, d

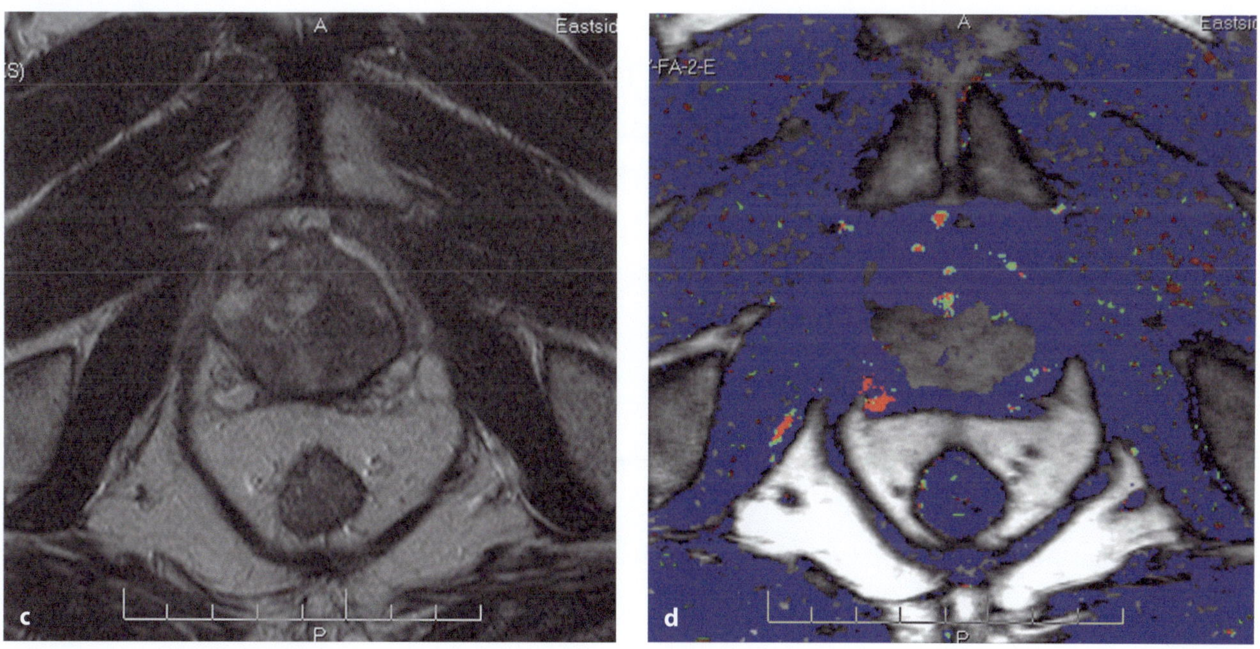

Fig. 7.4 c, d Post HIFU midgland

Fig. 7.4 e, f

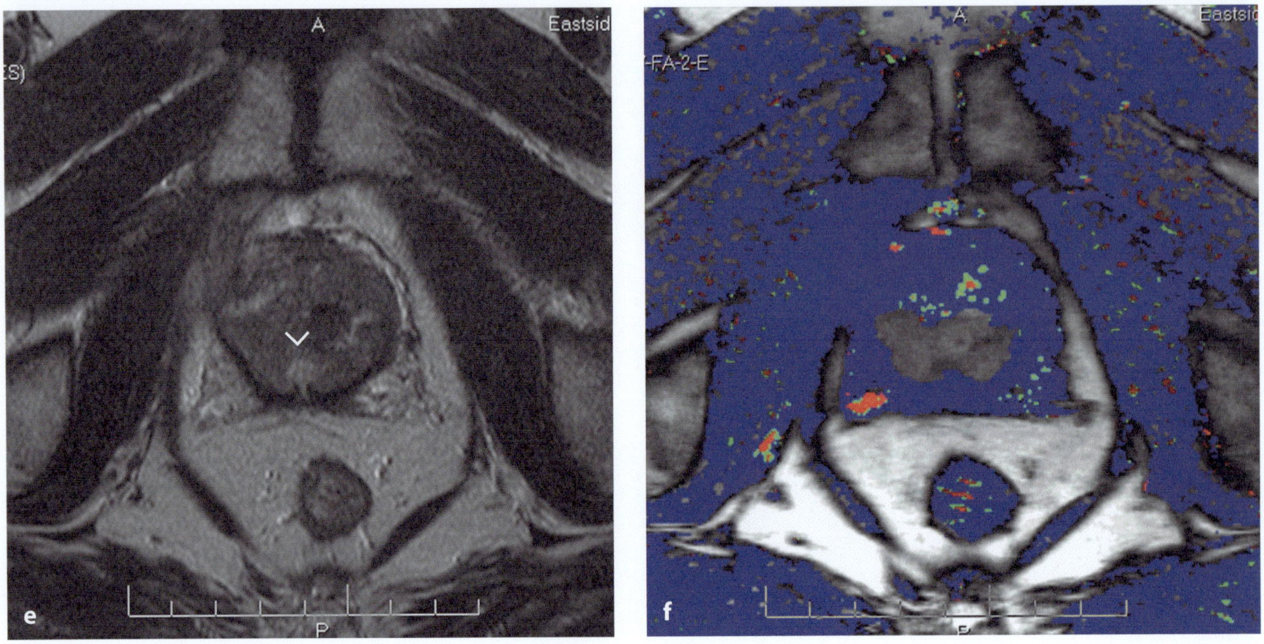

Fig. 7.4 e, f Post HIFU proximal midgland- note dilated urethra

Fig. 7.4 g, h

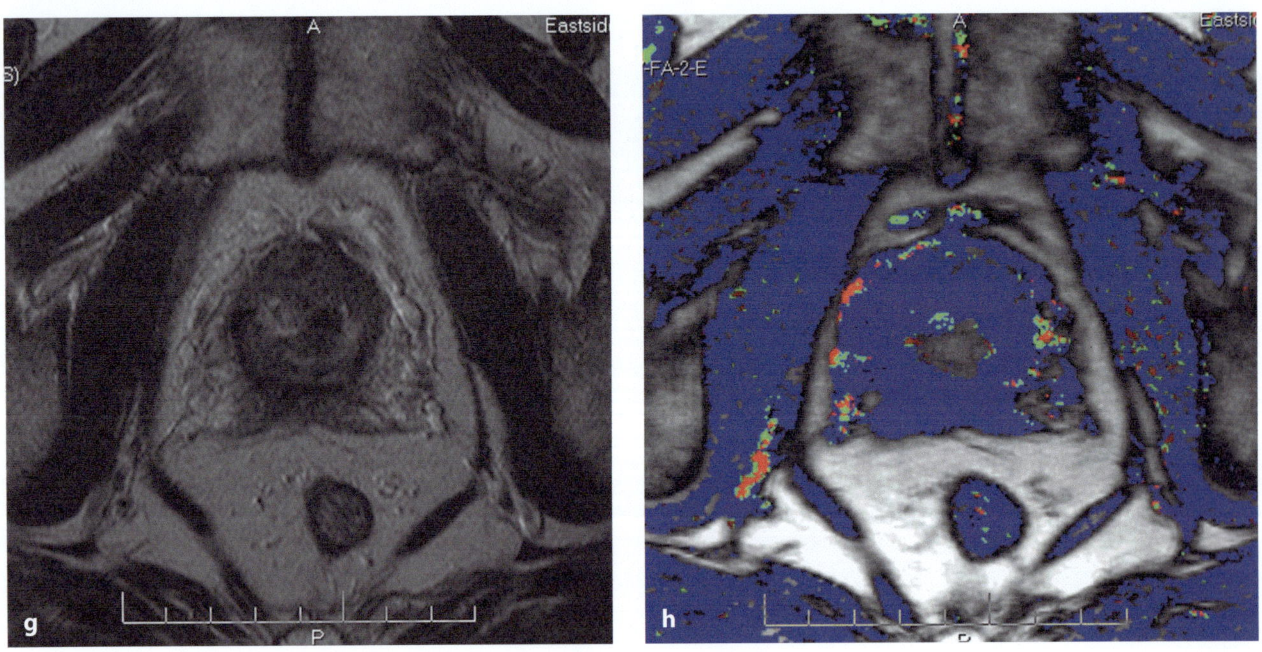

Fig. 7.4 g, h Post HIFU base-note flow in neurovascular bundles

Fig. 7.4 i, j

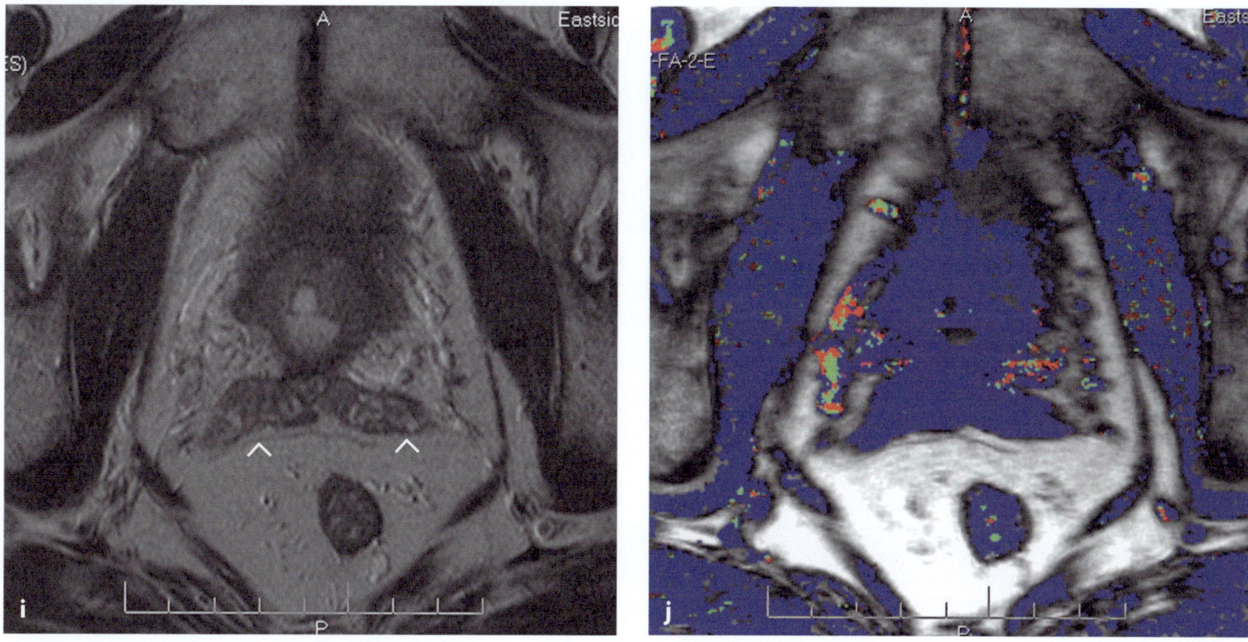

Fig. 7.4 i, j Post HIFU seminal vesicles

Fig. 7.5 a, b

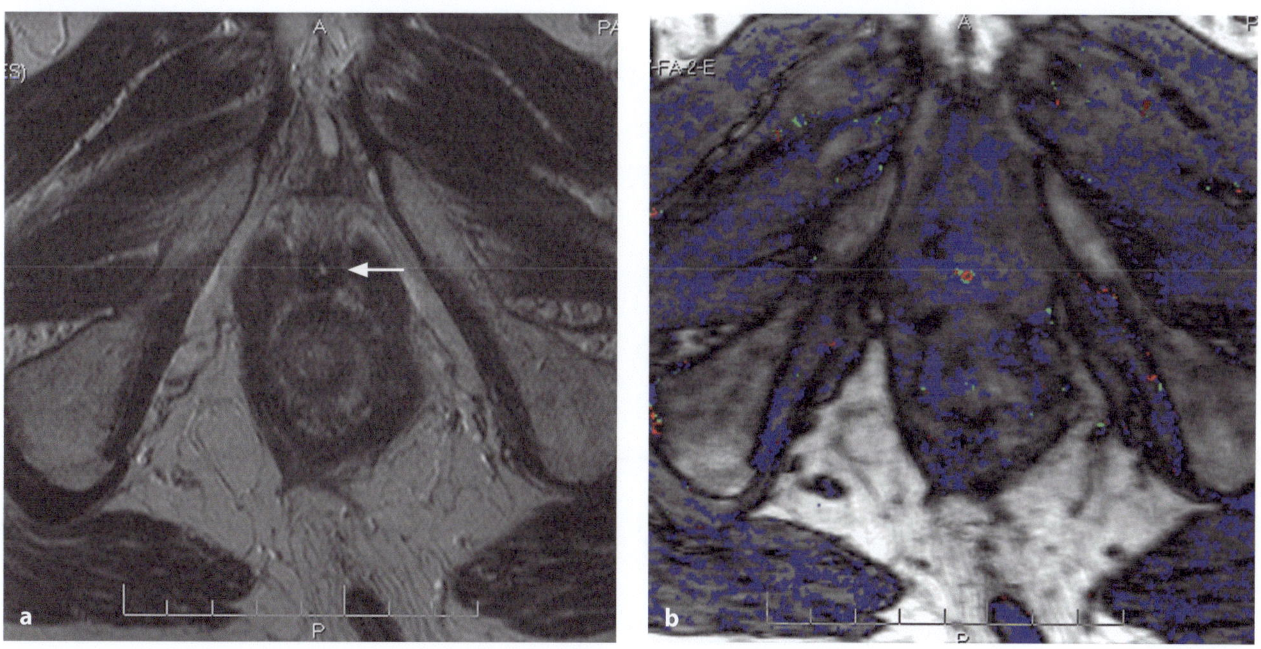

Fig. 7.5 a, b Post HIFU urethritis-note periurethral vascularity

Fig. 7.6 a, b

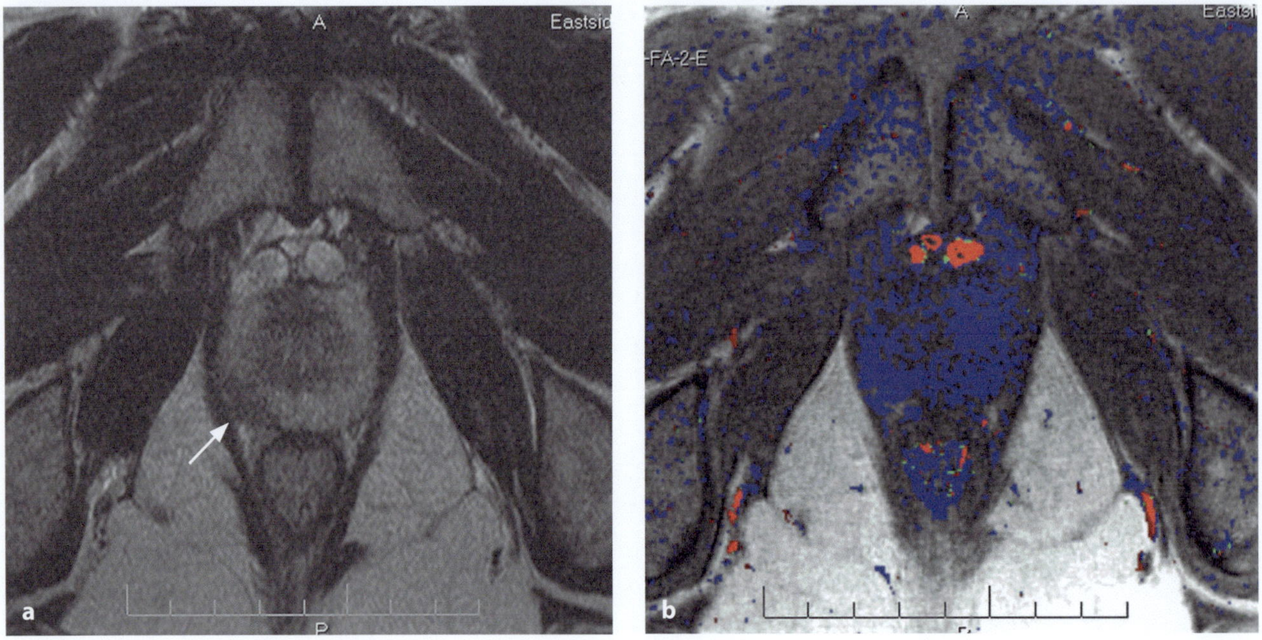

Fig. 7.6 a, b Antioxidant therapy-note right midgland avascular lesion

Fig. 7.7 a, b

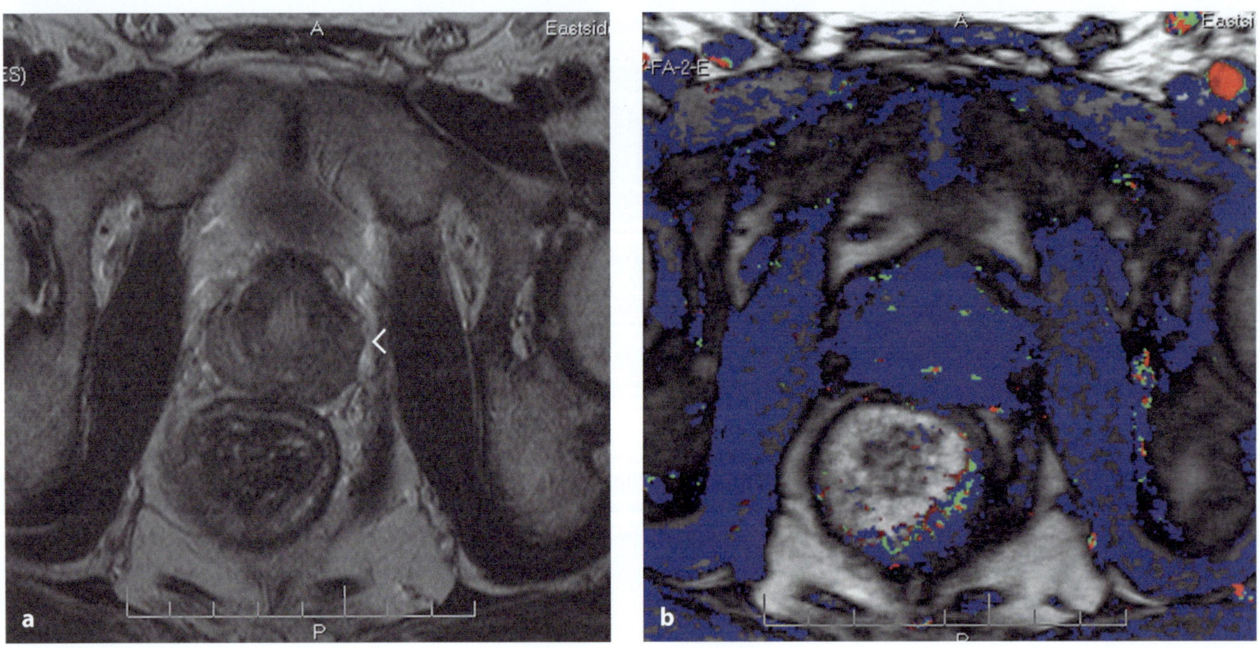

Fig. 7.7 a, b Antioxidant therapy-note avascular left extracapsular disease

Fig. 7.8 a, b

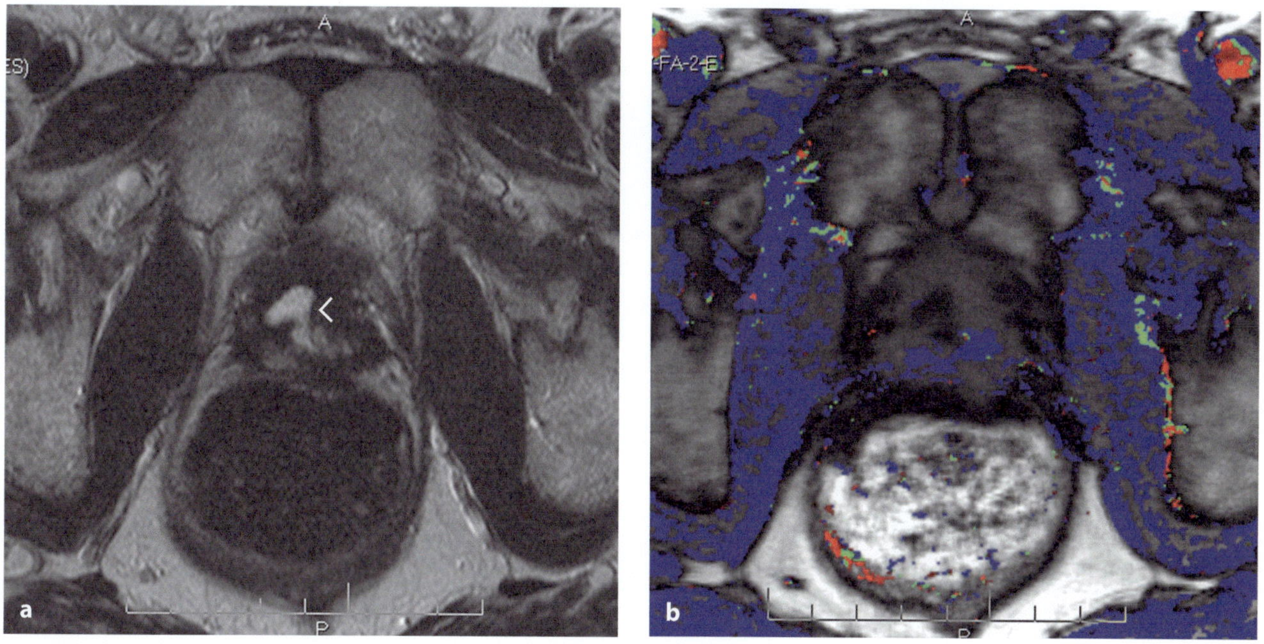

Fig. 7.8 a, b Post HIFU–note dilated urethra and no tumor vascularity

Fig. 7.9 a–d

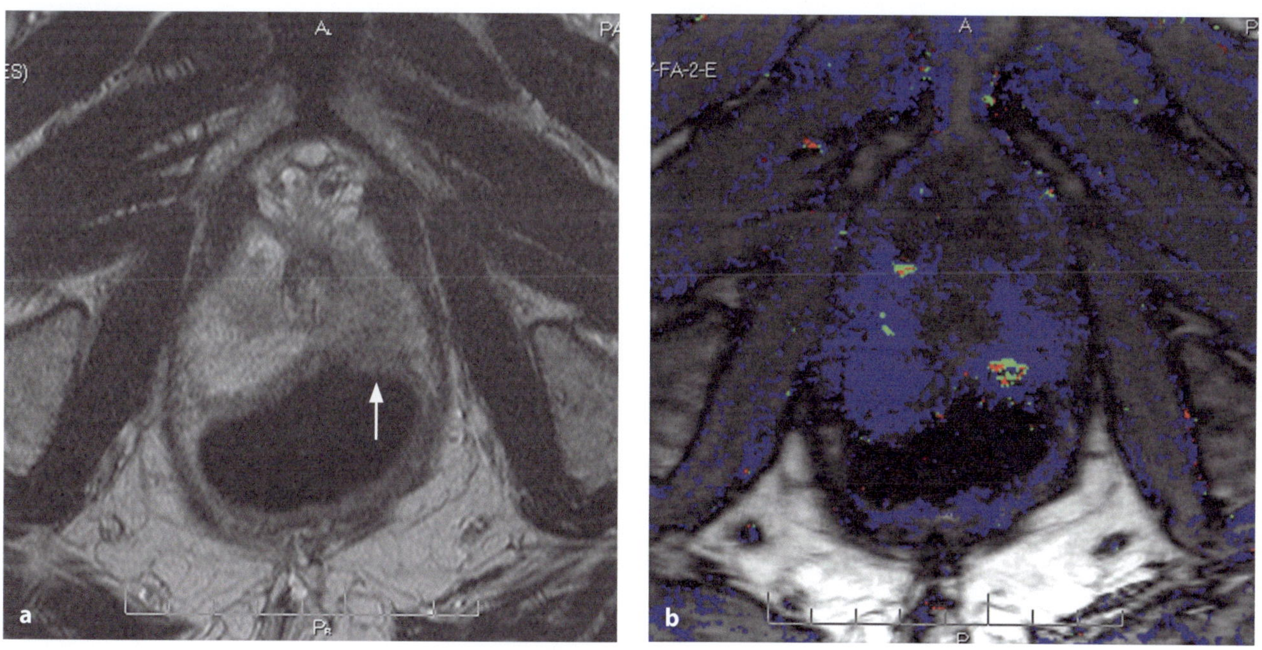

Fig. 7.9 a, b Post cryotherapy-note slight vascularity left apex

Fig. 7.9 c, d

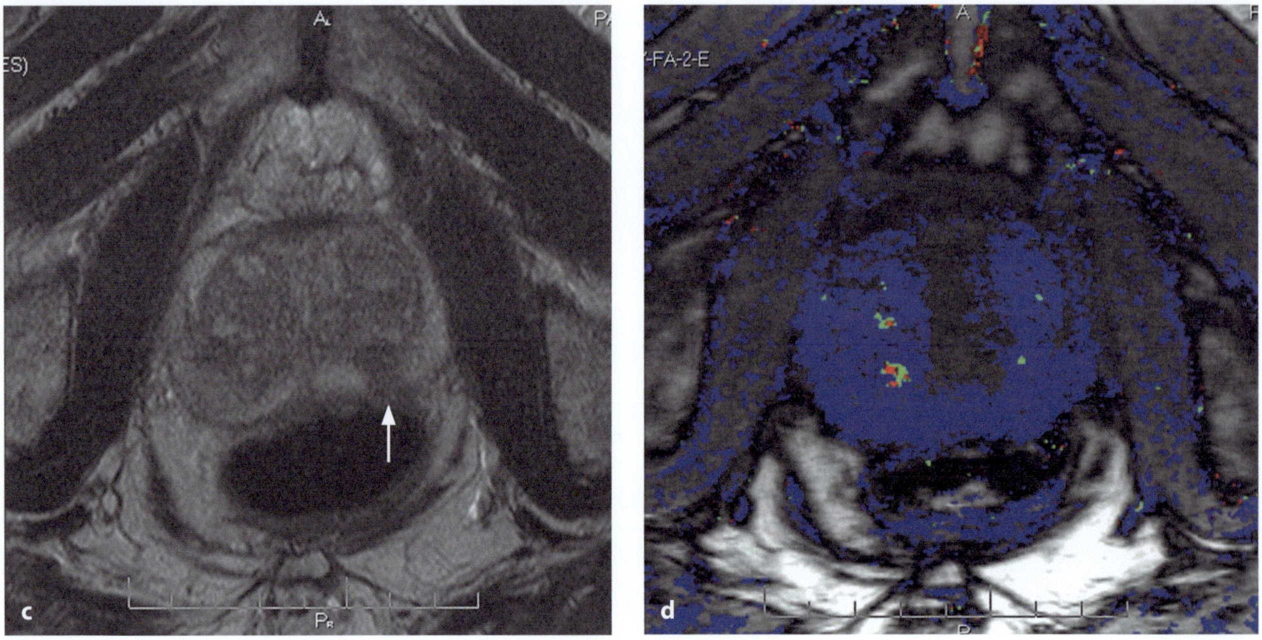

Fig. 7.9 c, d No vascularity in treated left midgland

Chapter

Post Treatment Recurrence

8

Recurrence from treatment(s) is common and appears more often with aggressive high grade cancers. Recurrent tumor is more accurately diagnosed by DCE-MRI than by repeat biopsy. Targeted biopsy based on imaging findings greatly improves tissue diagnosis.

Fig. 8.1 a, b

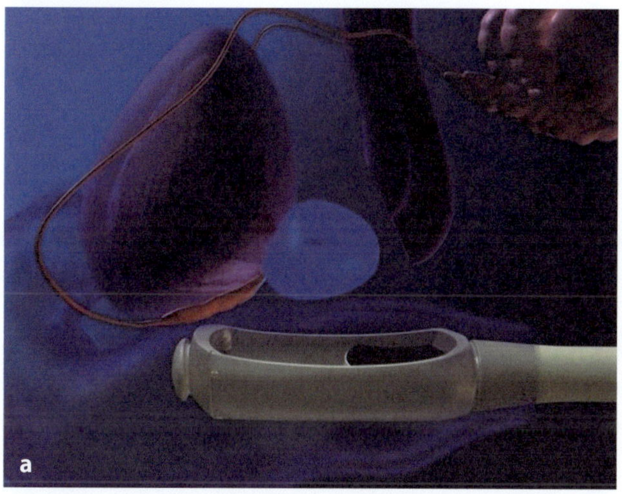

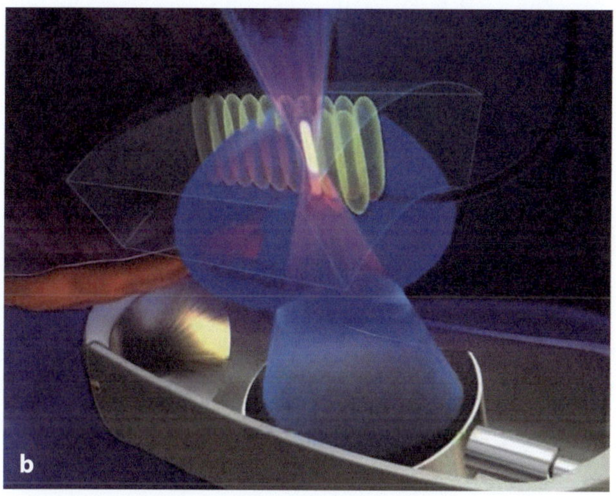

Fig. 8.1 a, b HIFU (high intensity focused ultrasound) treatment plan and insonation therapy. Focal sound beams destroy prostatic tumor under image guidance. This procedure is increasingly used due to low morbidity and ability to repeat treatment. It is used to perform salvage therapy when recurrence follows surgery or radiation.

Fig. 8.2 a–l

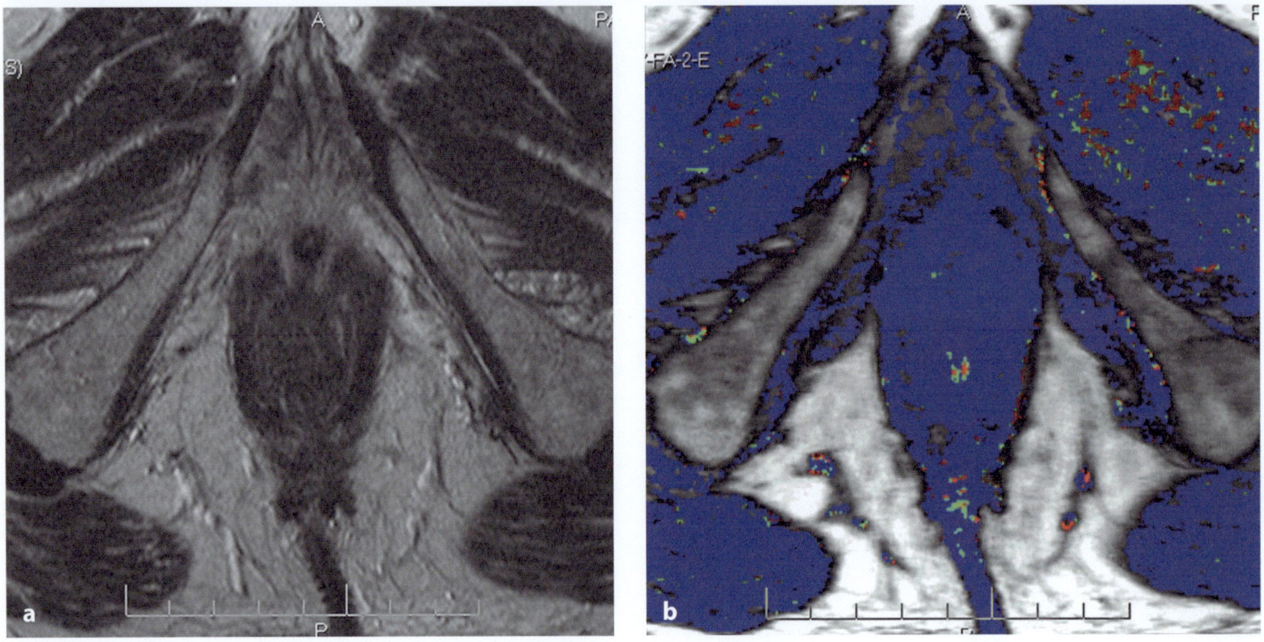

Fig. 8.2 a, b Post HIFU Gleason 4-apex shows no tumor

Fig. 8.2 c, d

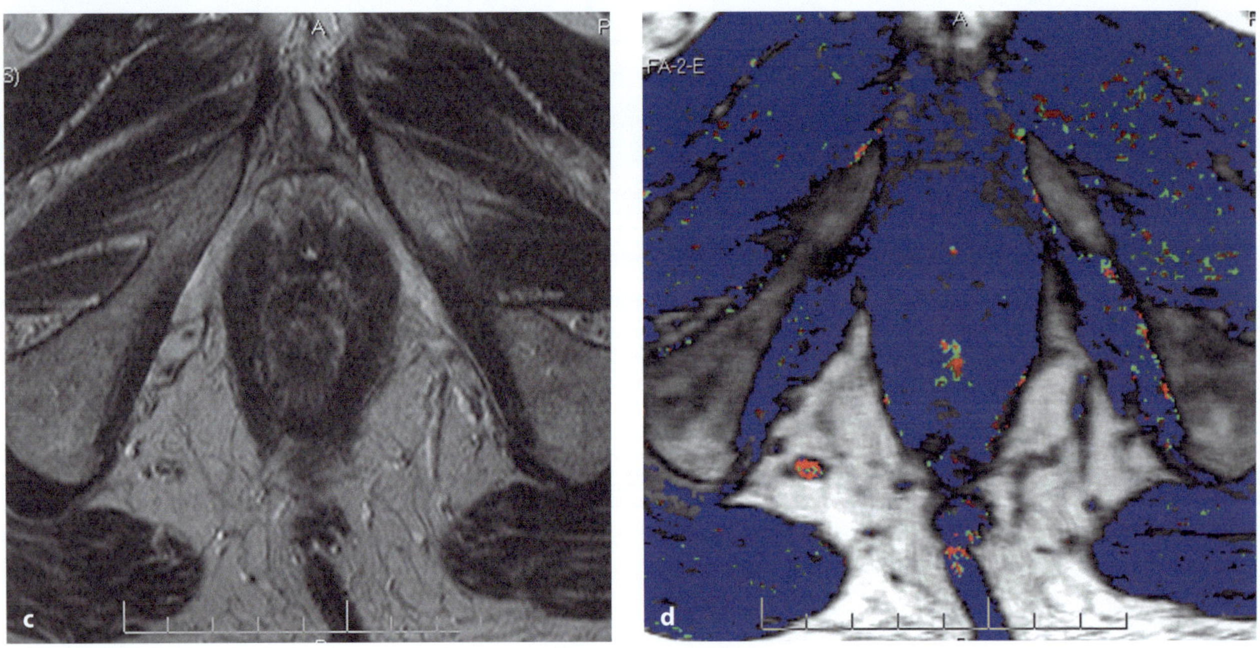

Fig. 8.2 c, d Distal midgland shows tumor vascularity as recurrence

Fig. 8.2 e, f

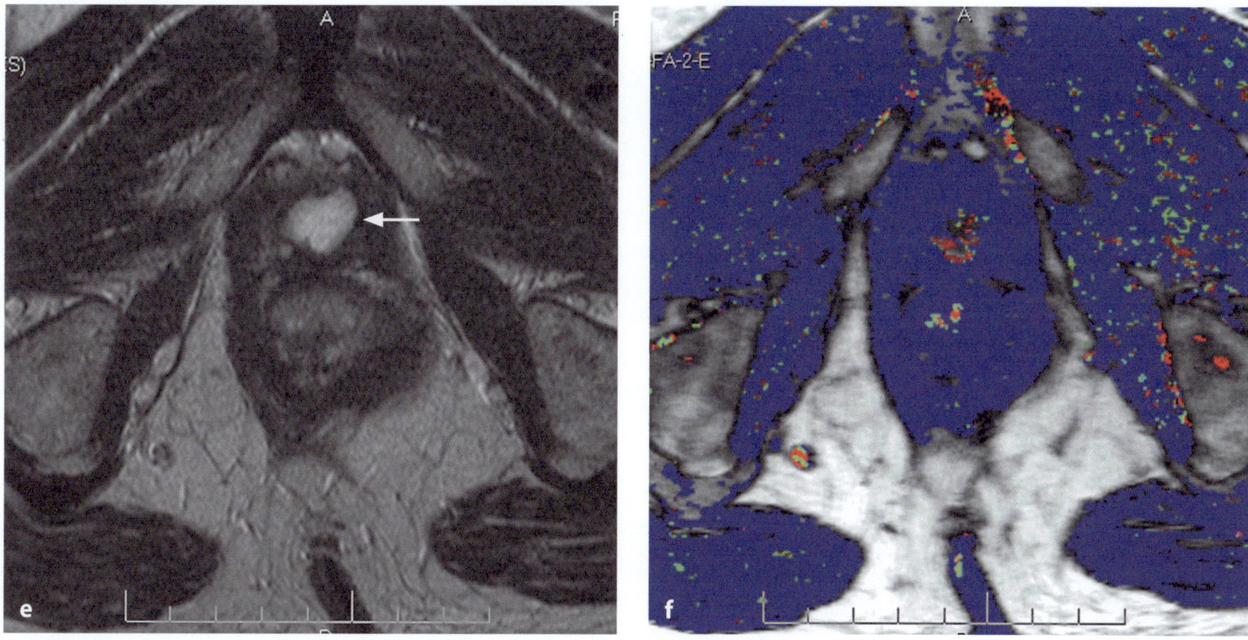

Fig. 8.2 e, f Proximal midgland shows prostatic urethral dilation

Fig. 8.2 g, h

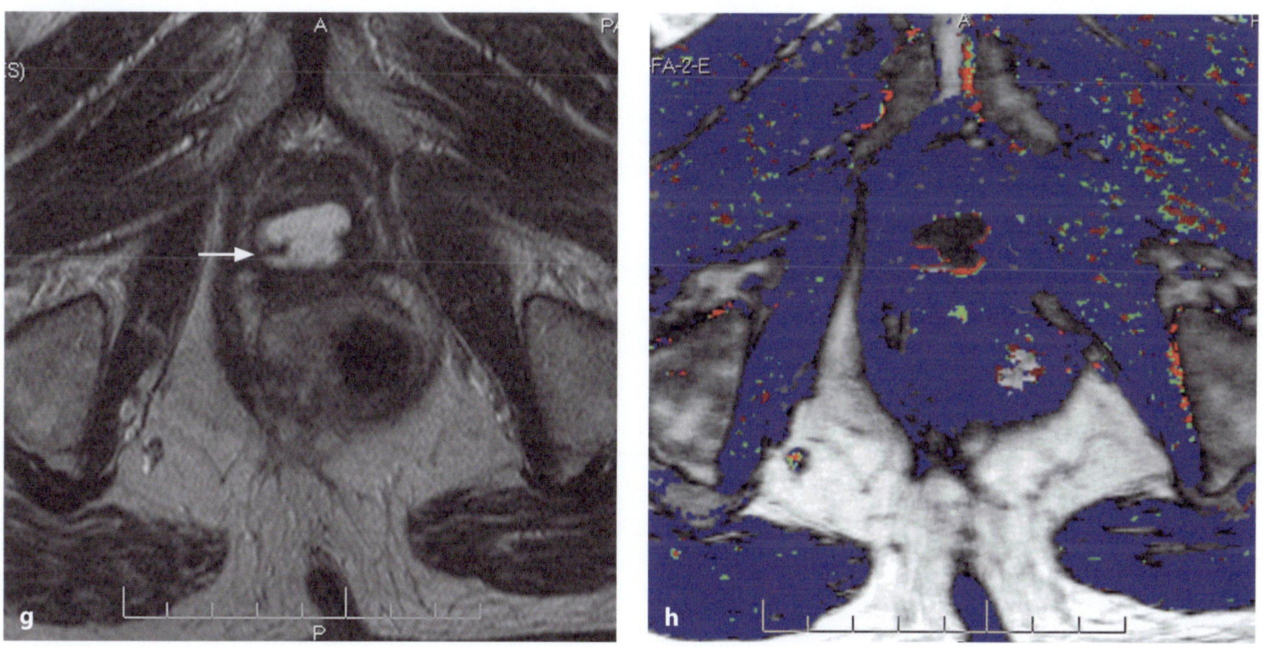

Fig. 8.2 g, h Midgland shows right ischial metastatic focus and mid urethral partial post procedure fold

Fig. 8.2 i, j

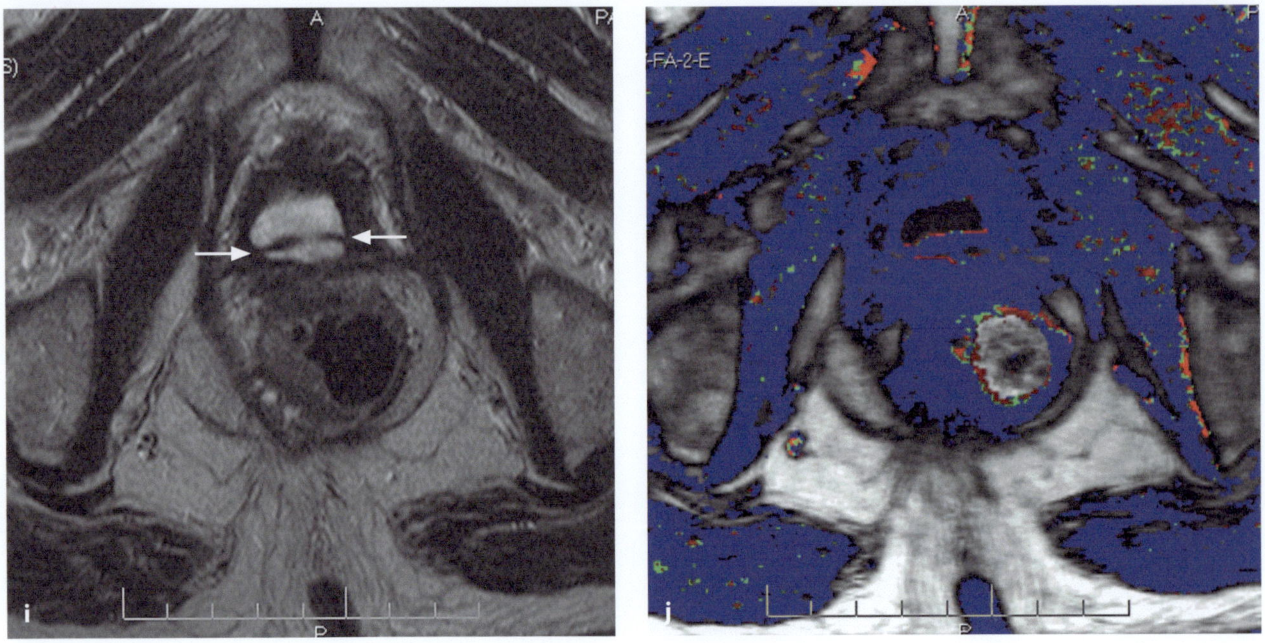

Fig. 8.2 i, j Base shows complete midurethral septum

Fig. 8.2 k, l

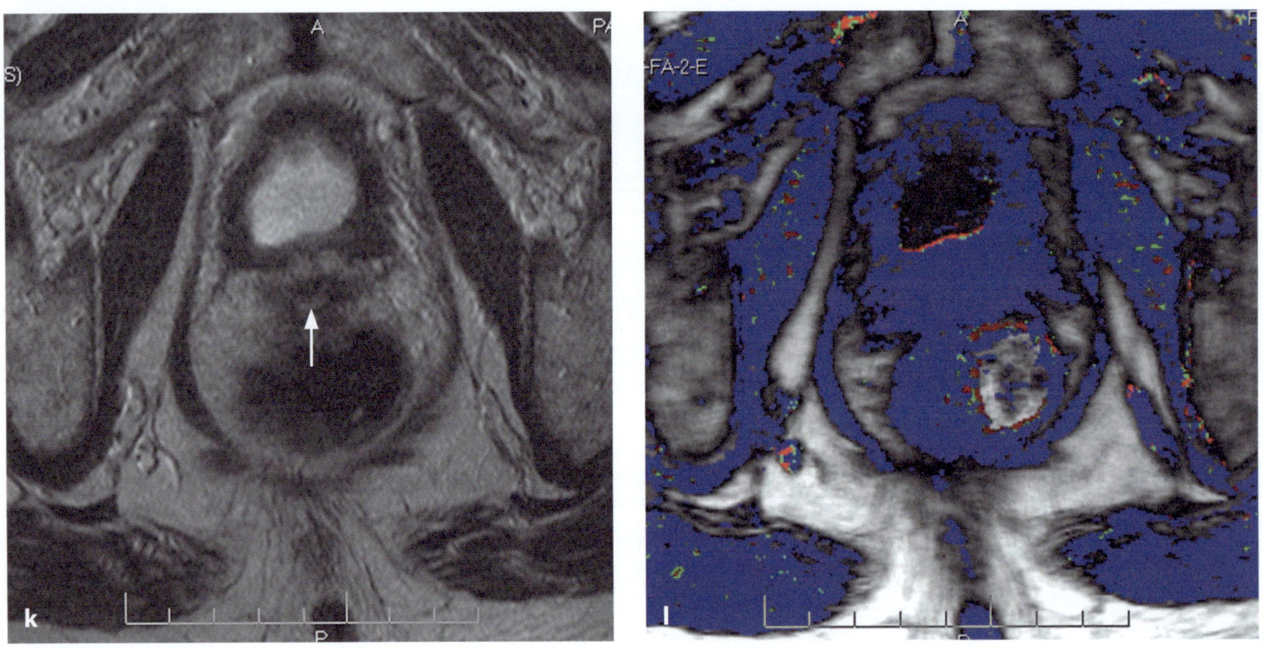

Fig. 8.2 k, l Seminal vesicles show no vascular tumor recurrence

Fig. 8.3 a–j

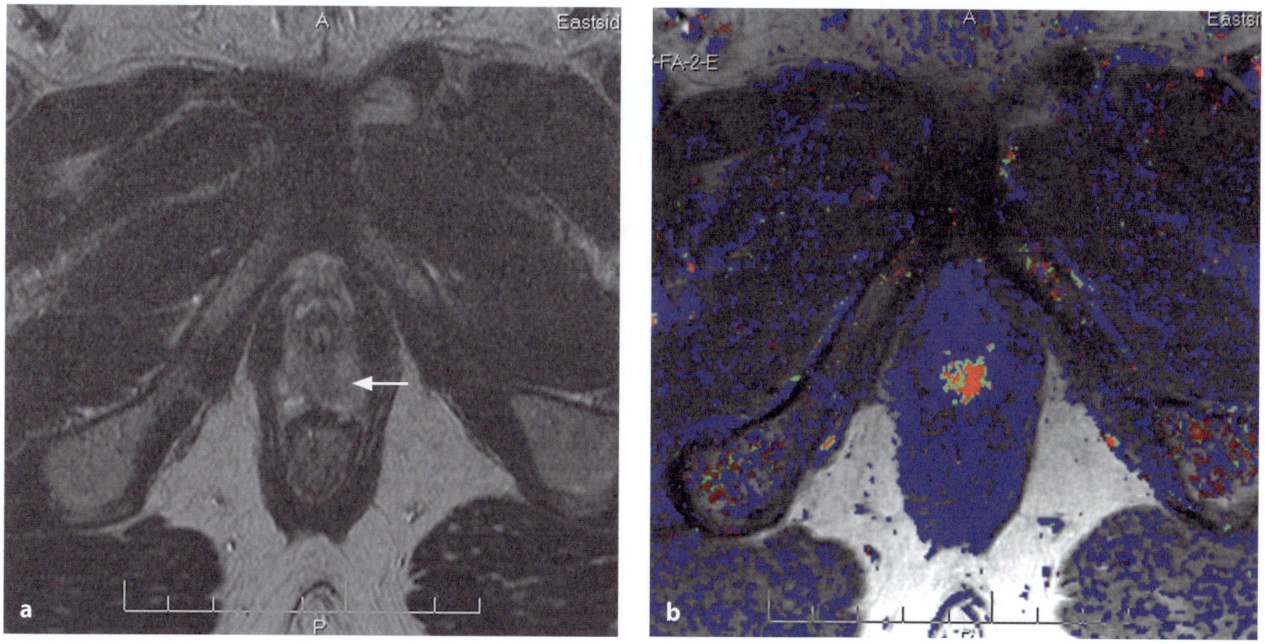

Fig. 8.3 a, b Gleason 4 in apex-hormone therapy produces signal loss

Fig. 8.3 c, d

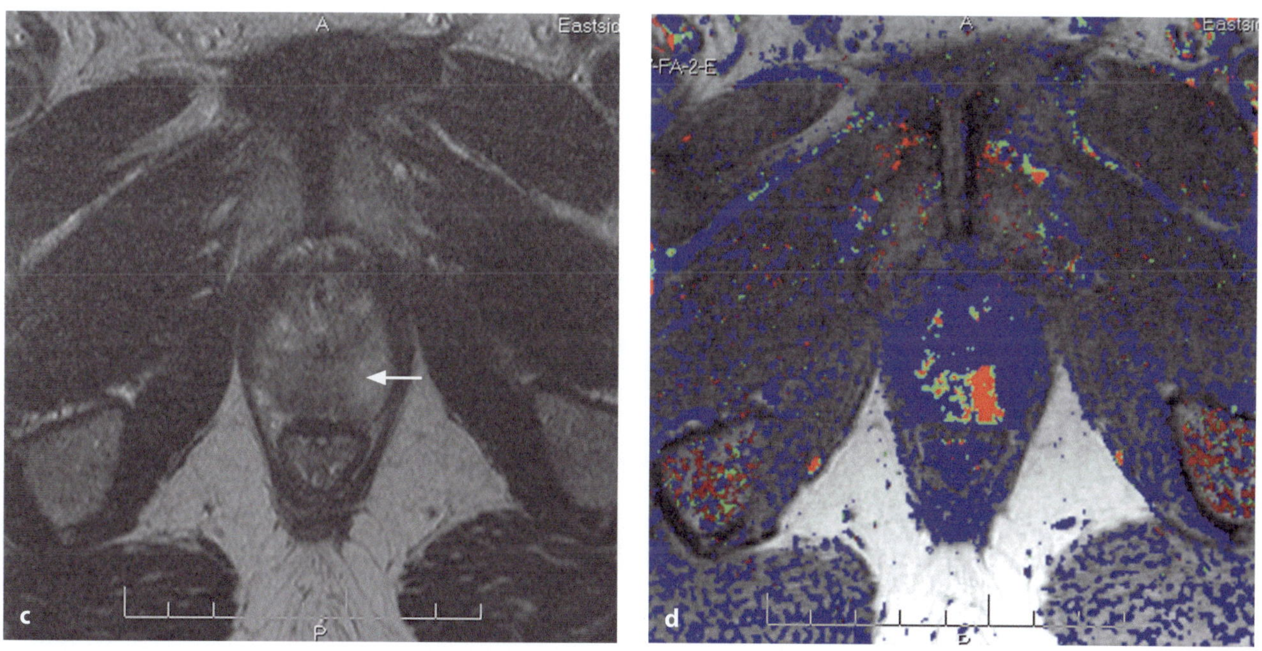

Fig. 8.3 c, d With extension into posterior midgland

Fig. 8.3 e, f

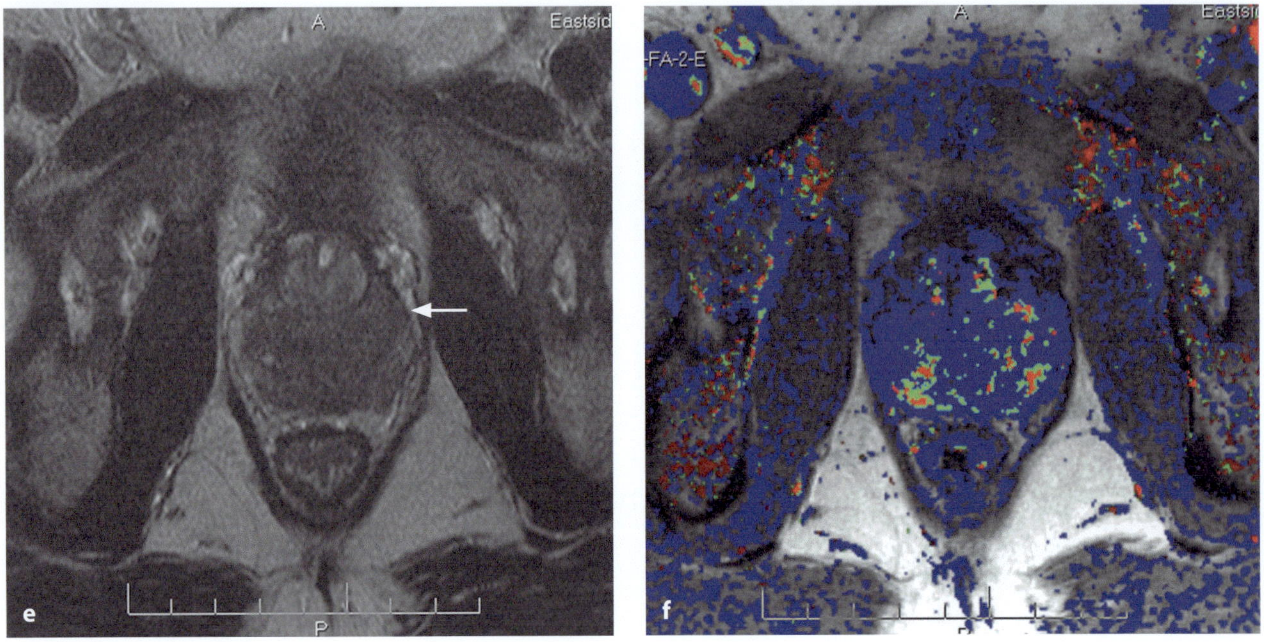

Fig. 8.3 e, f With extension into anterior midgland

Fig. 8.3 g, h

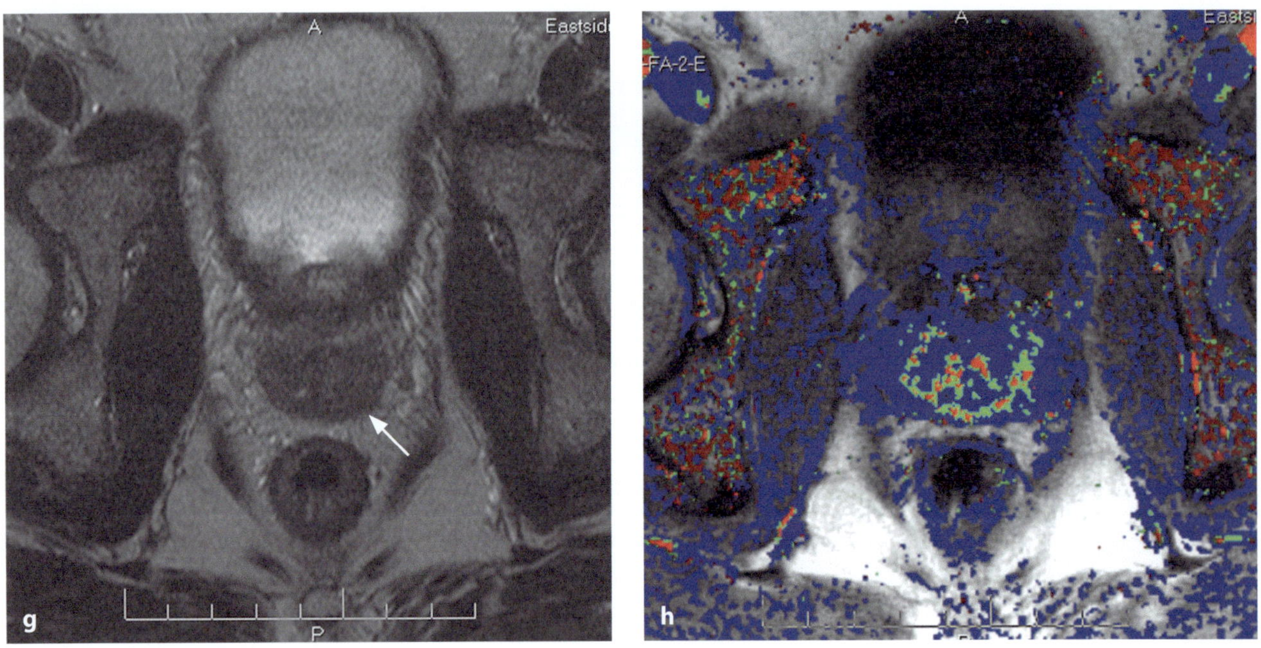

Fig. 8.3 g, h With extension into base

Fig. 8.3 i, j

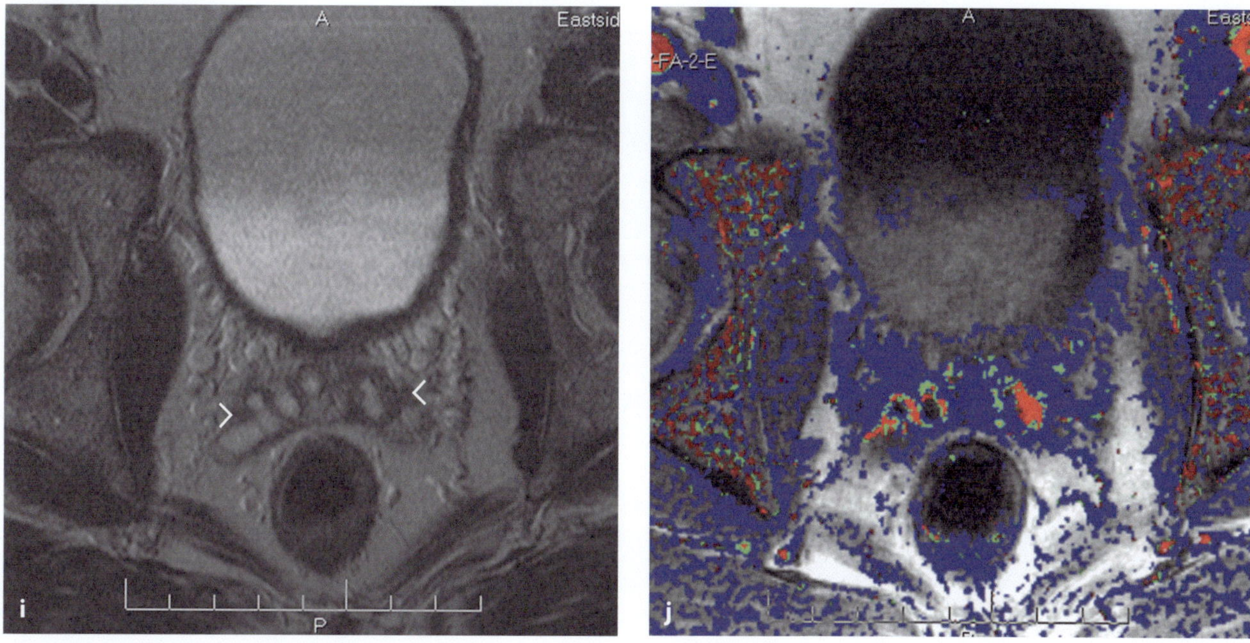

Fig. 8.3 i, j With extension into both proximal seminal vesicles

Fig. 8.4 a–h

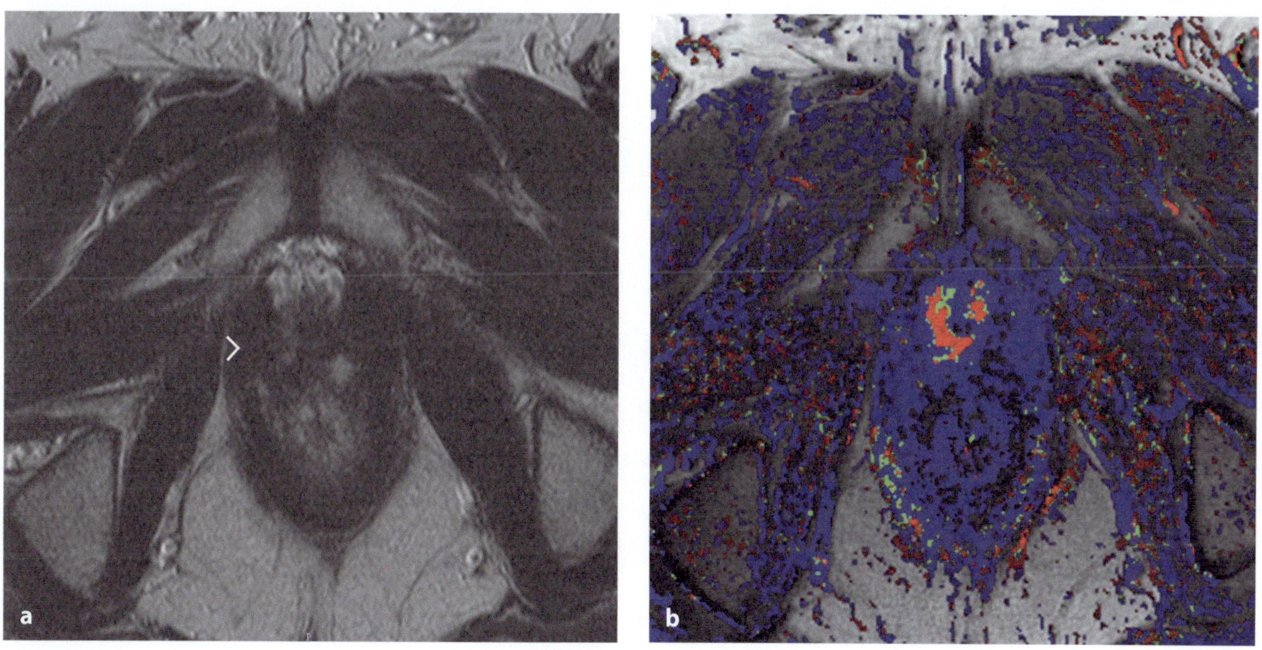

Fig. 8.4 a, b Post HIFU recurrence Gleason 5 in right apex

Fig. 8.4 c, d

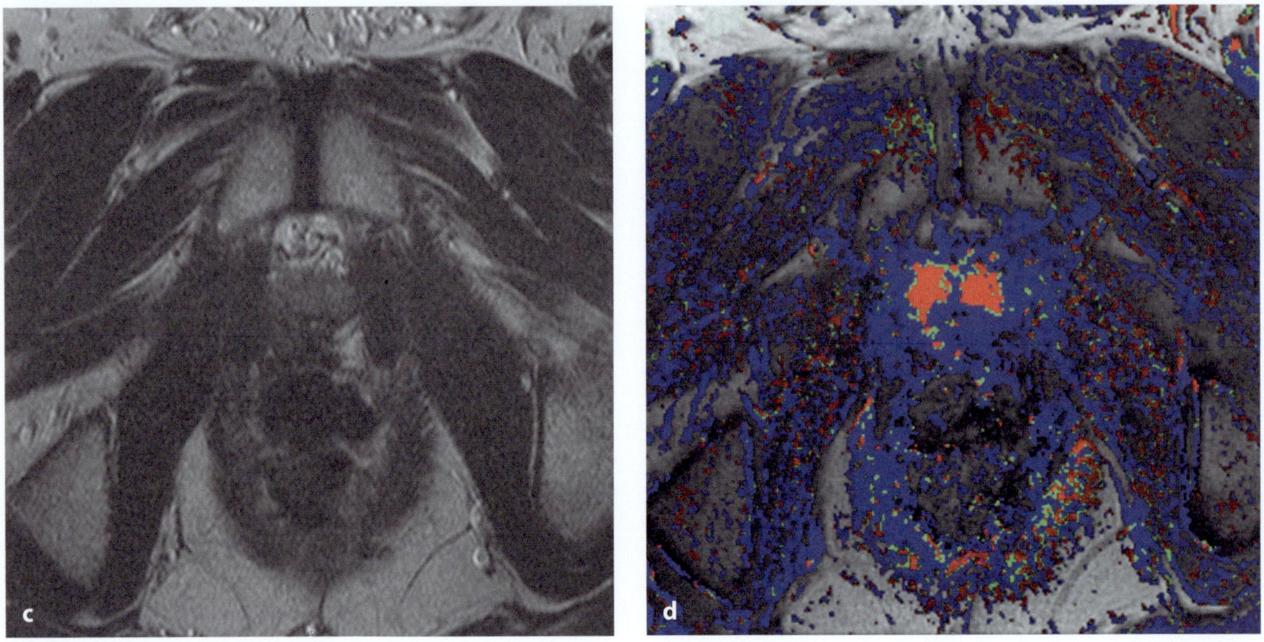

Fig. 8.4 c, d With extension into midgland

Fig. 8.4 e, f

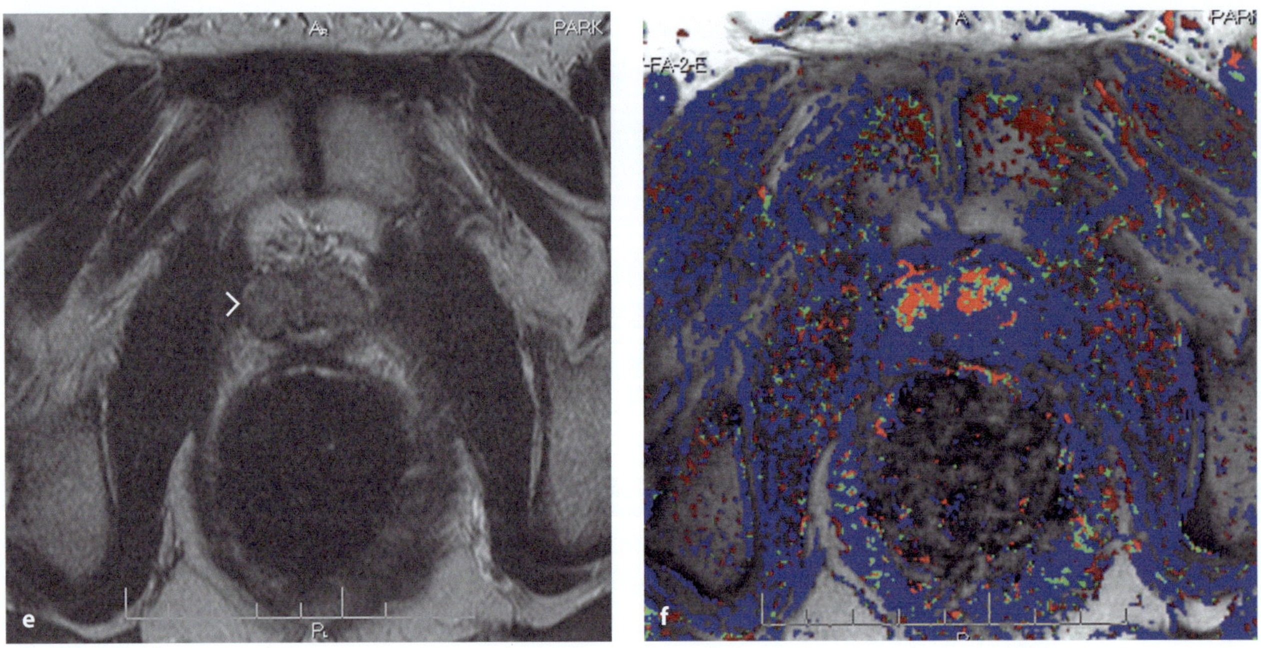

Fig. 8.4 e, f With lesser extension into proximal midgland

Fig. 8.4 g, h

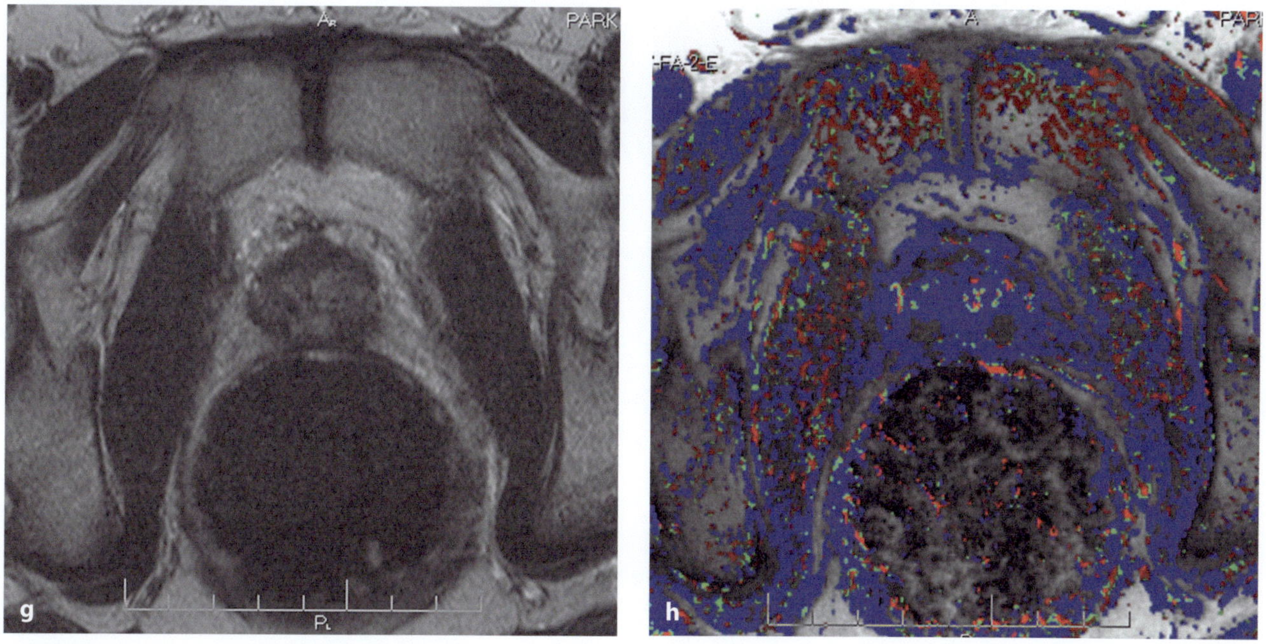

Fig. 8.4 g, h Without vascular extension into base

Fig. 8.5 a–h

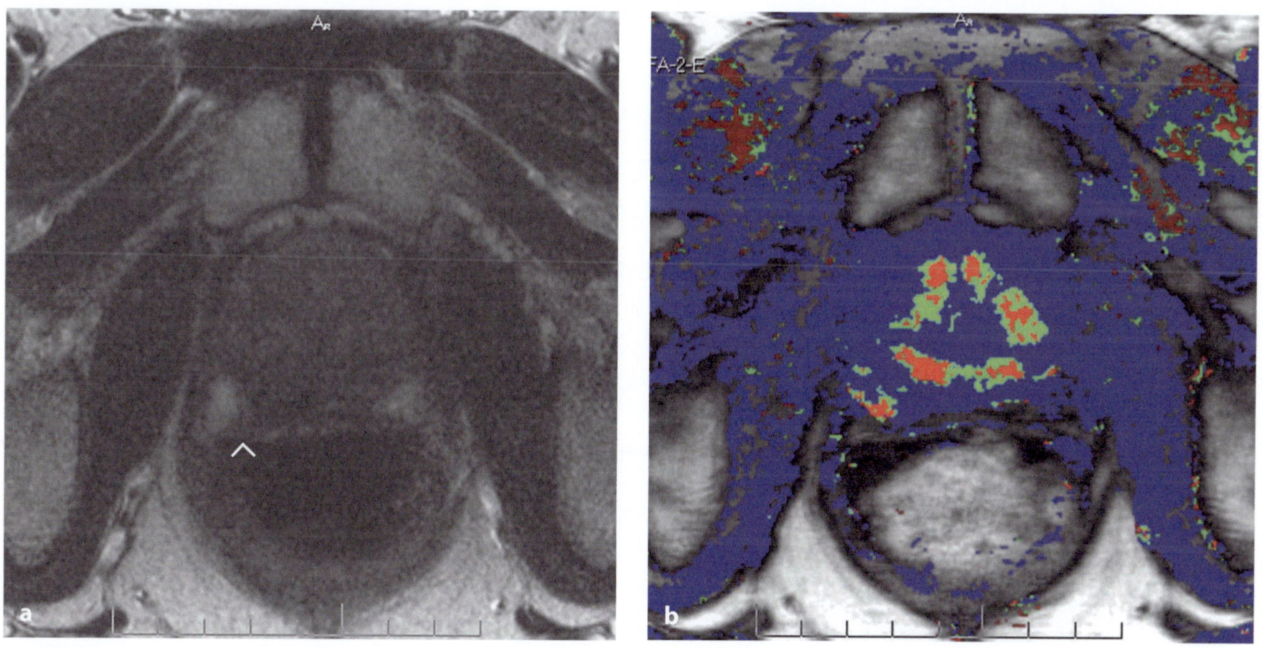

Fig. 8.5 a, b Post radiation with midgland central and right peripheral recurrence-note signal loss from radiation fibrosis

Fig. 8.5 c, d

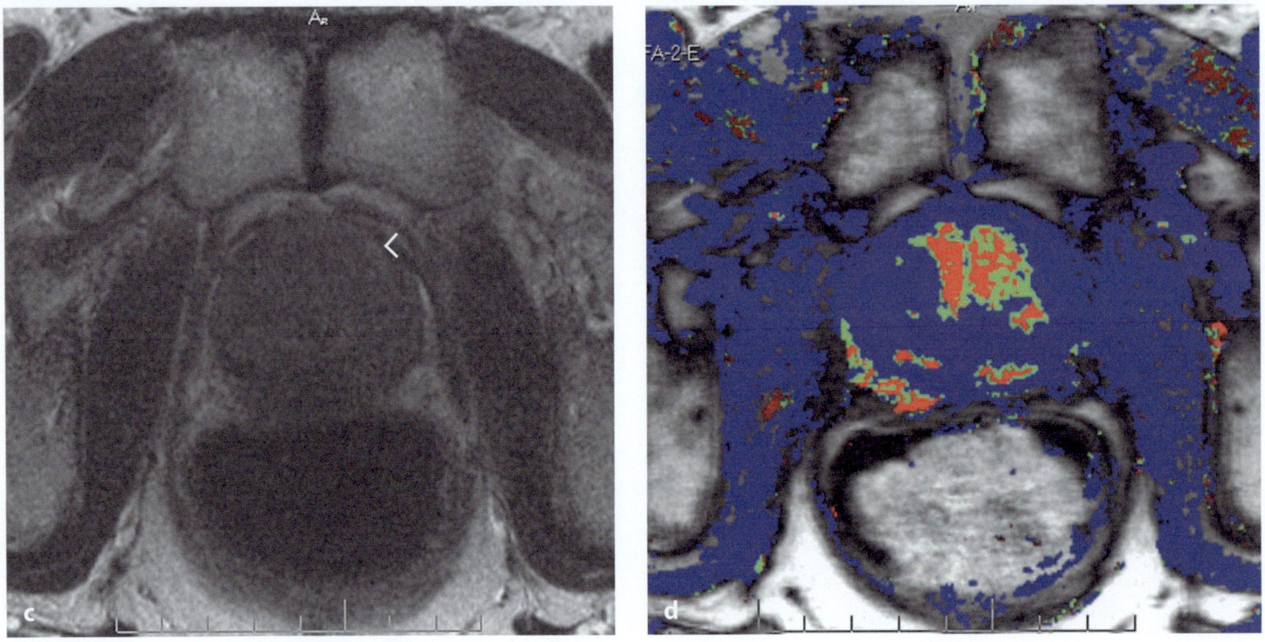

Fig. 8.5 c, d With extension into midgland anterior central zone

Fig. 8.5 e, f

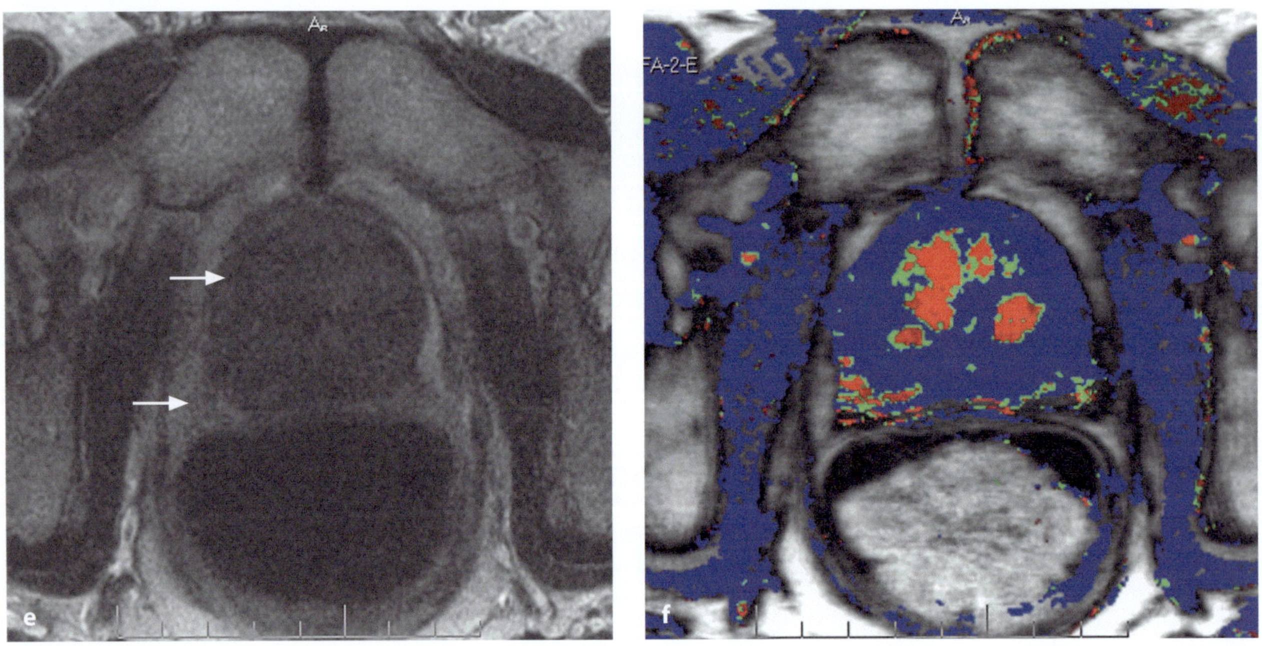

Fig. 8.5 e, f With extension into midgland left central zone and right lateral peripheral zone

Fig. 8.5 g, h

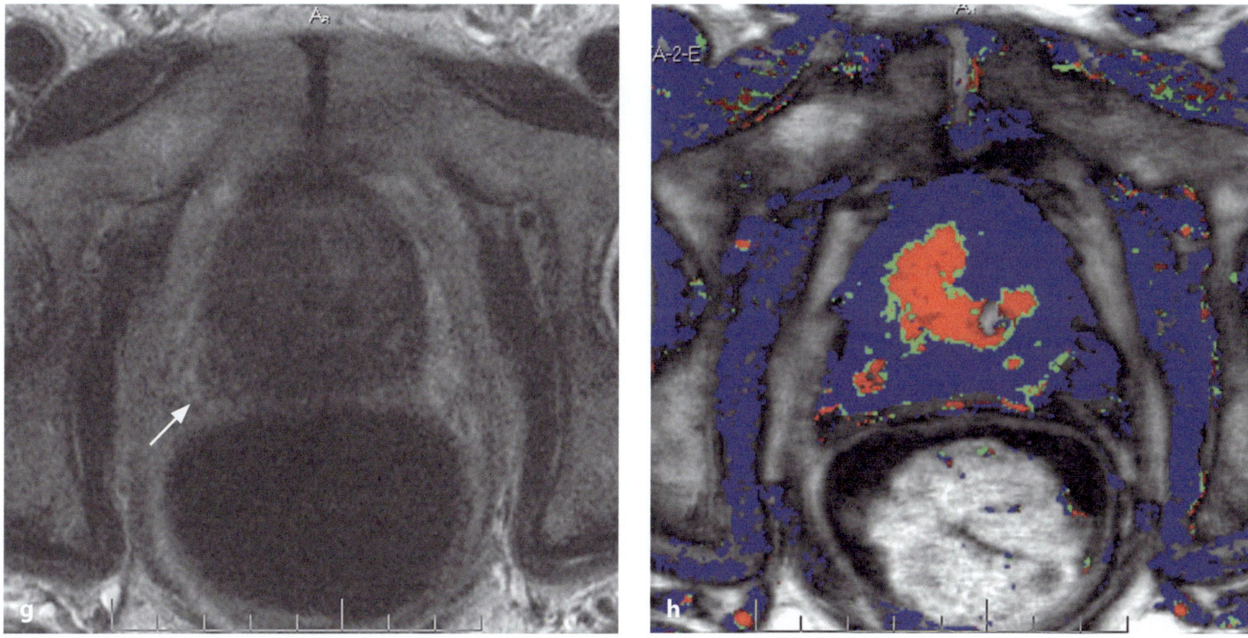

Fig. 8.5 g, h With extension into proximal right seminal vesicle

Fig. 8.6 a–d

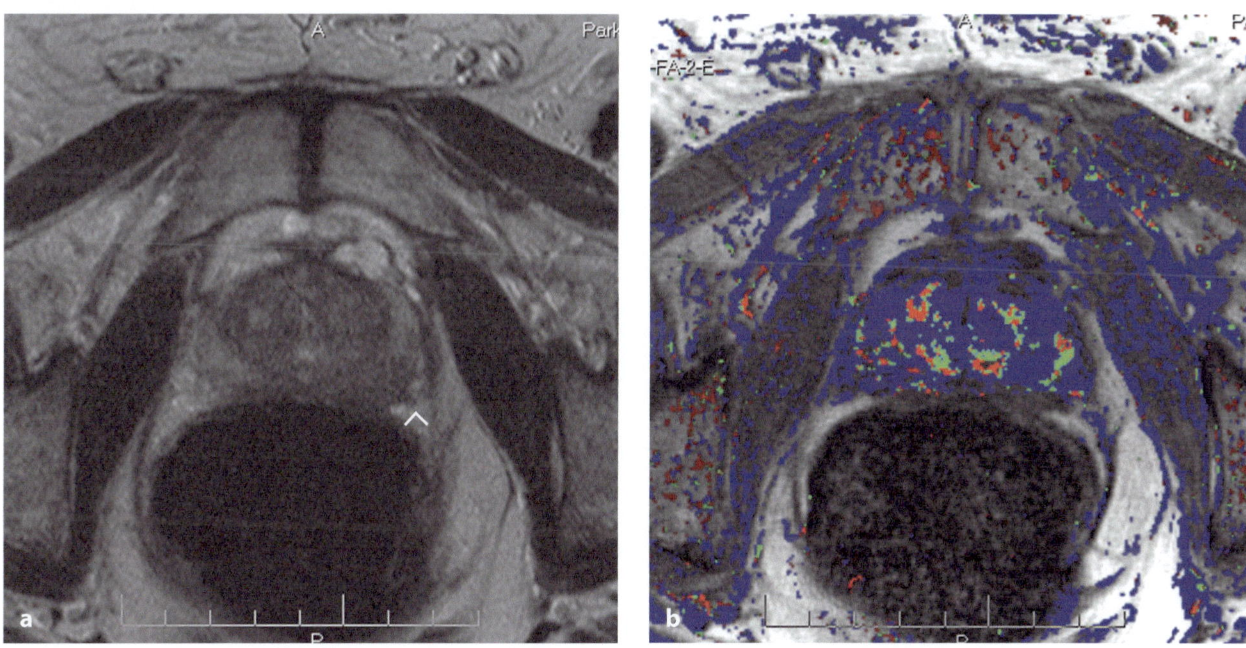

Fig. 8.6 a, b Post hormone therapy Gleason 4 with left midgland extracapsular extension

Fig. 8.6 c, d

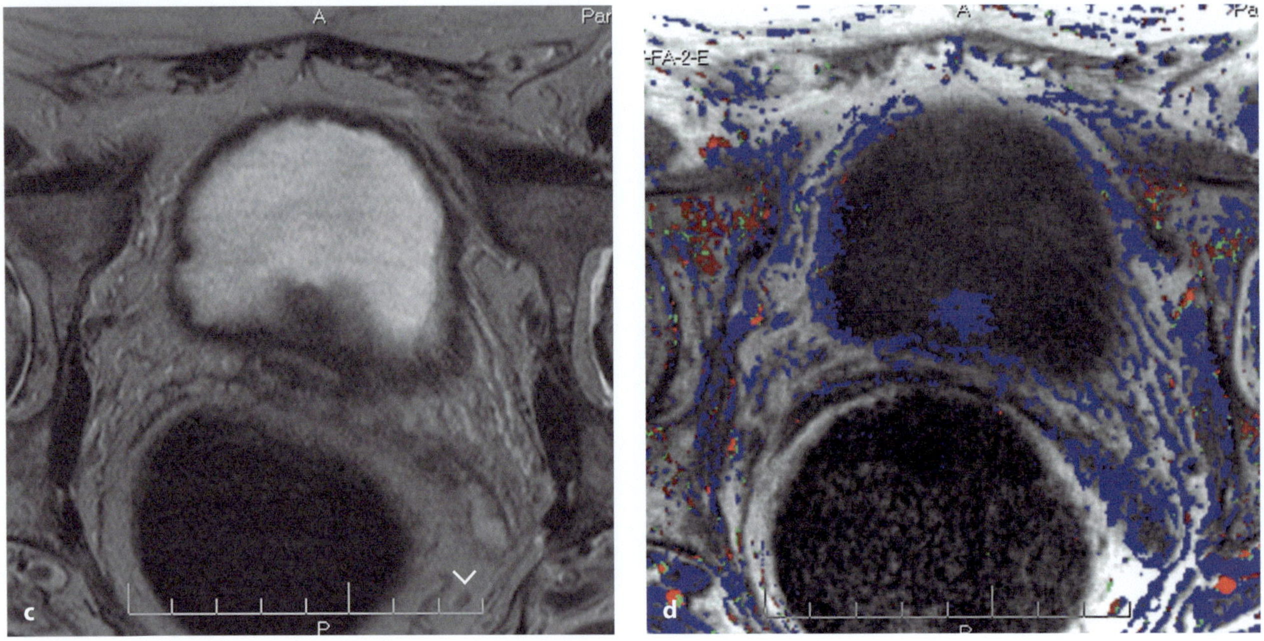

Fig. 8.6 c, d With vascular left 3x5 mm perirectal node

Fig. 8.7 a, b

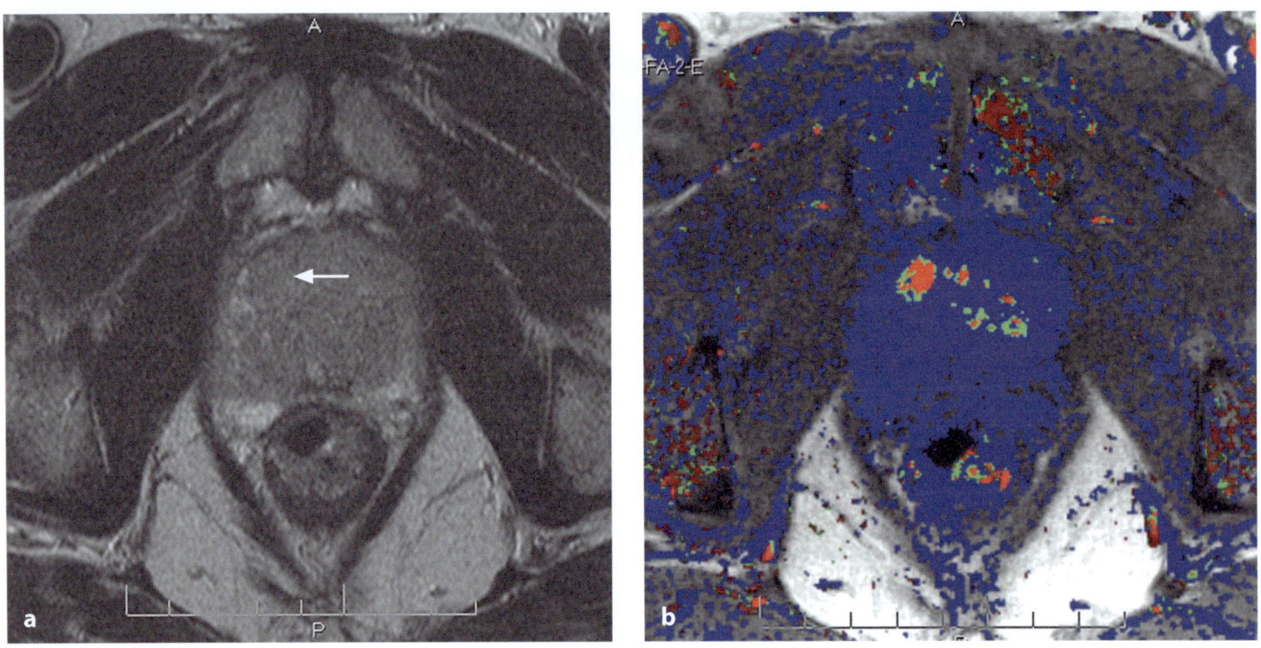

Fig. 8.7 a, b Post hormone therapy Gleason 3 with right anterior midgland recurrence biopsied as Gleason 4

Fig. 8.8 a, h

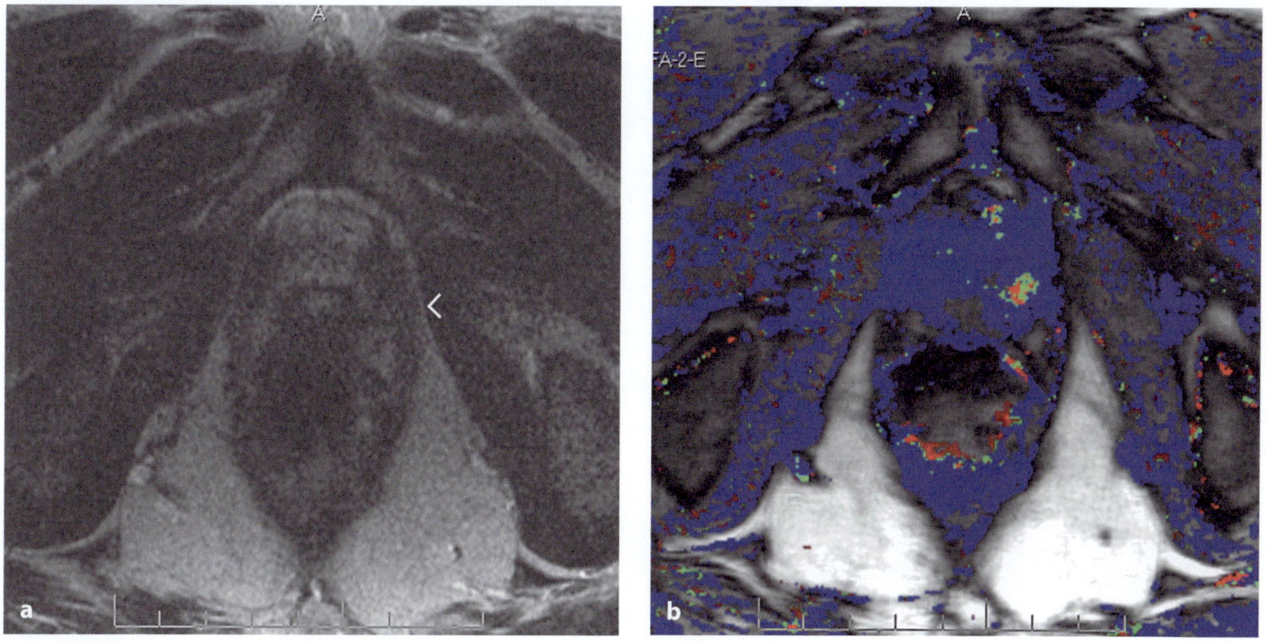

Fig. 8.8 a, b Post HIFU recurrence in left apex

Fig. 8.8 c, d

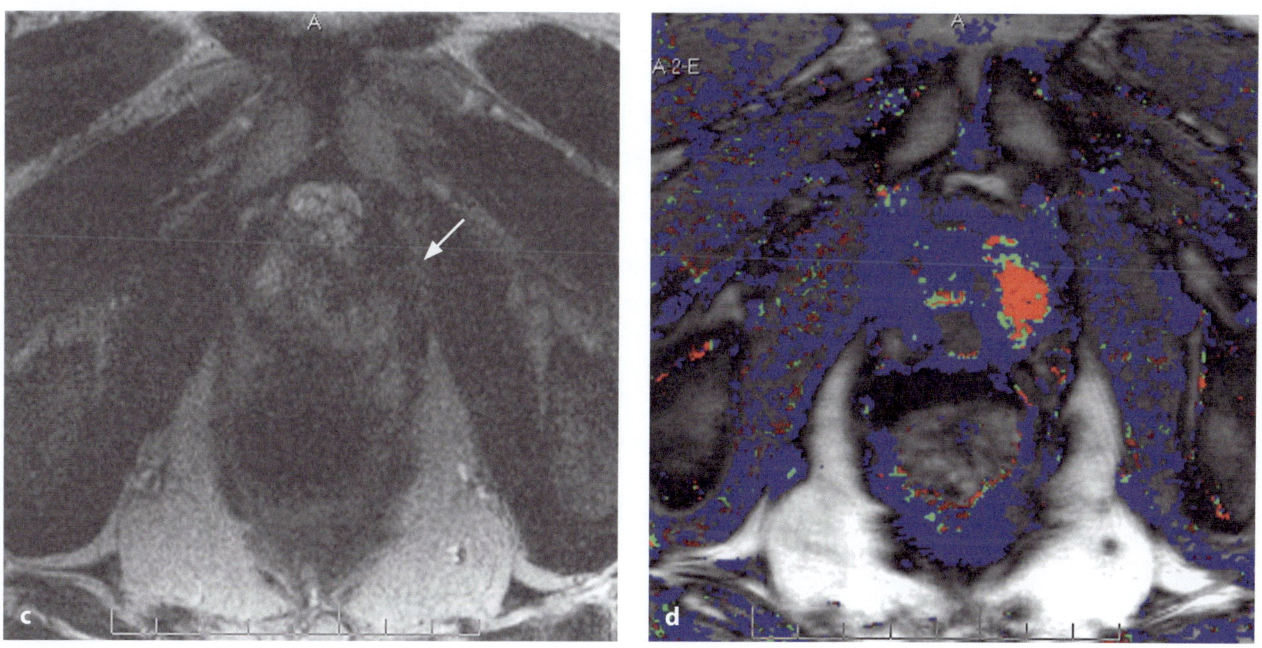

Fig. 8.8 c, d With extension into left midgland

Fig. 8.8 e, f

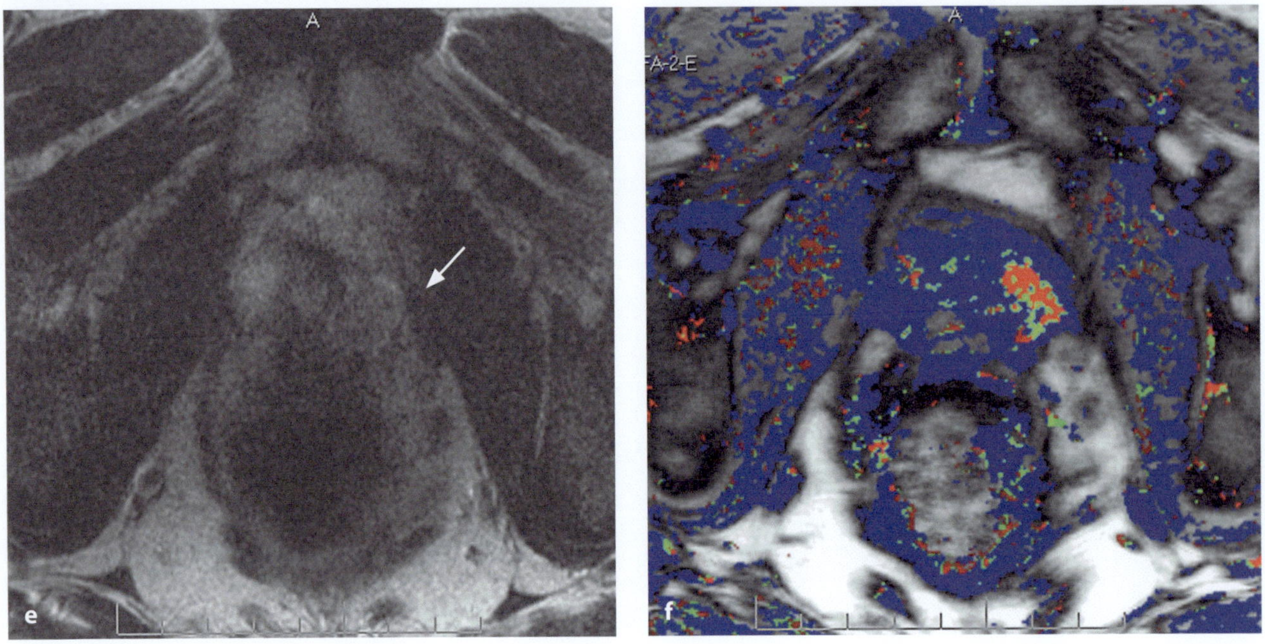

Fig. 8.8 e, f With extension into left base

Fig. 8.8 g, h

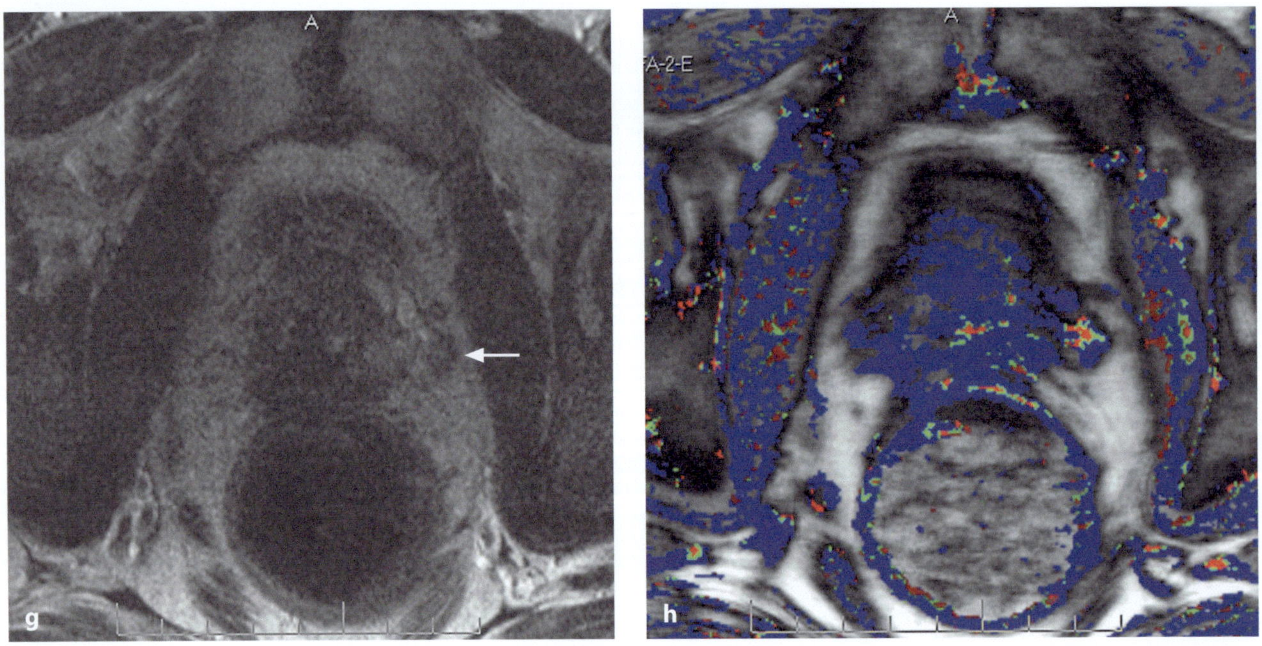

Fig. 8.8 g, h With left lateral extracapsular extension

Fig. 8.9 a–j

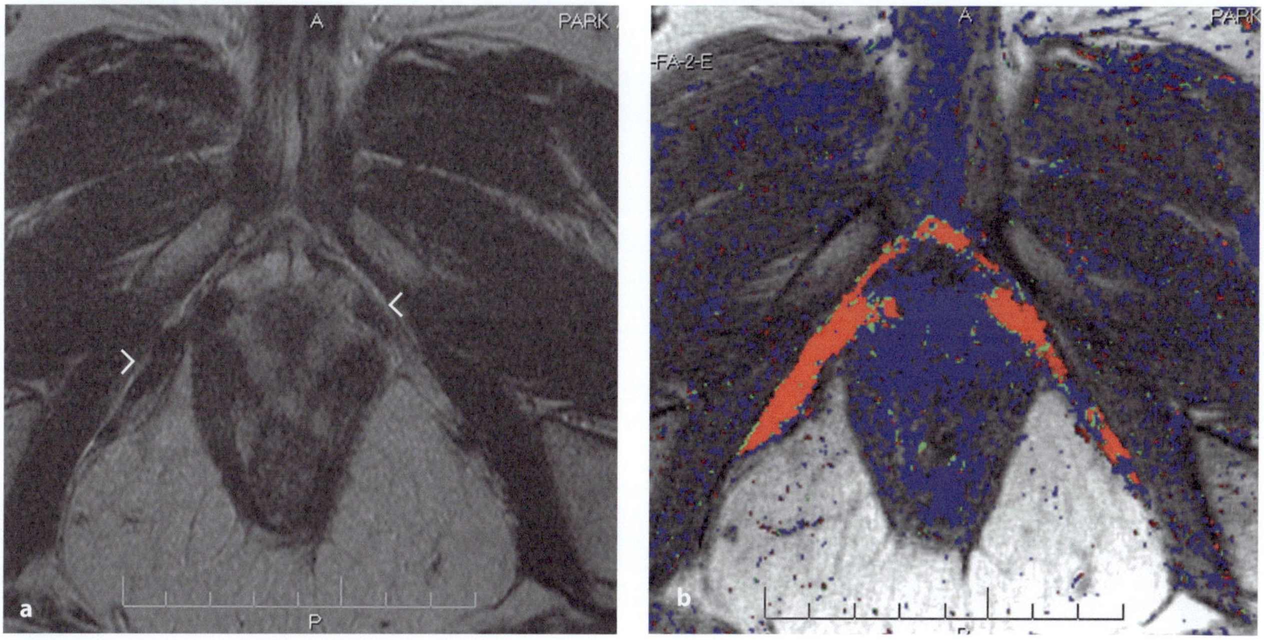

Fig. 8.9 a, b Post HIFU with dilated apical veins

Fig. 8.9 c, d

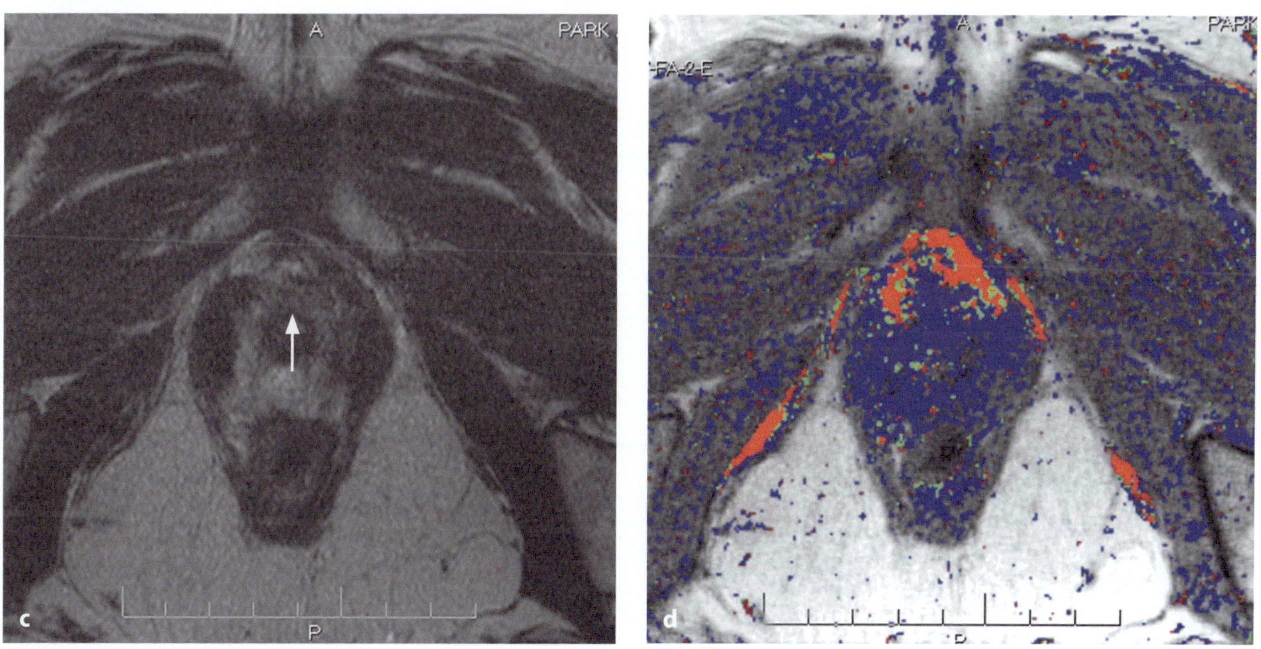

Fig. 8.9 c, d With apical recurrence

Fig. 8.9 e, f

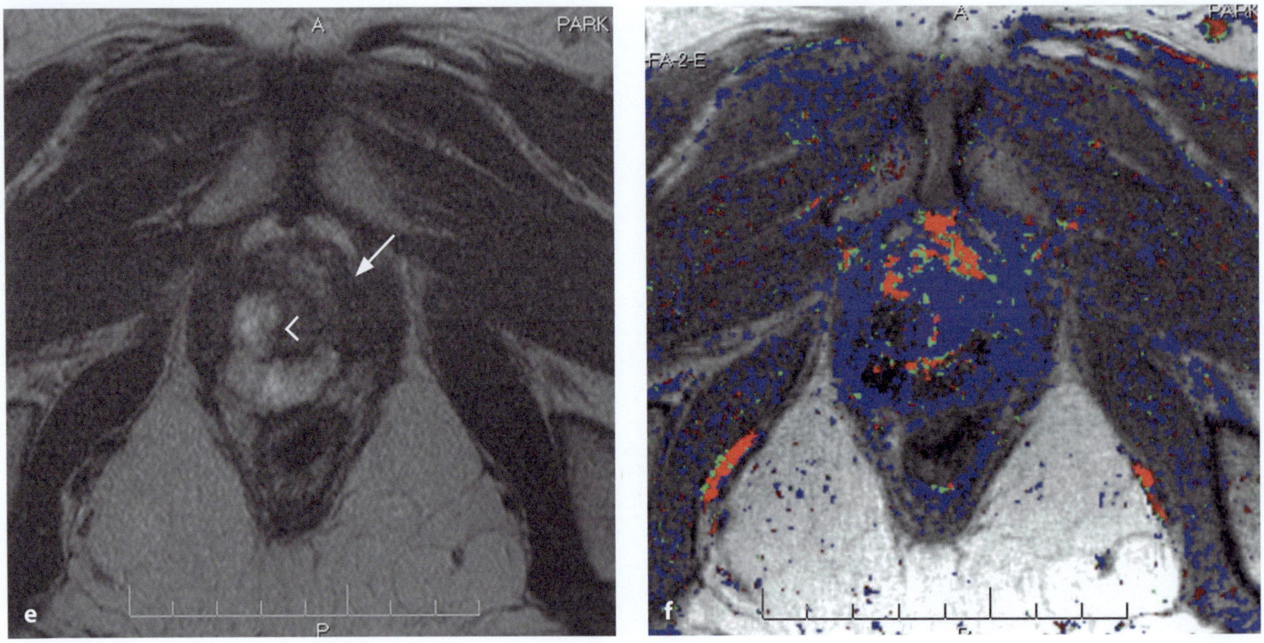

Fig. 8.9 e, f With midgland recurrence and prostatic urethral dilation

Fig. 8.9 g, h

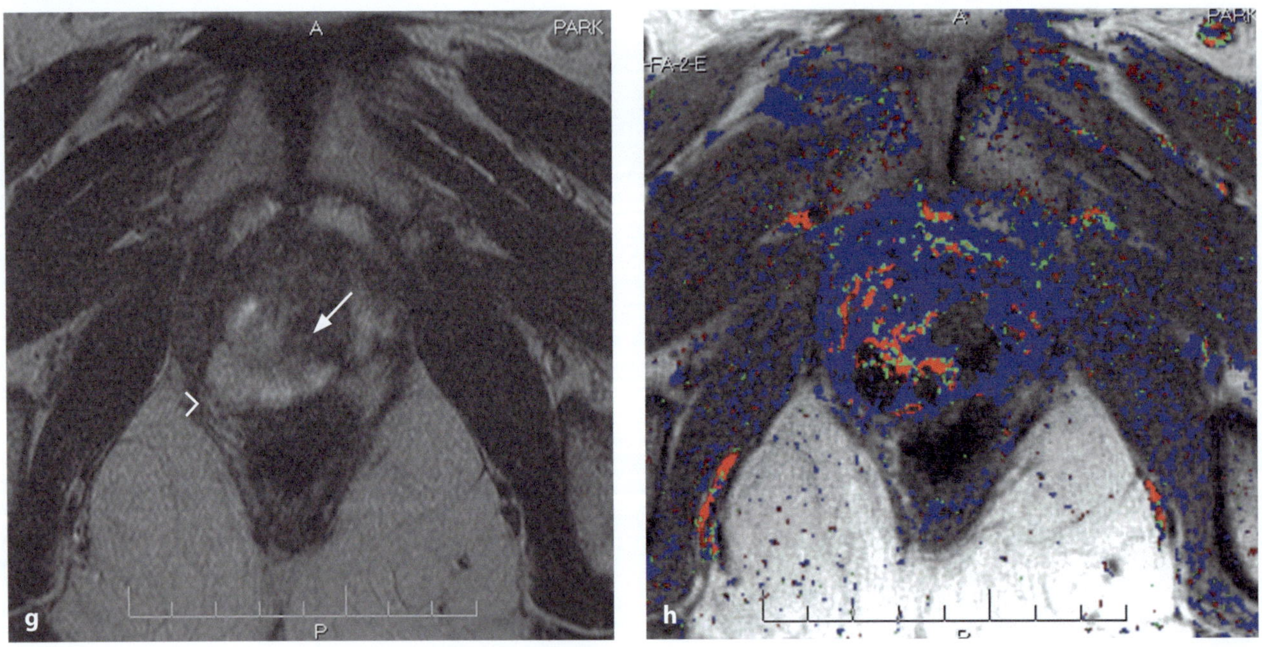

Fig. 8.9 g, h With basal recurrence and urethral diverticulum

Fig. 8.9 i, j

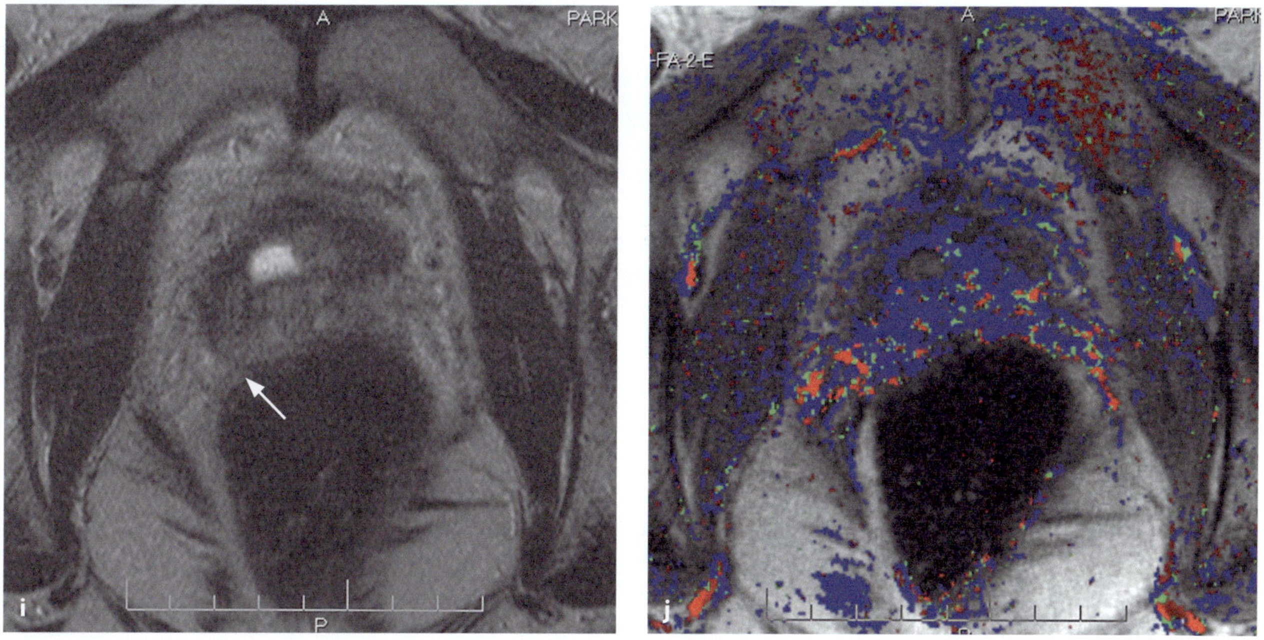

Fig. 8.9 i, j With dilated proximal urethra and seminal vesicle invasion

Fig. 8.10 a, b

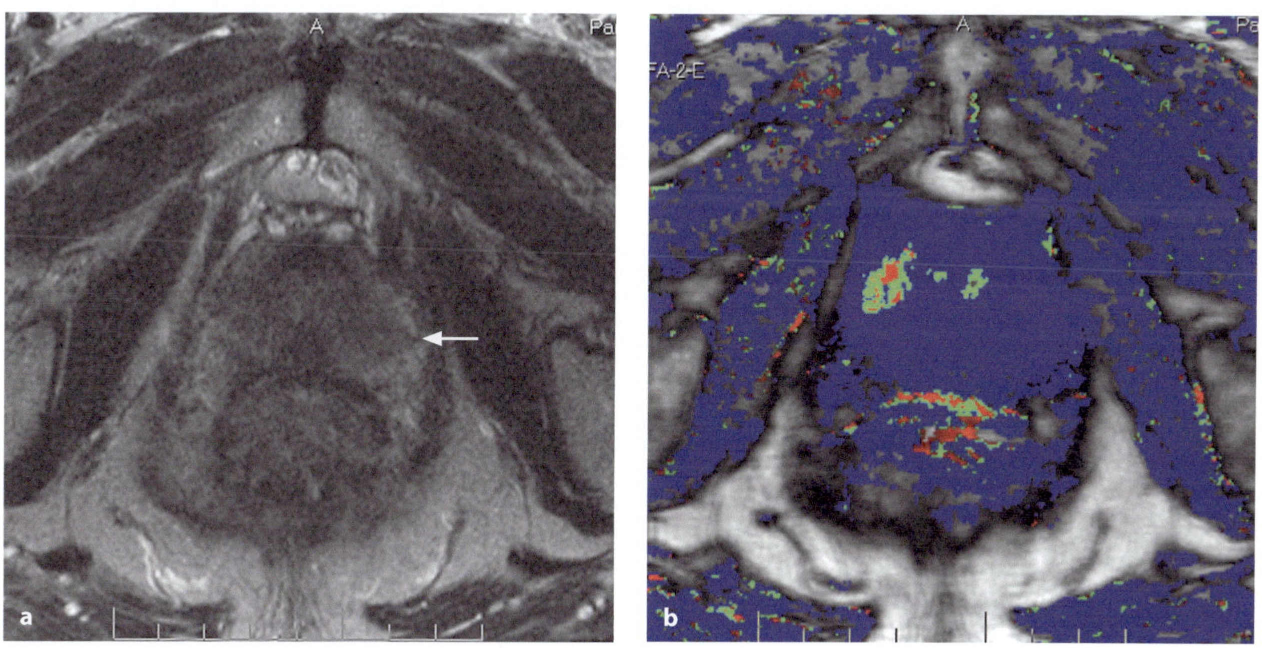

Fig. 8.10 a, b Gleason 4 hormonally treated-note avascular left midgland extracapsular extension

Fig. 8.10 c, d

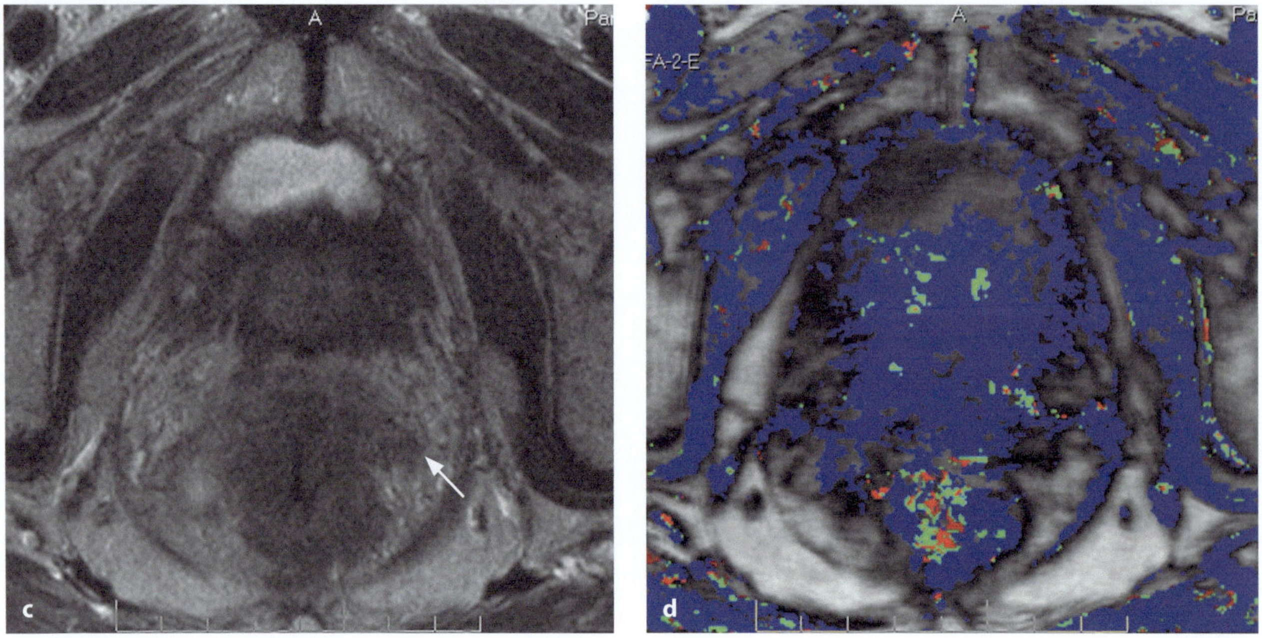

Fig. 8.10 c, d New left seminal vesical invasion

Fig. 8.11 a–h

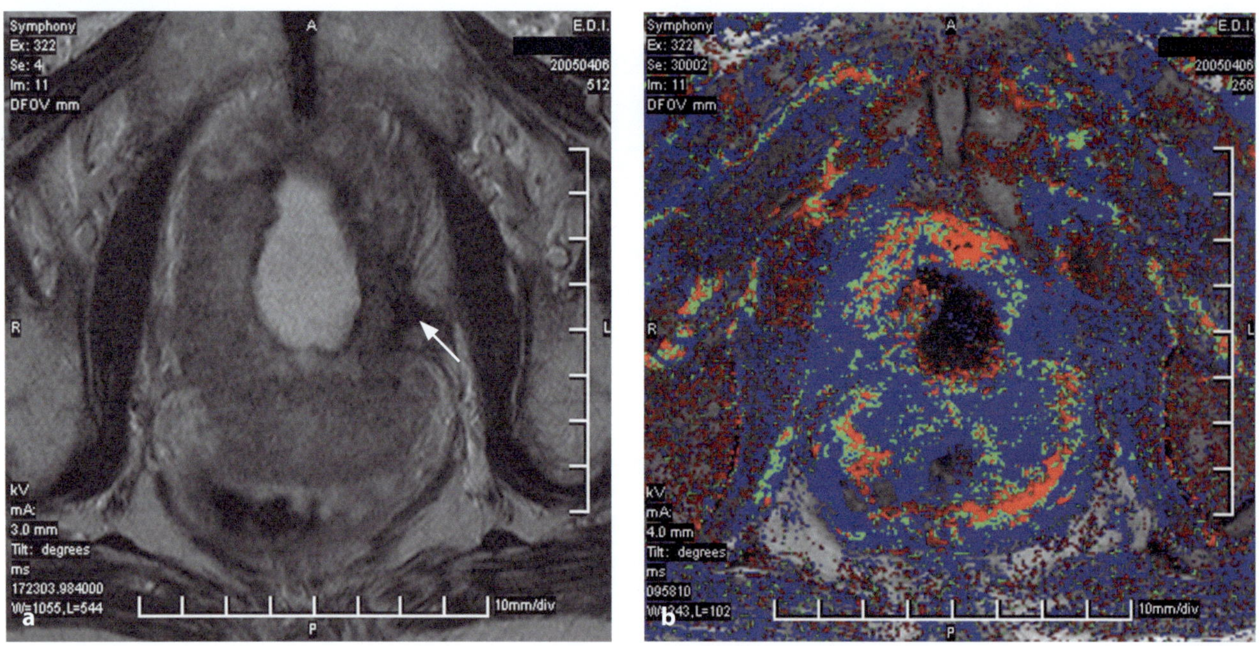

Fig. 8.11 a, b Squamous cell carcinoma following transurethral resection of prostate (TURP) and radiation-note tumor surrounds TURP

Fig. 8.11 c, d

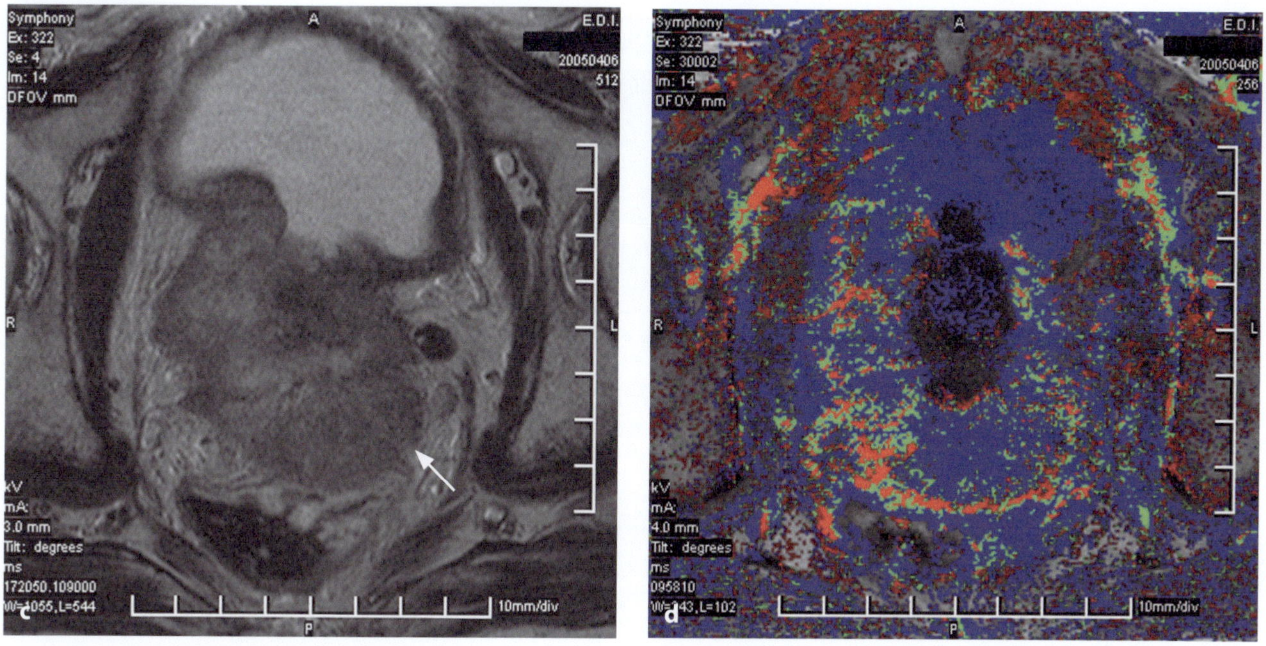

Fig. 8.11 c, d Massive tumor infiltration of left seminal vesicle with peripheral vascularity identified-note artifacts due to early experience with DCE-April 2005 study

Fig. 8.11 e, f

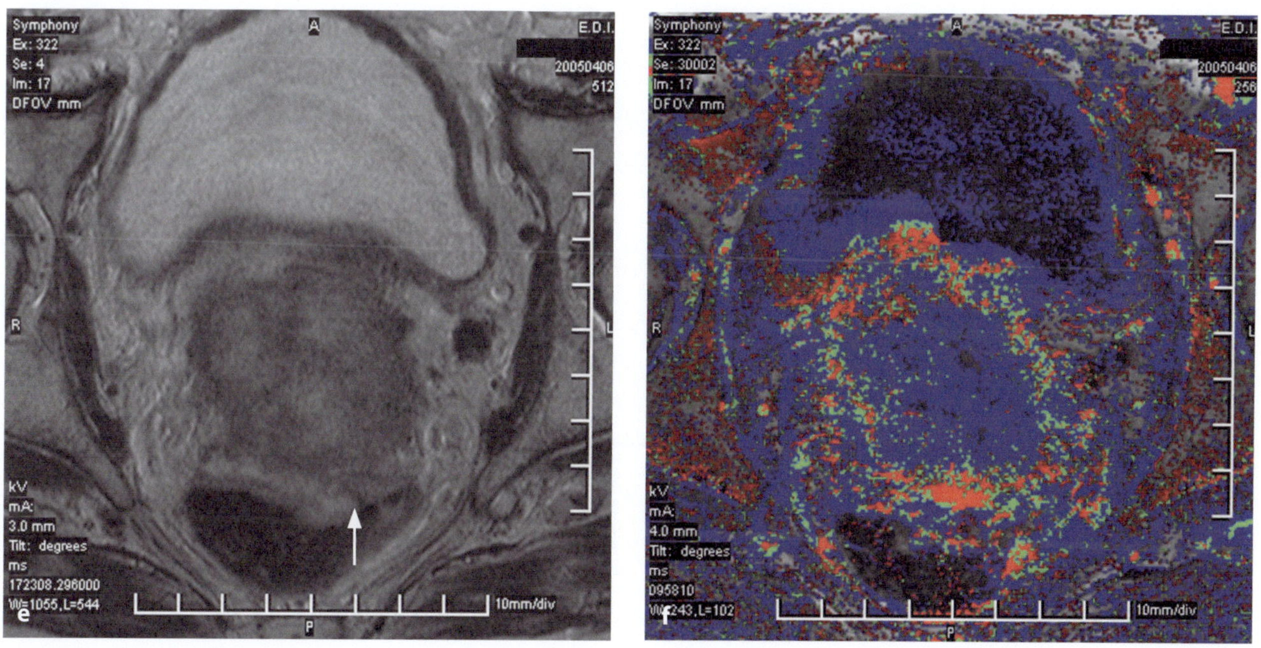

Fig. 8.11 e, f Peripheral vascularity due to massive internal necrosis-note hyperemic tumor margins invade bladder anteriorly and rectum posteriorly

Fig. 8.11 g, h

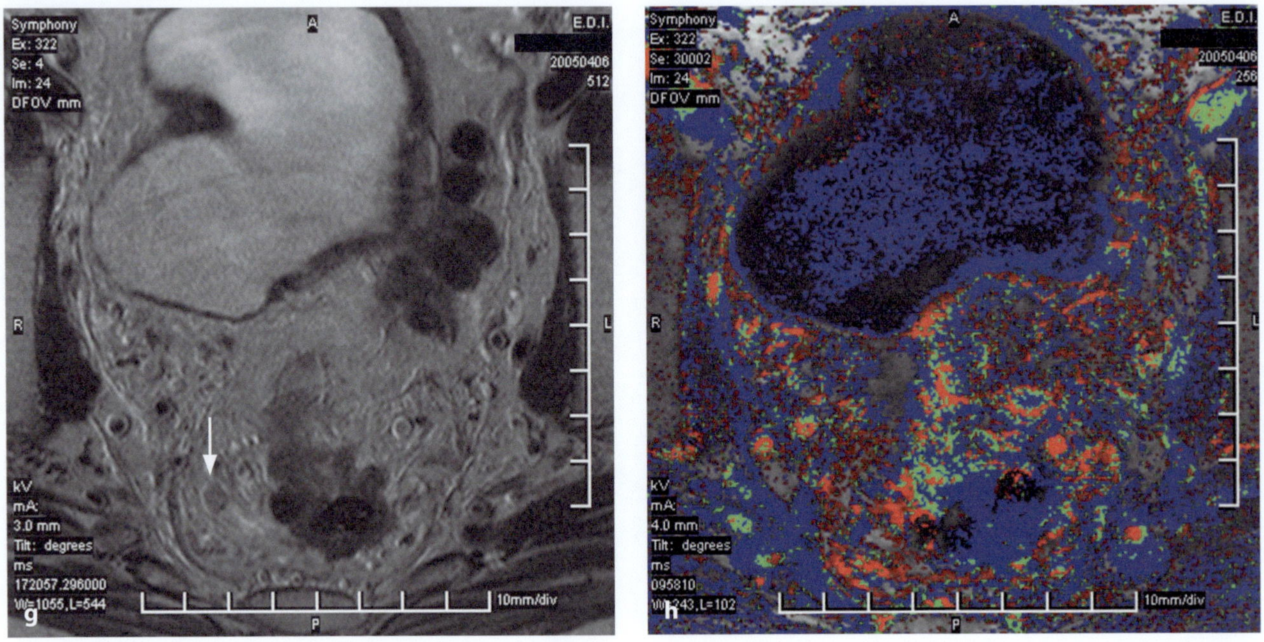

Fig. 8.11 g, h Right perirectal node with massive rectal invasion

Fig. 8.12 a, b

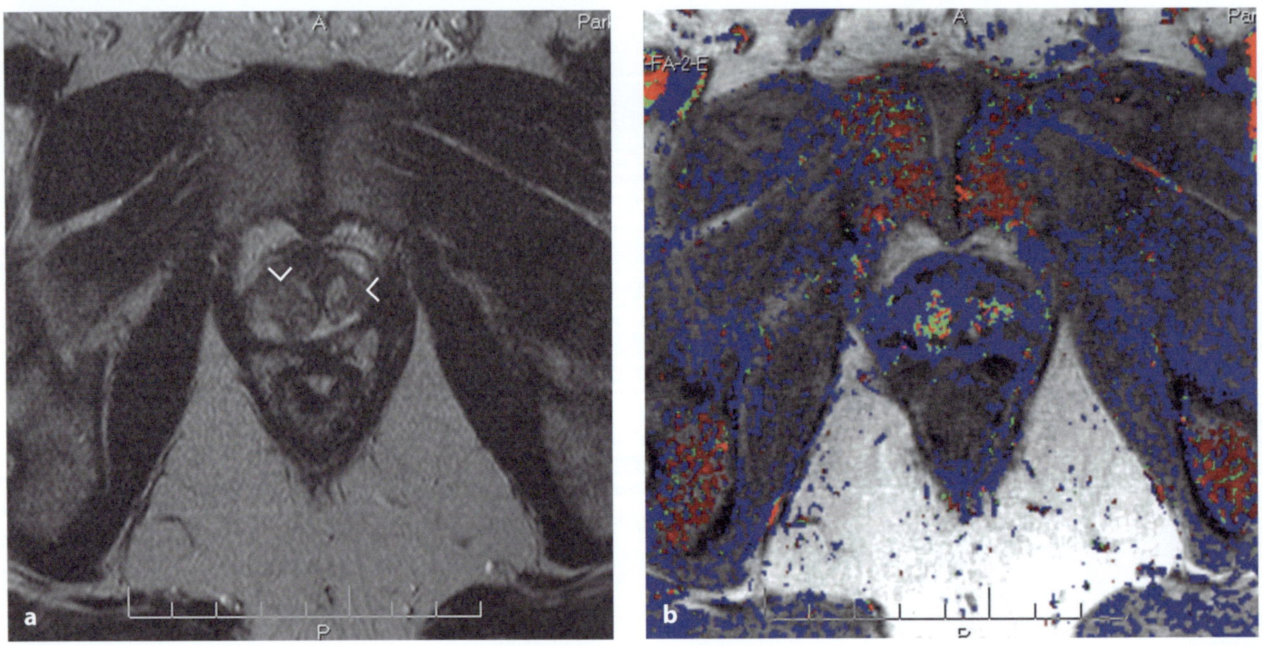

Fig. 8.12 a, b Post HIFU with bilateral apical recurrence

Fig. 8.13 a, b

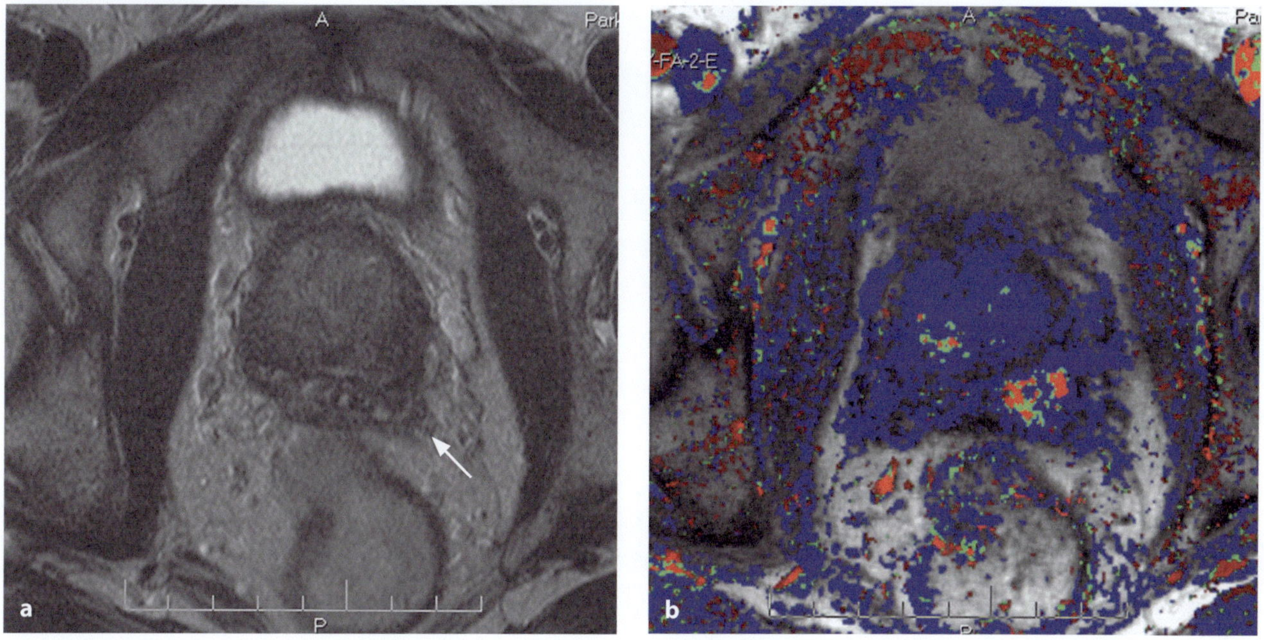

Fig. 8.13 a, b Post hormone treatment with left seminal vesicle recurrence

Fig. 8.14 a–f

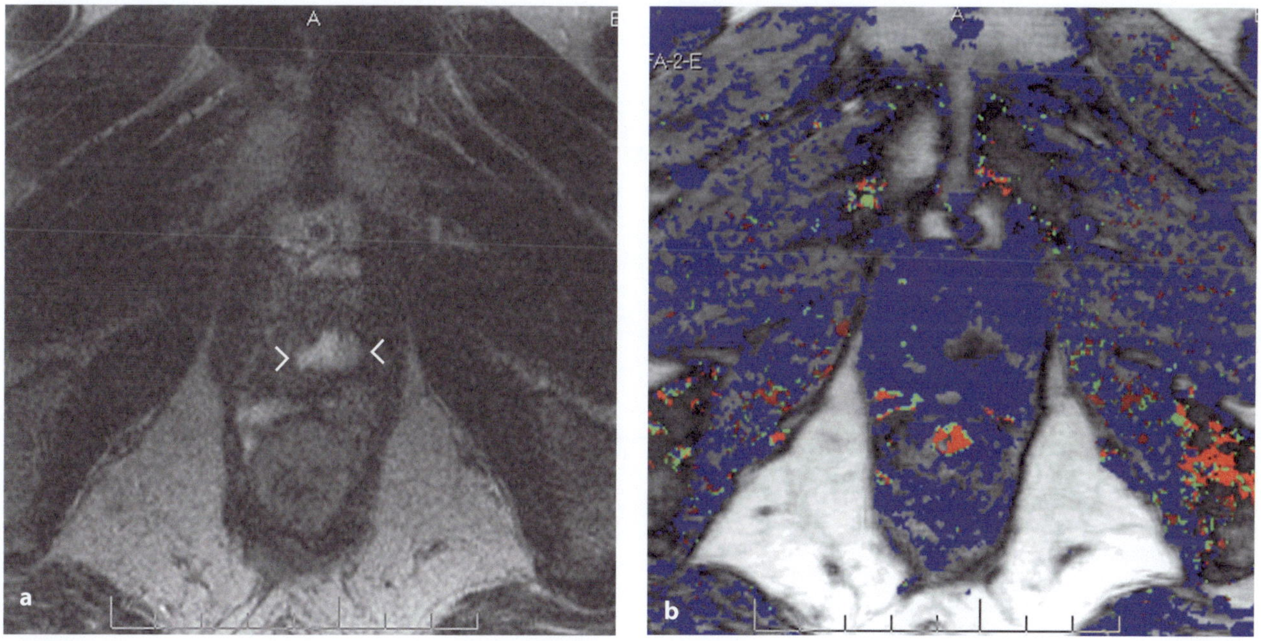

Fig. 8.14 a, b Post HIFU with dilated prostatic urethra

Fig. 8.14 c, d

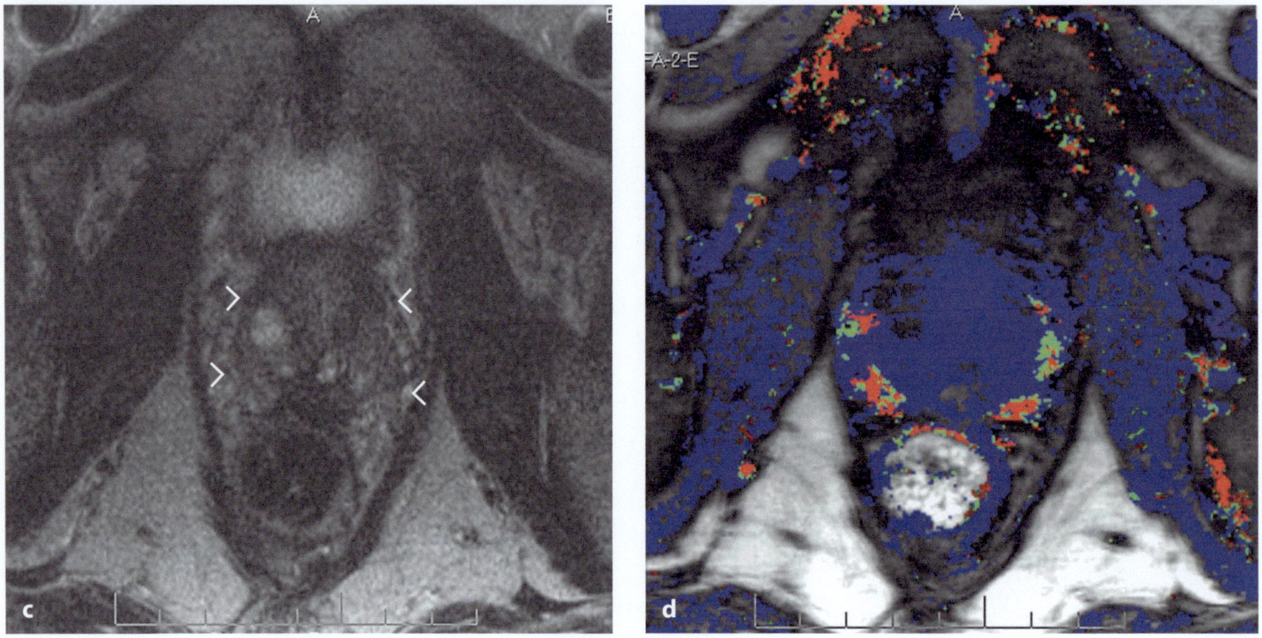

Fig. 8.14 c, d With bilateral anterior and posterior focal recurrences

Fig. 8.14 e, f

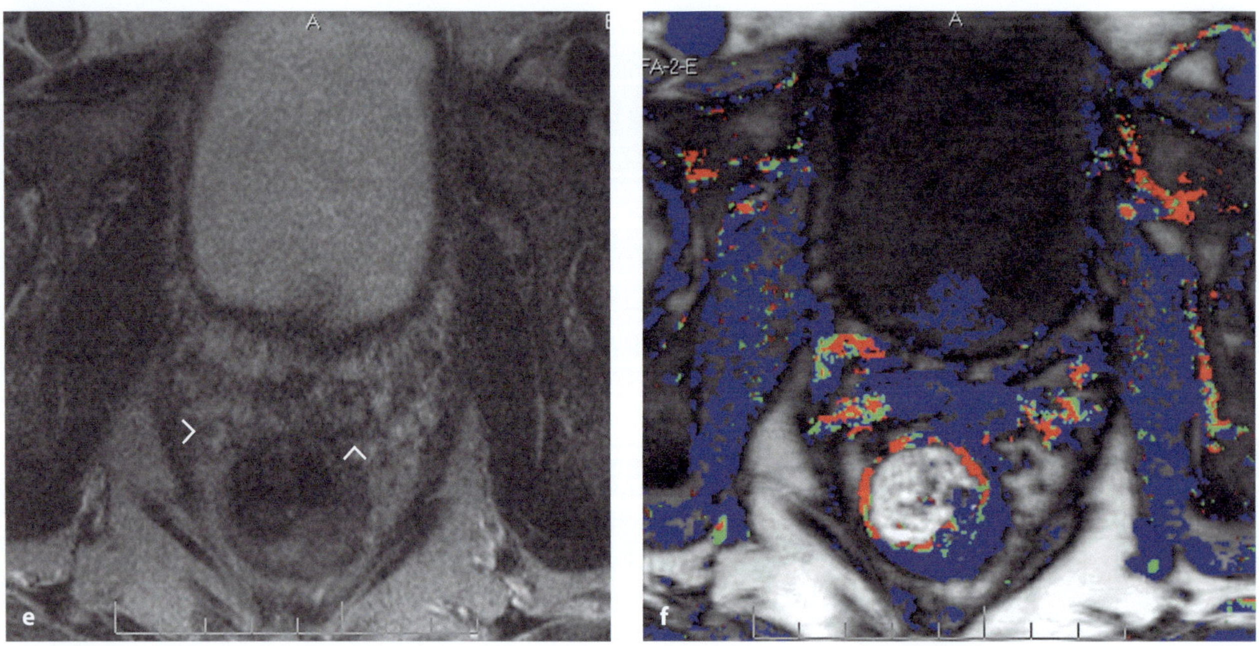

Fig. 8.14 e, f With bilateral seminal vesicle invasion

Fig. 8.15 a, b

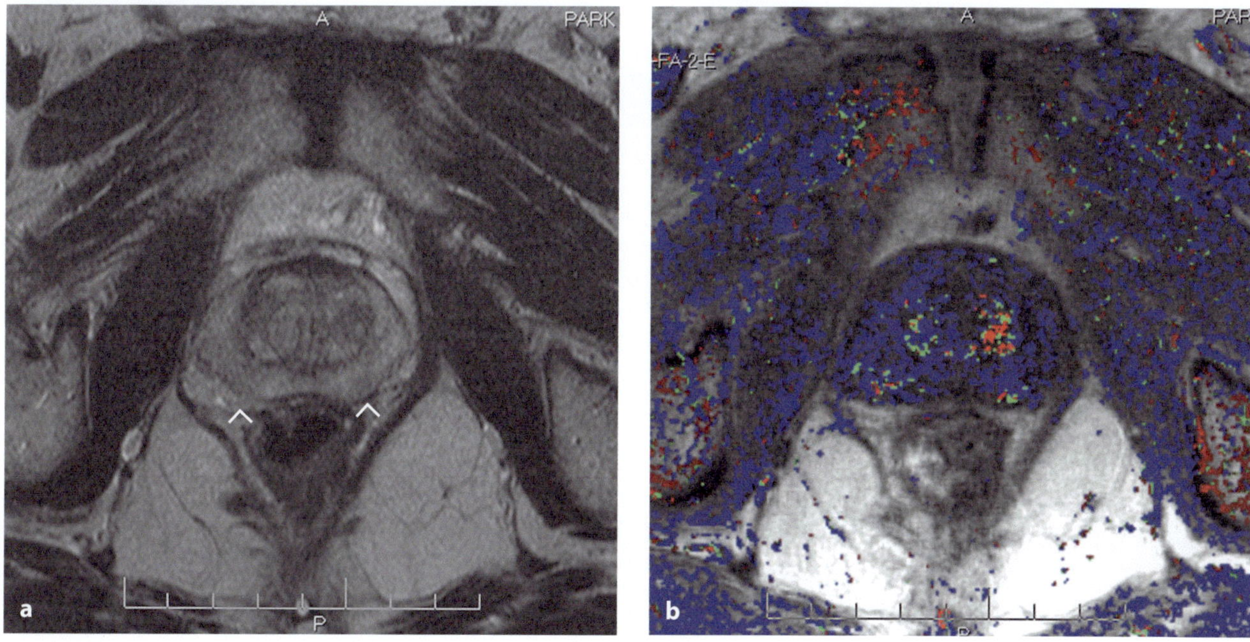

Fig. 8.15 a, b Post HIFU with focal posterior bilateral recurrences

Fig. 8.16 a, b

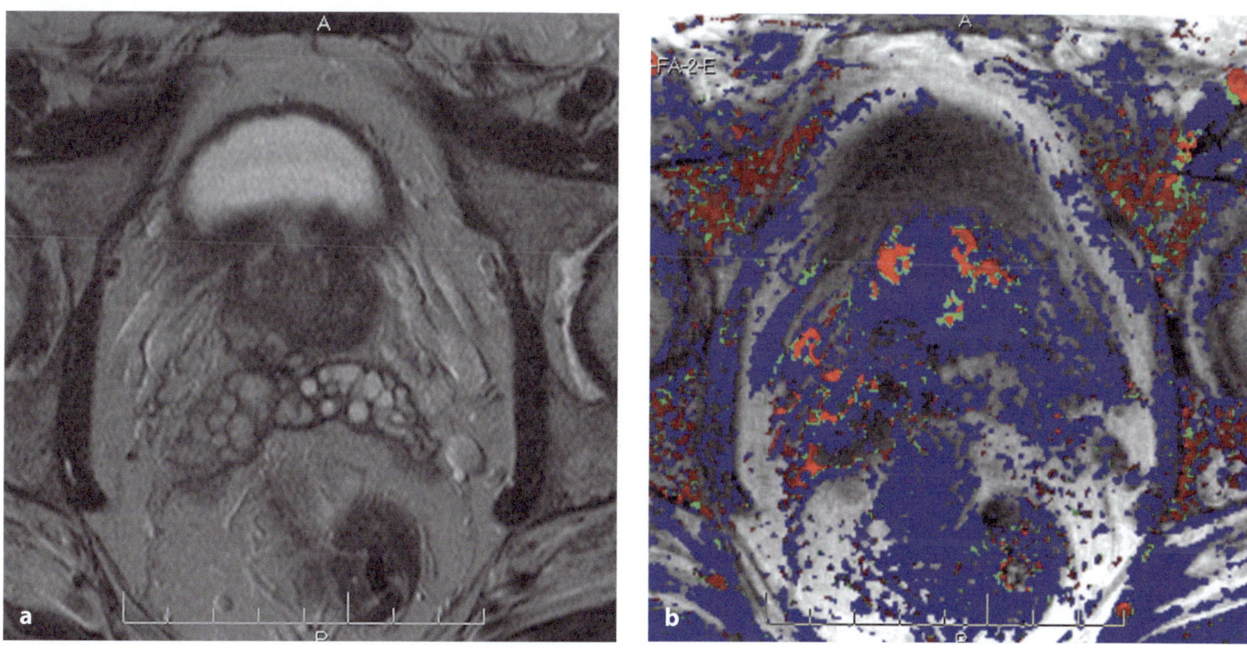

Fig. 8.16 a, b Post HIFU focal with anterior bilateral recurrence

Fig. 8.17 a–d

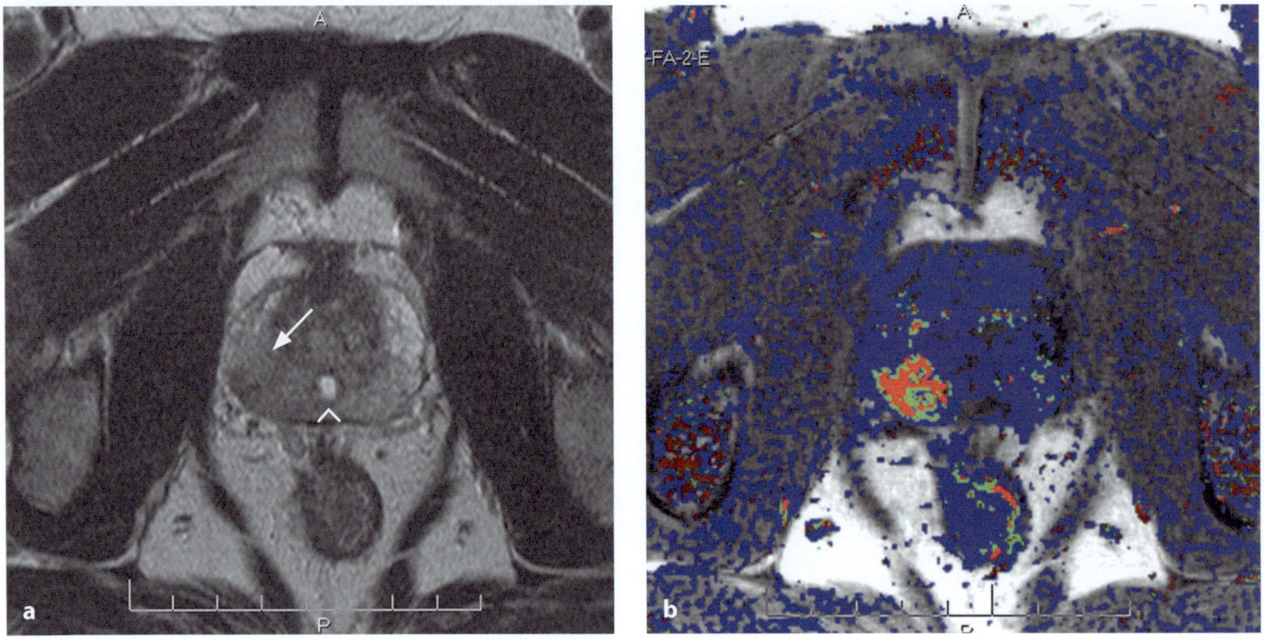

Fig. 8.17 a, b Gl 4 r midgland without extracapsular extension-note midline cyst

Fig.8.17 c, d

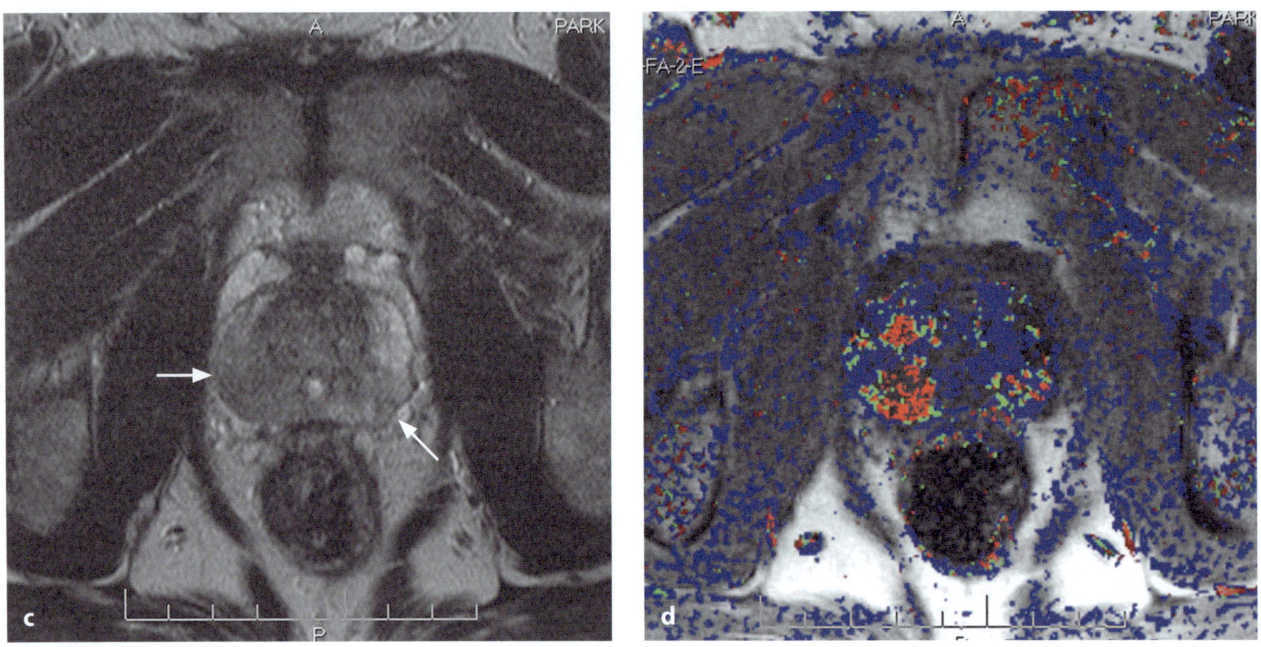

Fig. 8.17 c, d 11 mo post hormone therapy neovascular recurrences in left midgland and right anterior midgland

Fig. 8.18 a, b

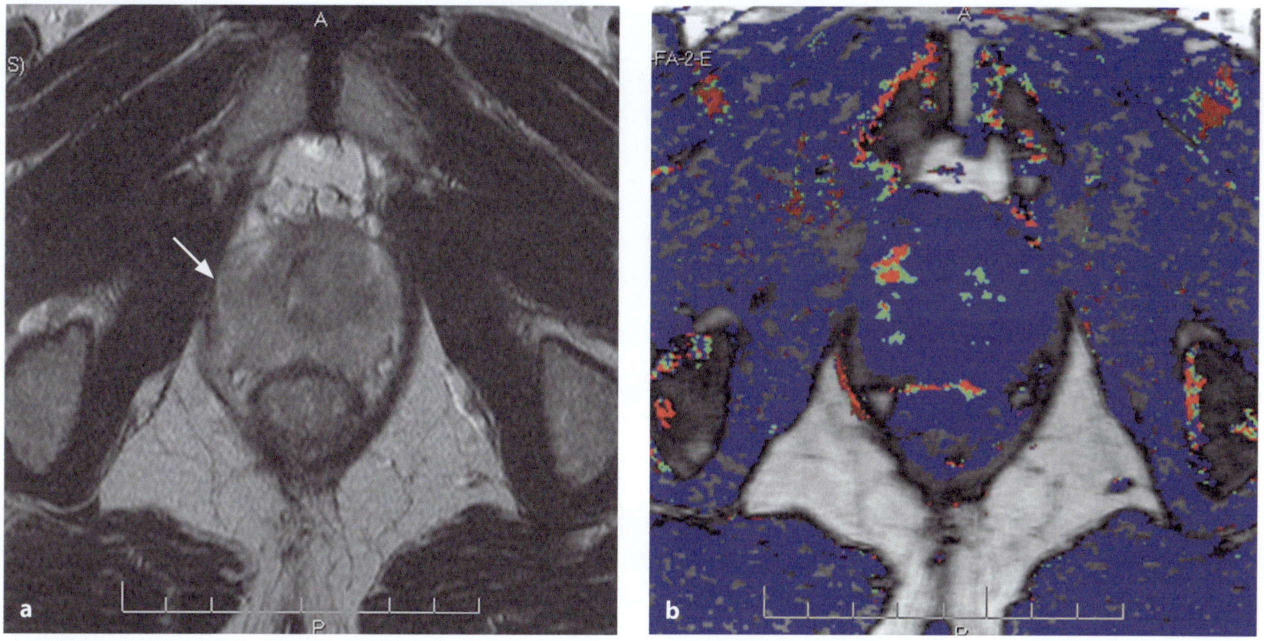

Fig. 8.18 a, b Recurrent Gleason 4 mid right anterior midgland

Fig. 8.19 a–f

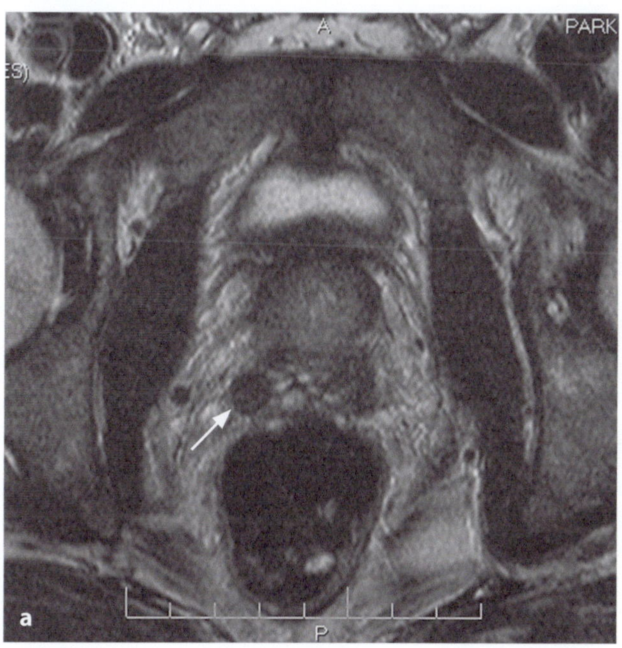

Fig. 8.19 a Post radiation for Gleason 4 in September 2005

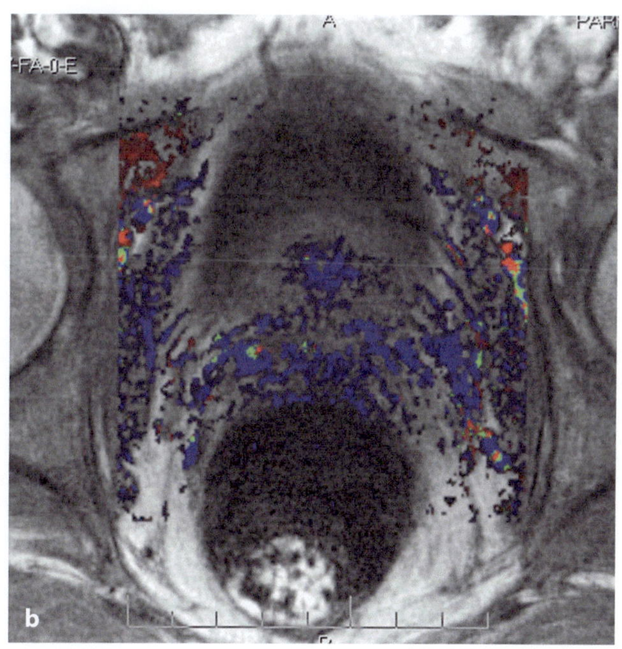

Fig. 8.19 b February 2006 avascular gland with right SV invasion

Fig. 8.19 c, d

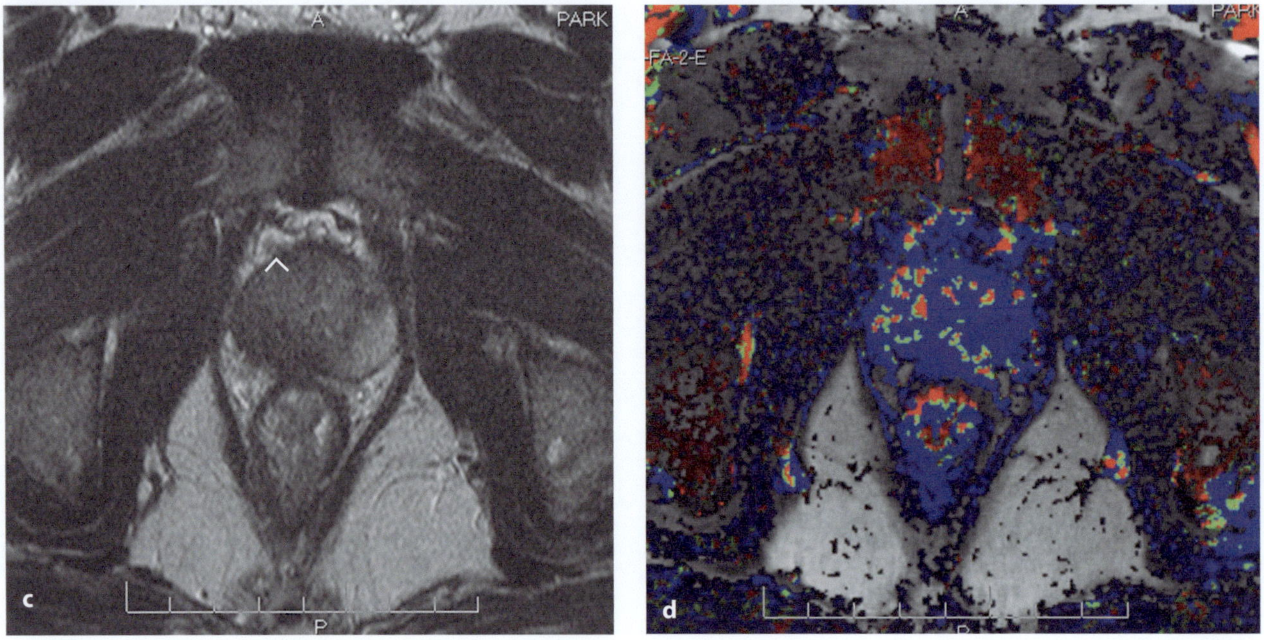

Fig. 8.19 c, d September 2006 avascular retropubic 4 mm R anterior lymph node

Fig. 8.19 e, f

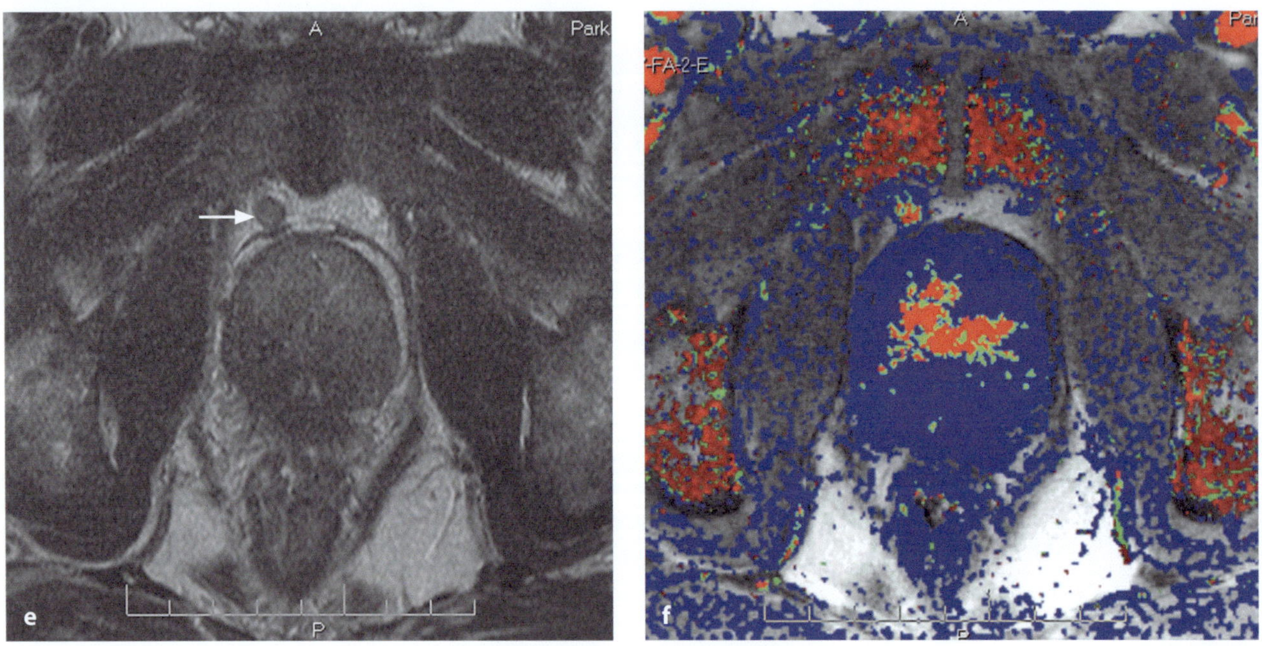

Fig. 8.19 e, f June 2008 retropubic node increased to 6 mm with neovascularity

Fig. 8.19 g, h

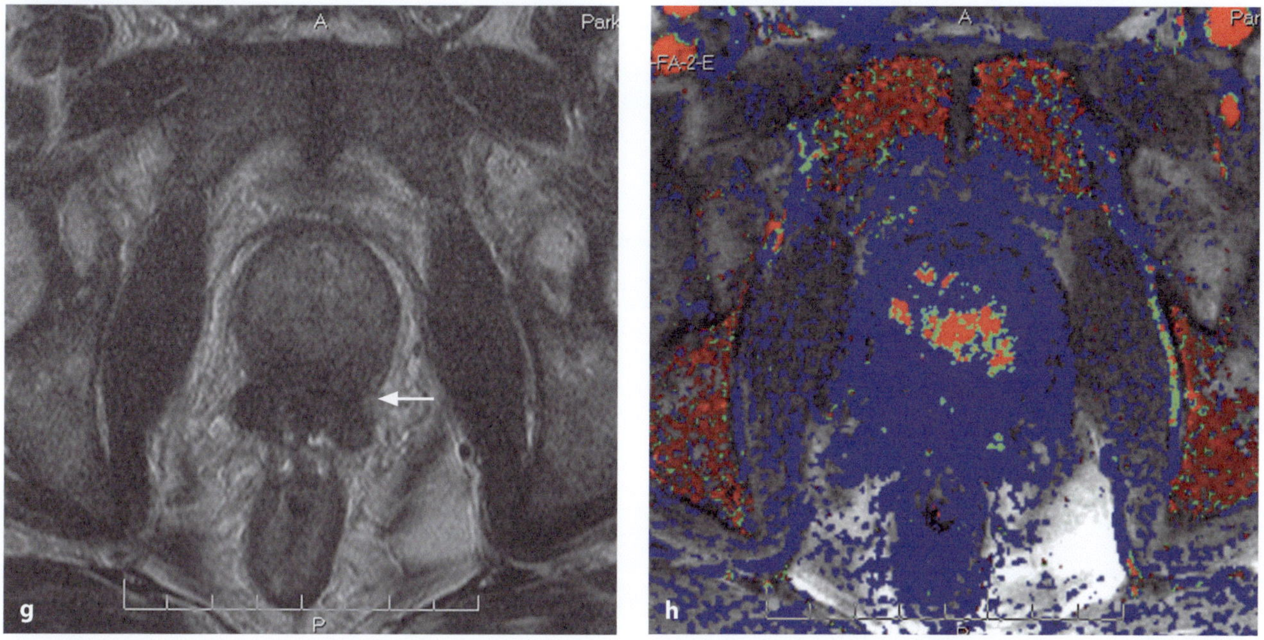

Fig. 8.19 g, h Increased left seminal vesicle involvement and boney pubic symphysis metastatic disease

Chapter

9 Case Studies

Fig. 9.1 a,–j

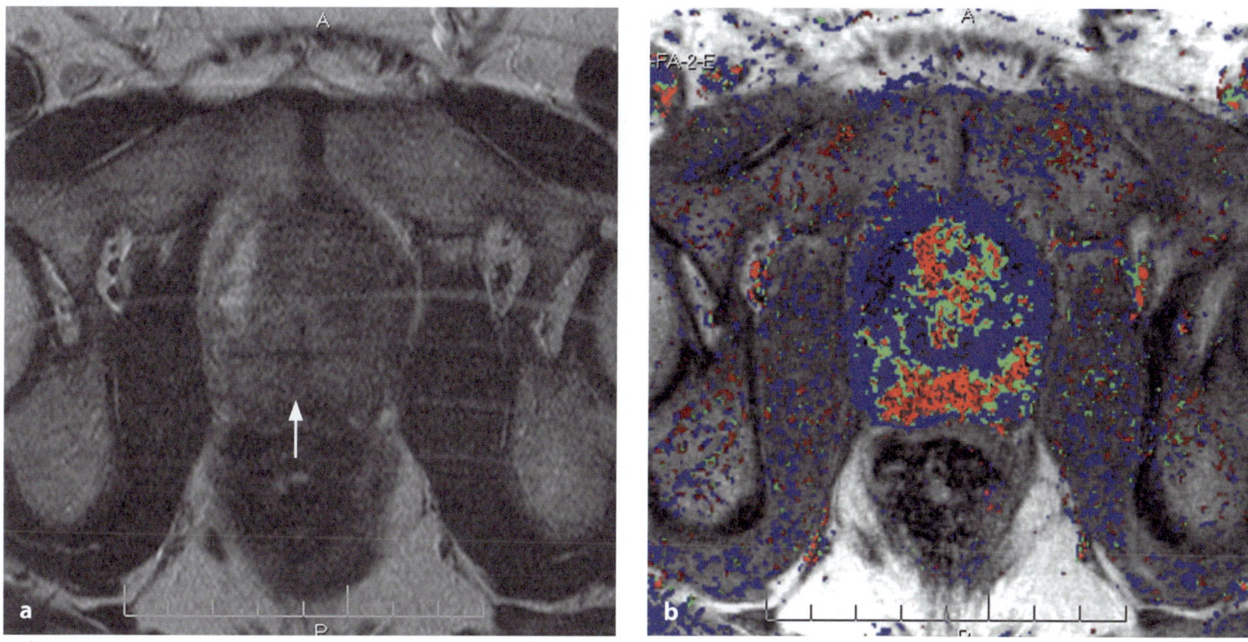

Fig. 9.1 a, b Posterior midgland Gleason 4 lesion

Fig. 9.1 c, d

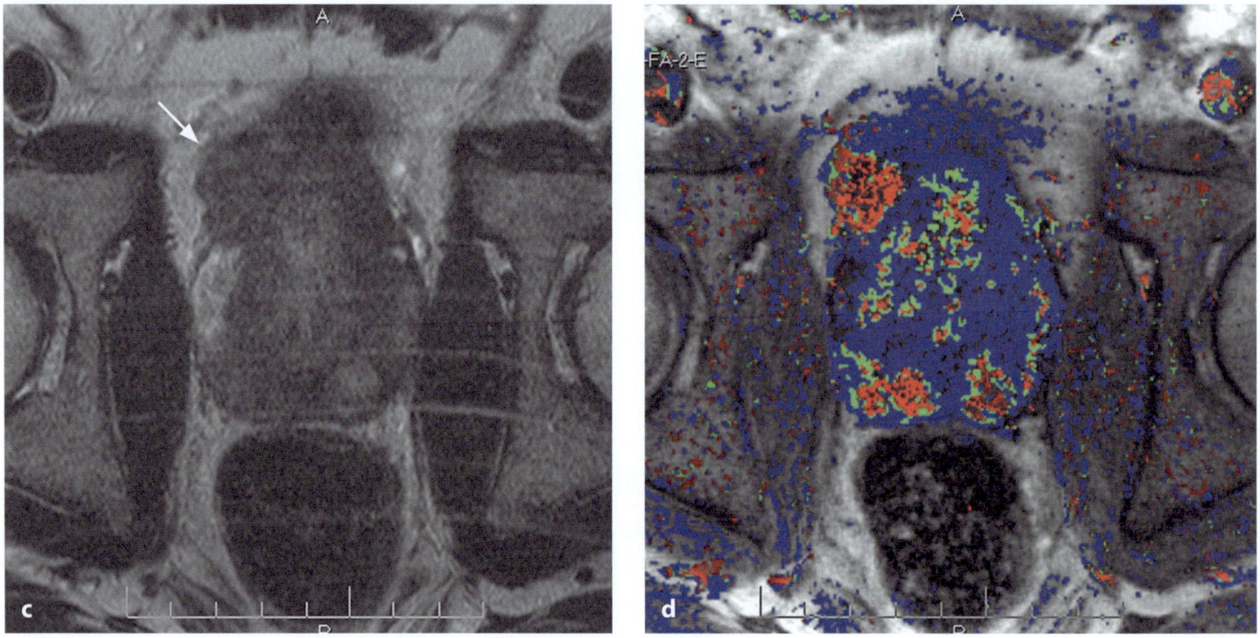

Fig. 9.1 c, d With anterior base Gleason 5 lesion with capsular erosion

Fig. 9.1 e, f

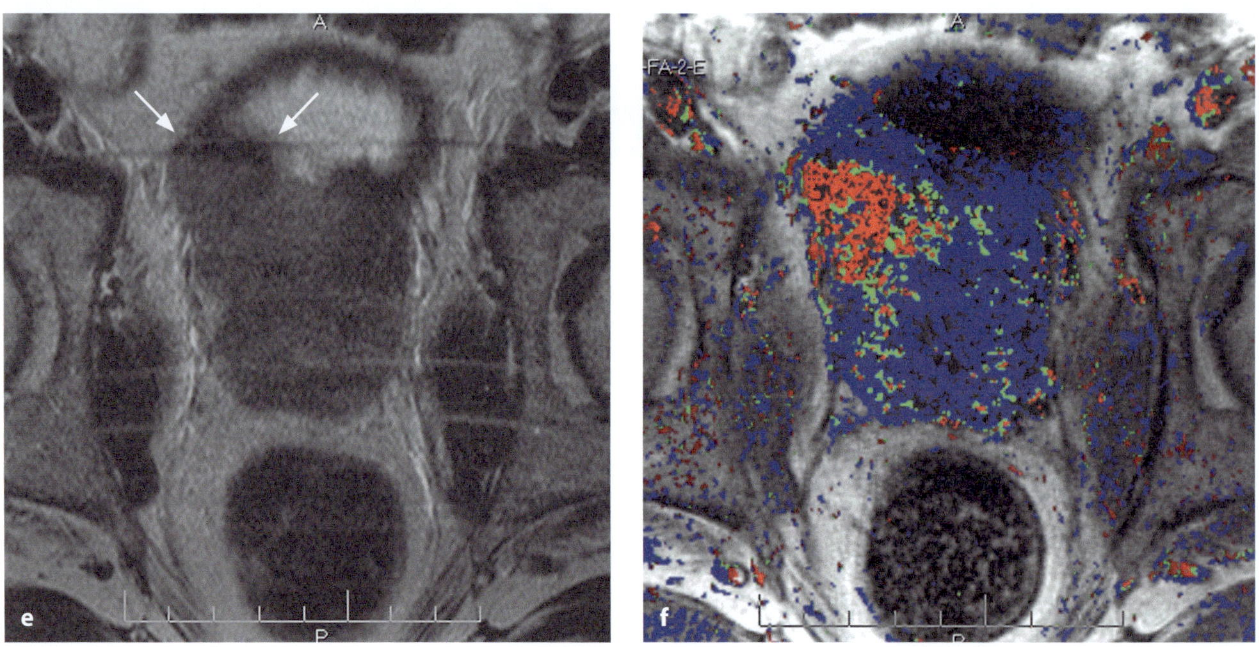

Fig. 9.1 e, f With right bladder invasion and extension through wall

Fig. 9.1 g, h

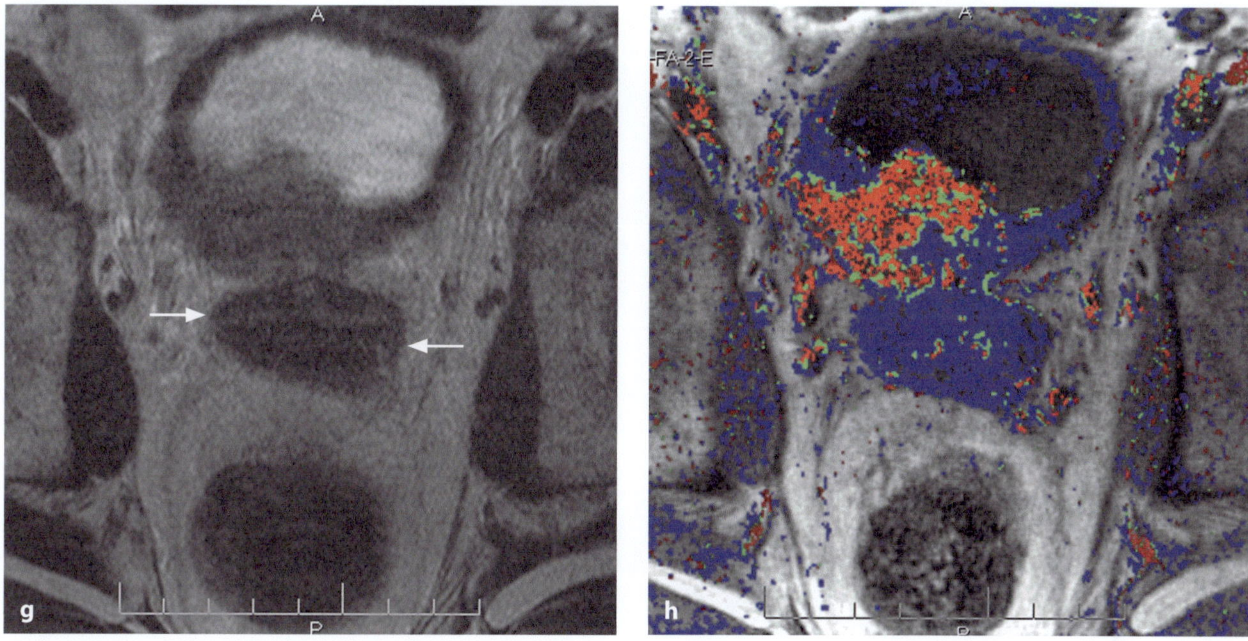

Fig. 9.1 g, h With bilateral seminal vesicle invasion

Fig. 9.1 i, j

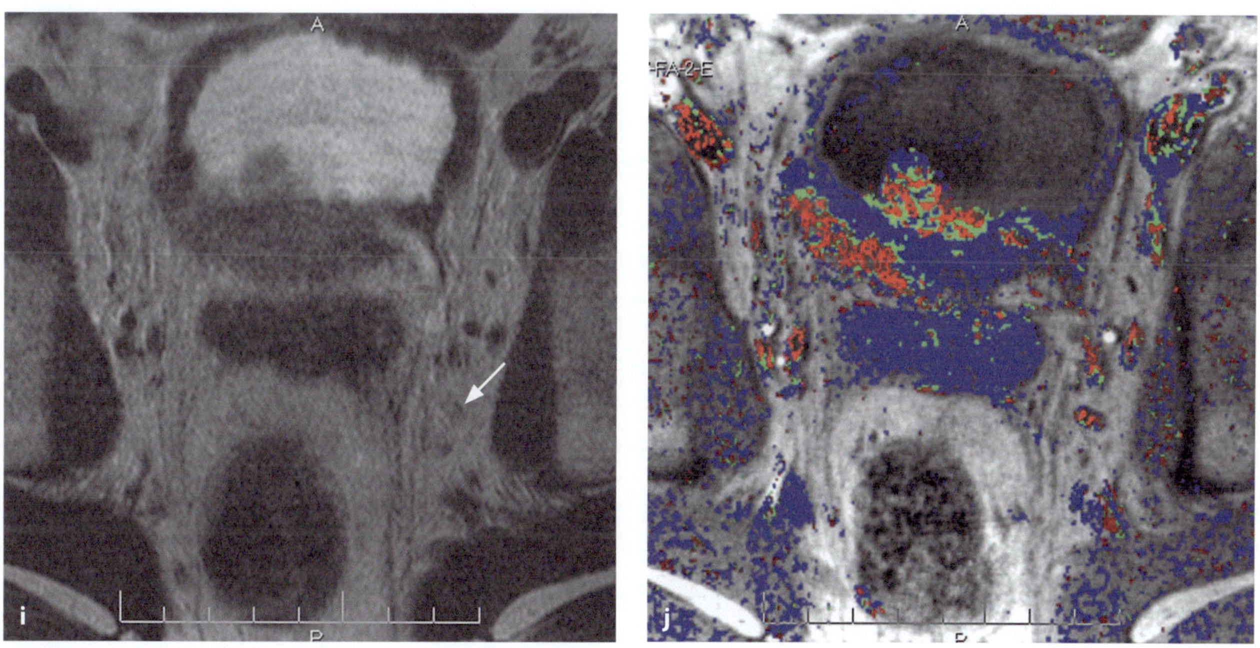

Fig. 9.1 i, j With left obturator node and bladder mass

Fig. 9.2 a–x

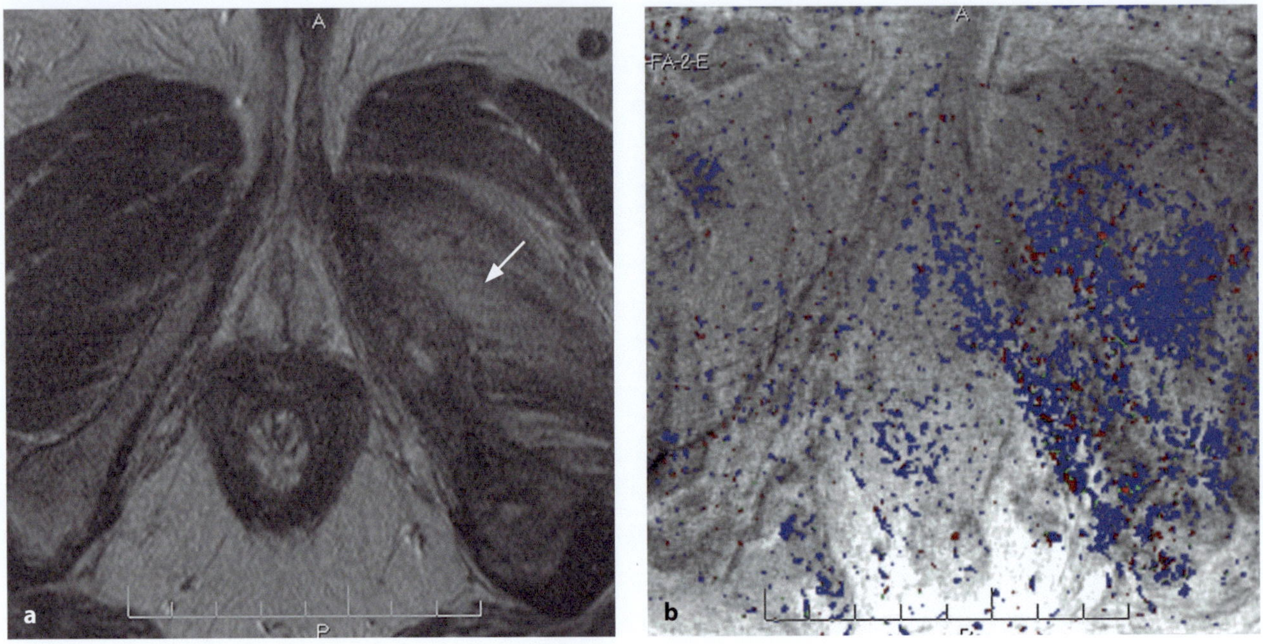

Fig. 9.2 a, b Abnormal signal left levator ani and adductor muscles-low grade prostate and high grade bladder cancers

Fig. 9.2 c, d

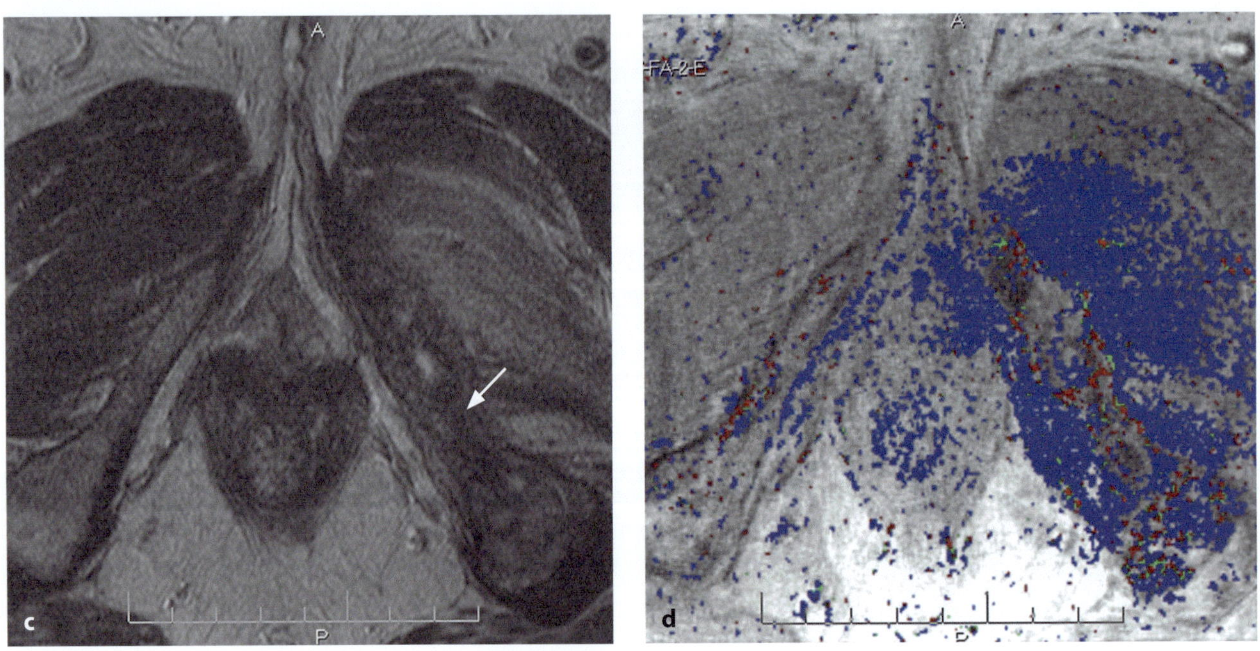

Fig. 9.2 c, d With abnormal left pubic ramus signal extending into muscle

Fig. 9.2 e, f

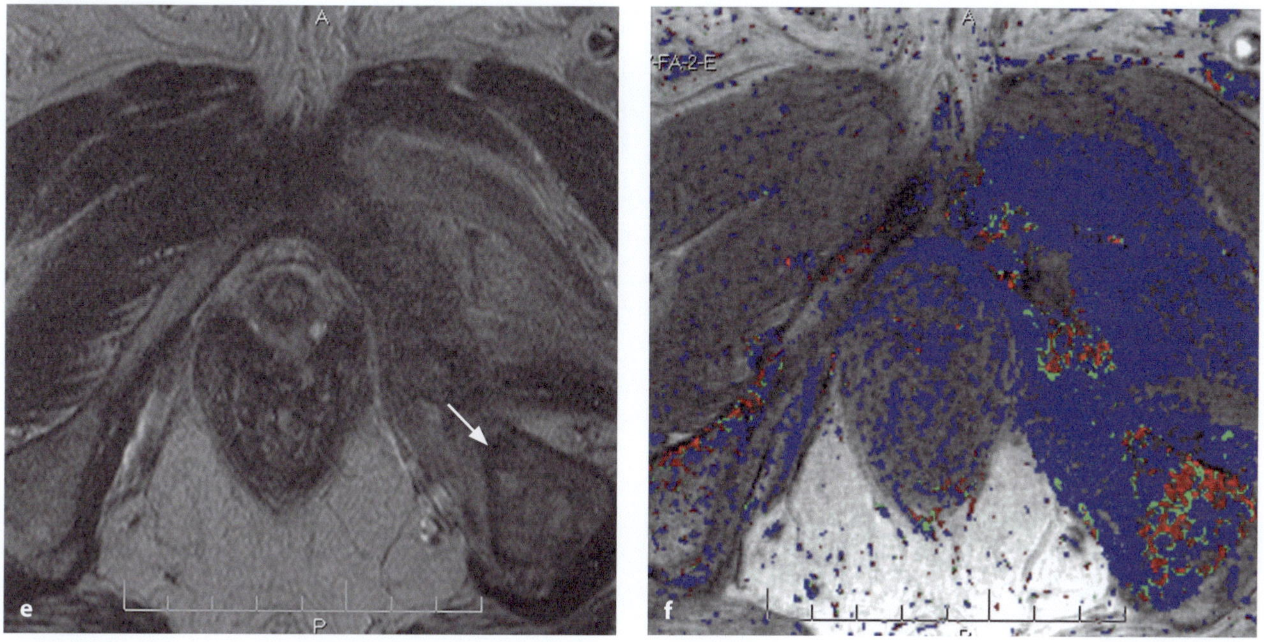

Fig. 9.2 e, f With abnormal left pubis and ischial signal

Fig. 9.2 g, h

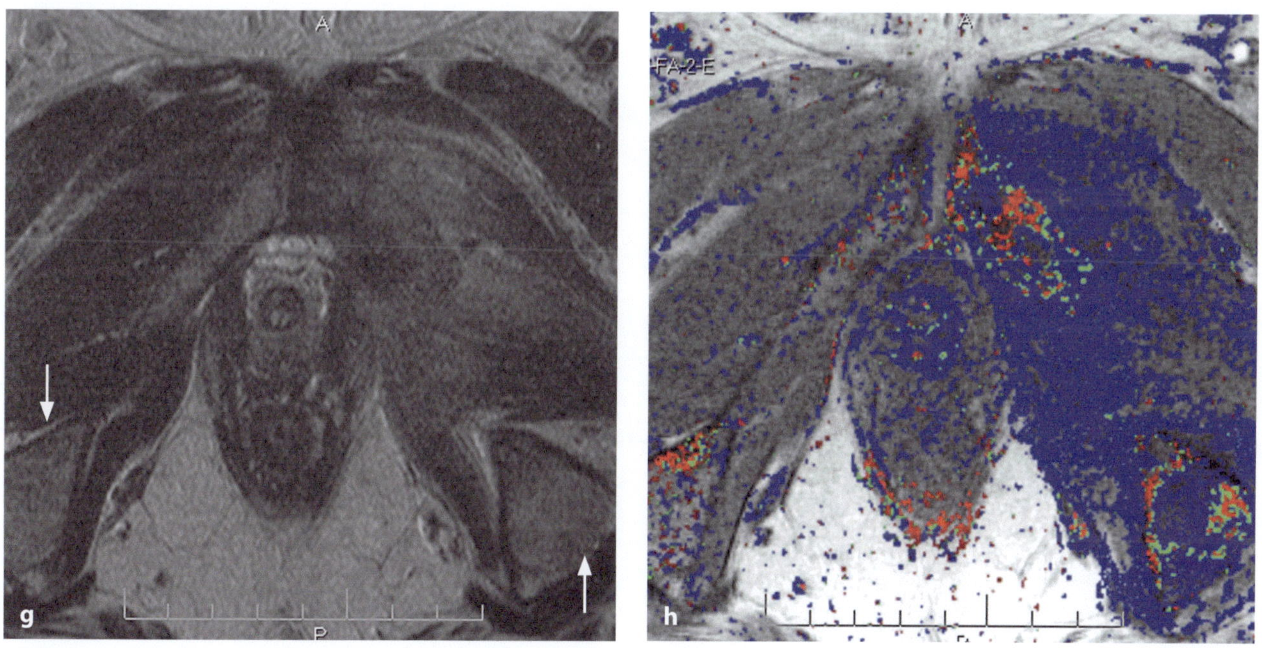

Fig. 9.2 g, h With abnormal right ischial signal

Fig. 9.2 i, j

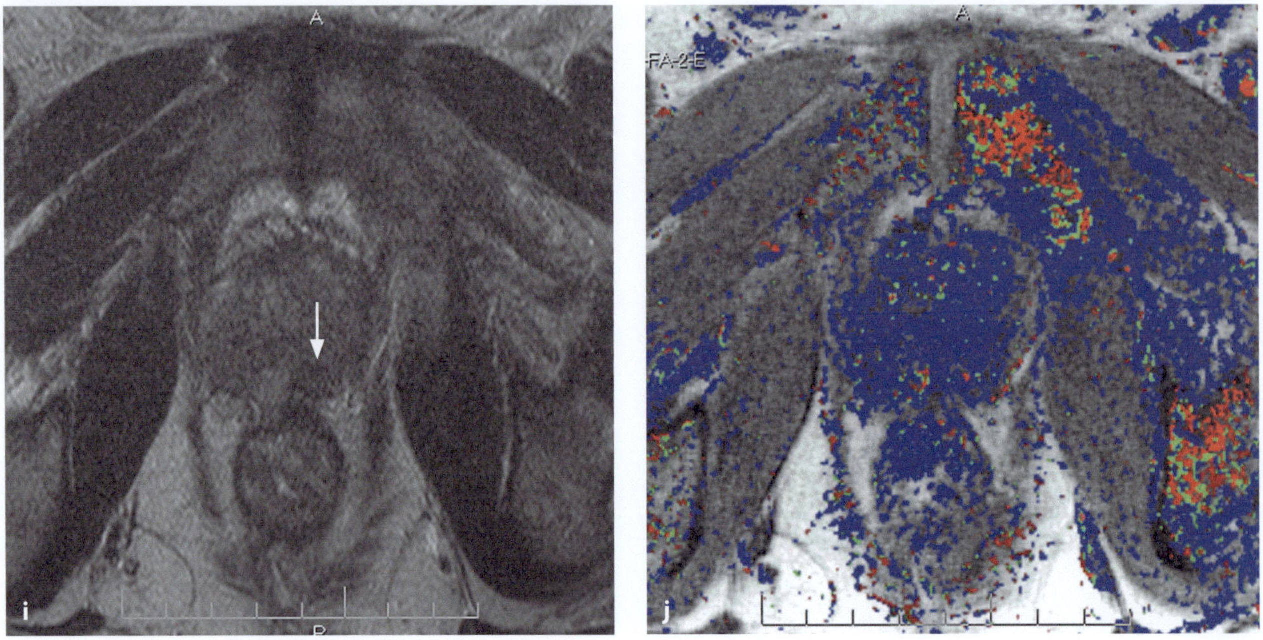

Fig. 9.2 i, j With lesion left posterior prostate gland

Fig. 9.2 k, l

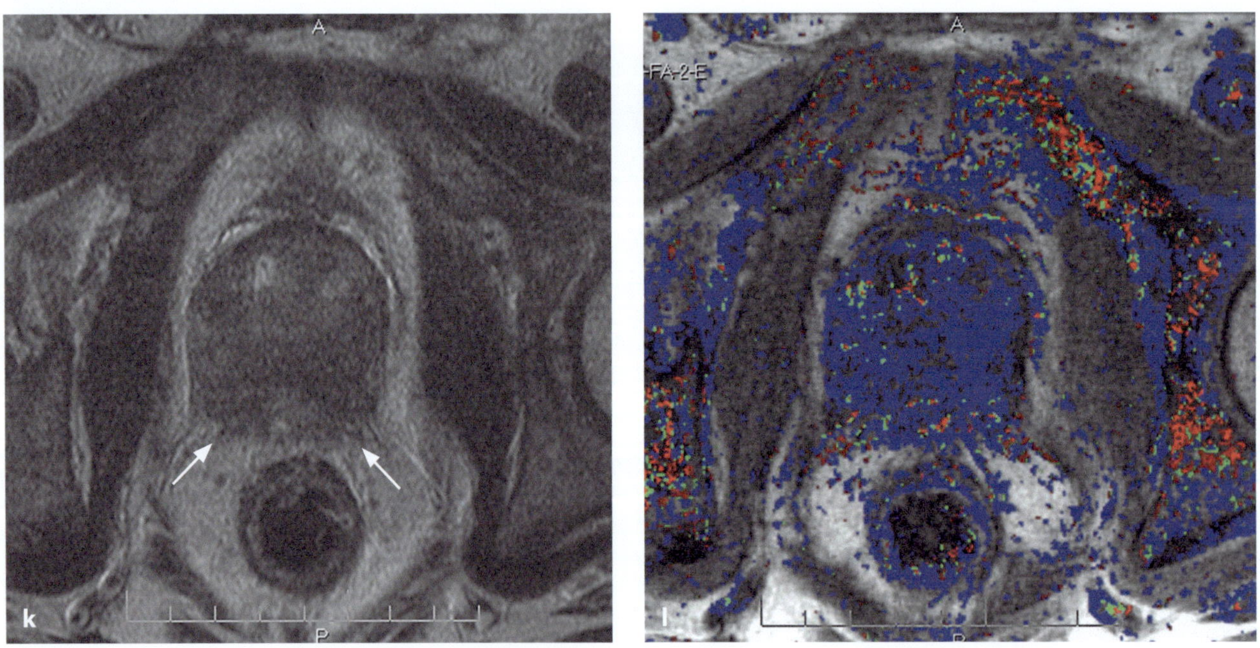

Fig. 9.2 k, l With abnormal right and left seminal vesicles

Fig. 9.2 m, n

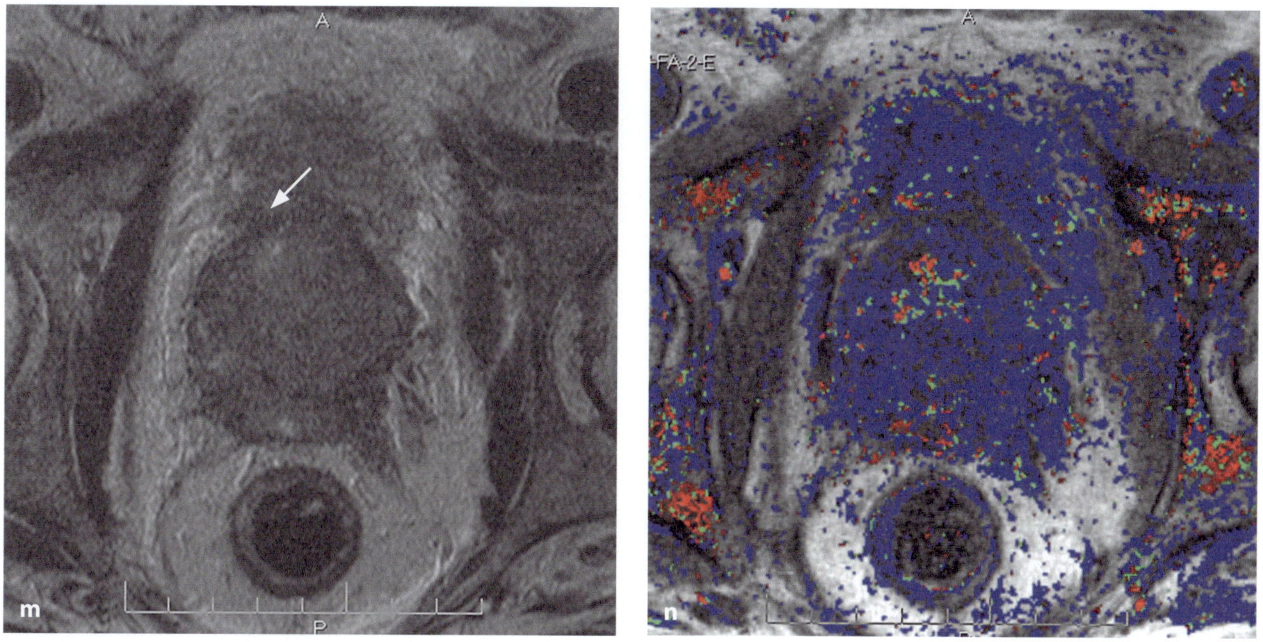

Fig. 9.2 m, n With right bladder wall mass

Fig. 9.2 o, p

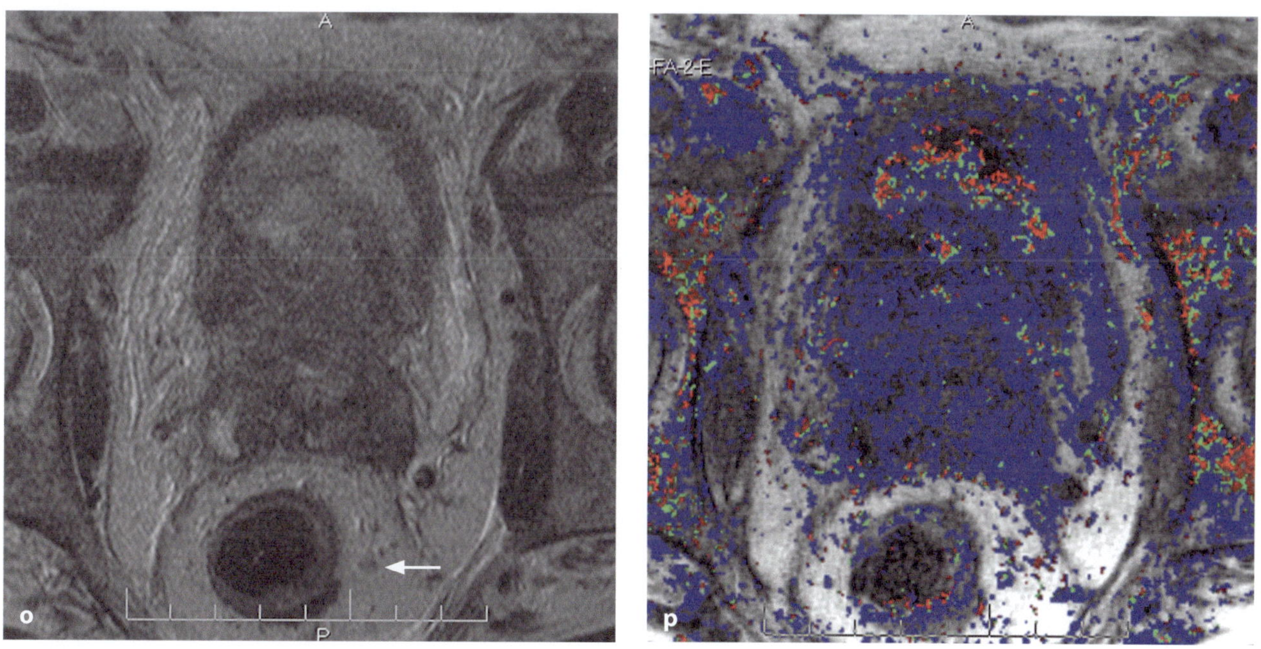

Fig. 9.2 o, p With left perirectal nodes

Fig. 9.2 q, r

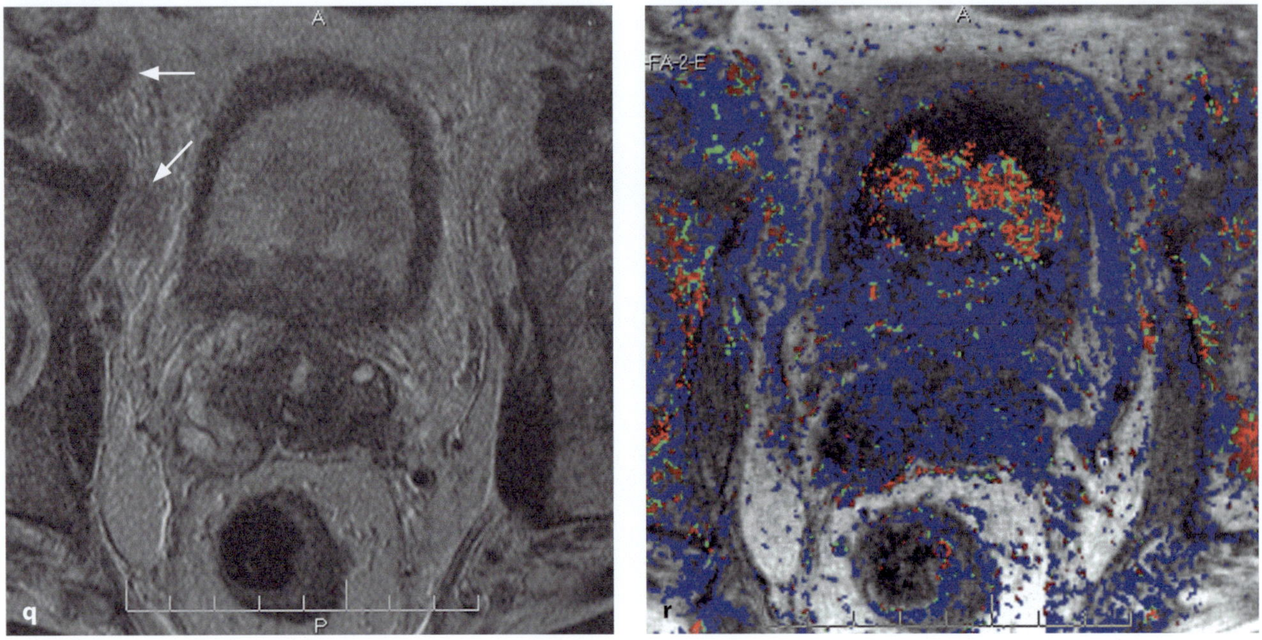

Fig. 9.2 q, r With right obturator nodes

Fig. 9.2 s, t

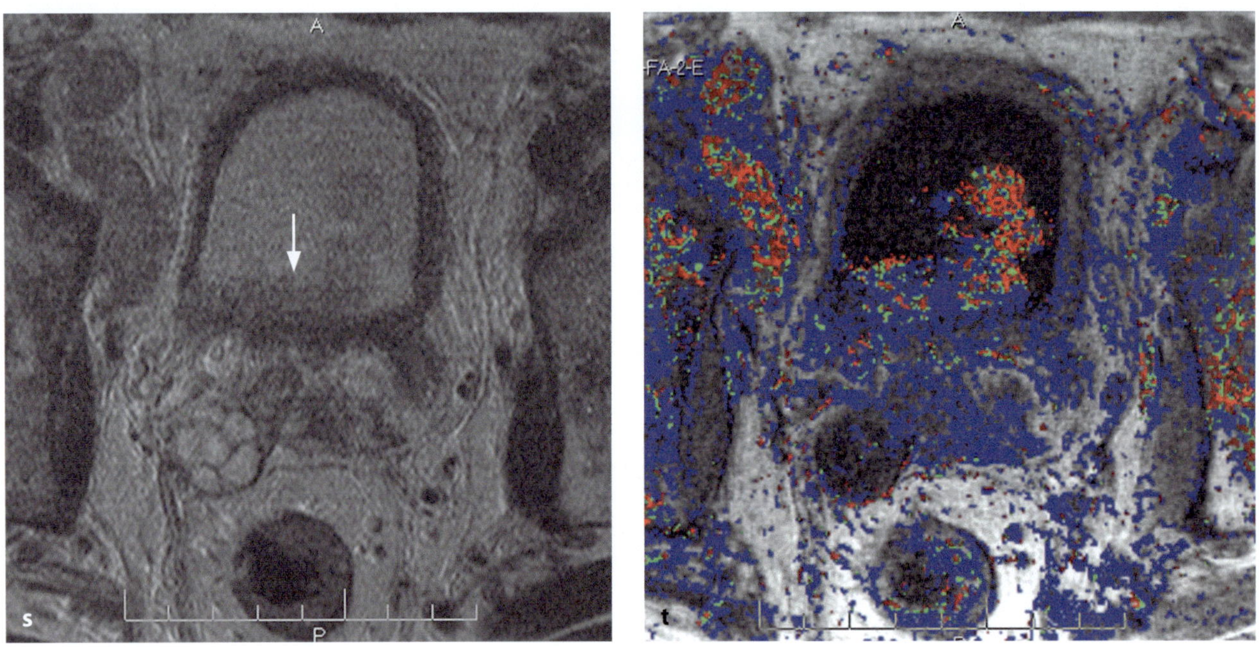

Fig. 9.2 s, t With left bladder base mass

Fig. 9.2 u, v

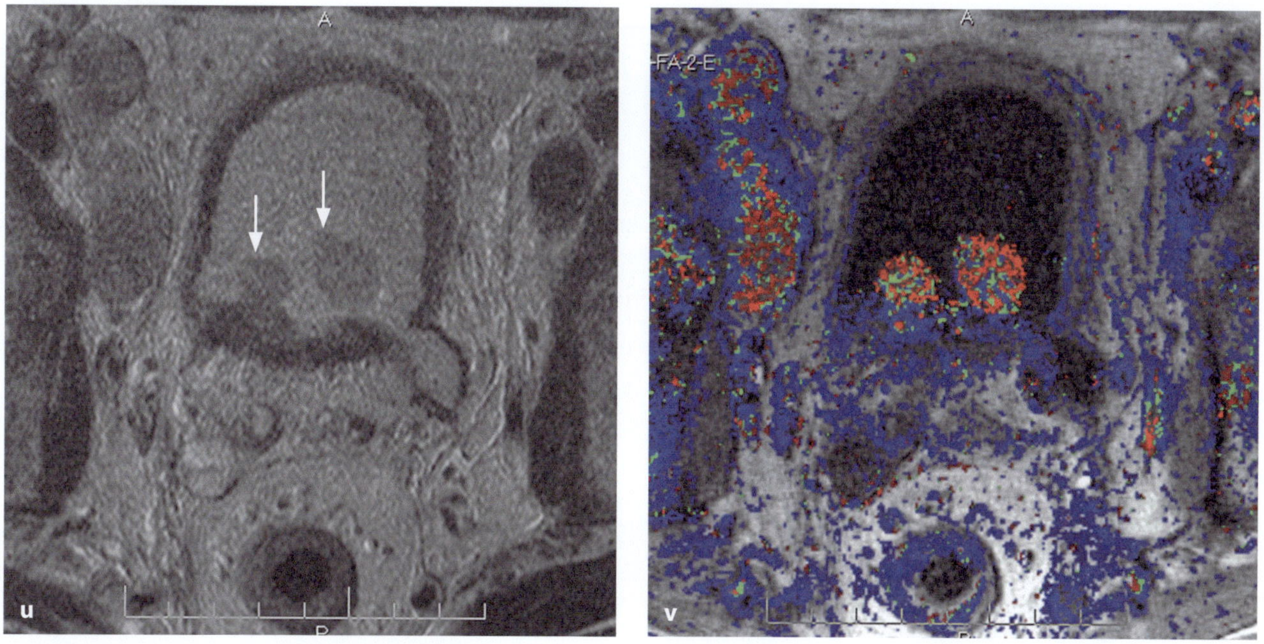

Fig. 9.2 u, v With bilobed mid bladder mass

Fig. 9.2 w, x

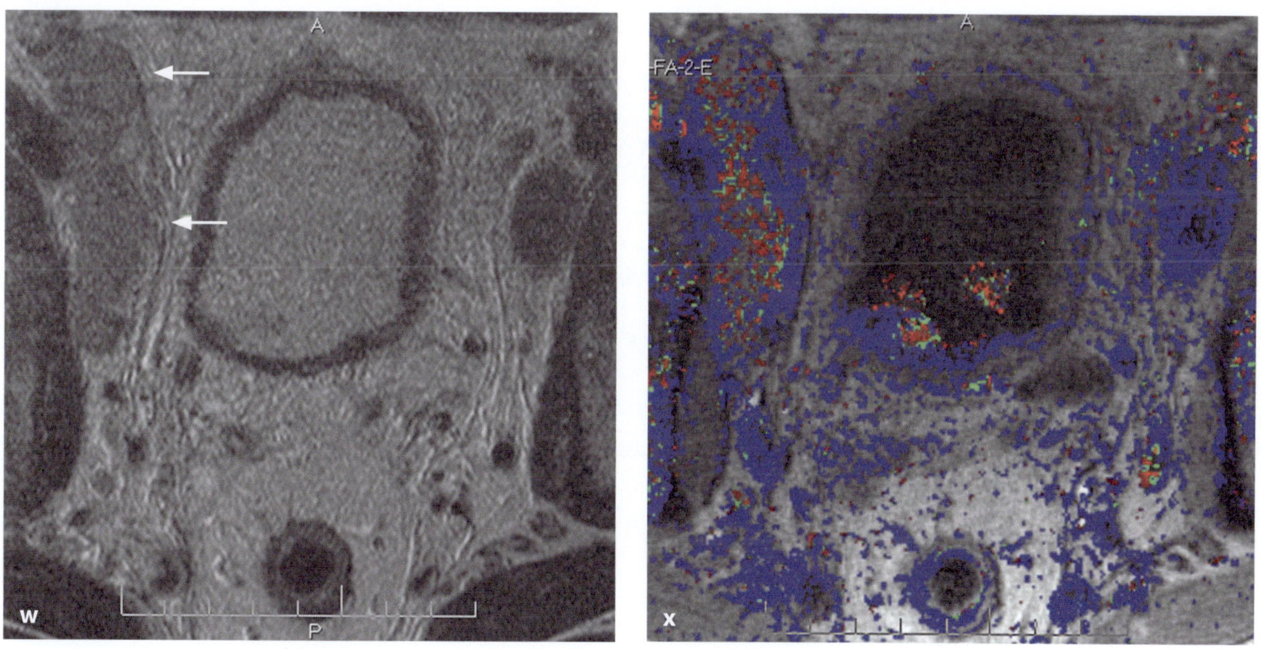

Fig. 9.2 w, x With pelvic sidewall nodes

Fig. 9.3 a–j

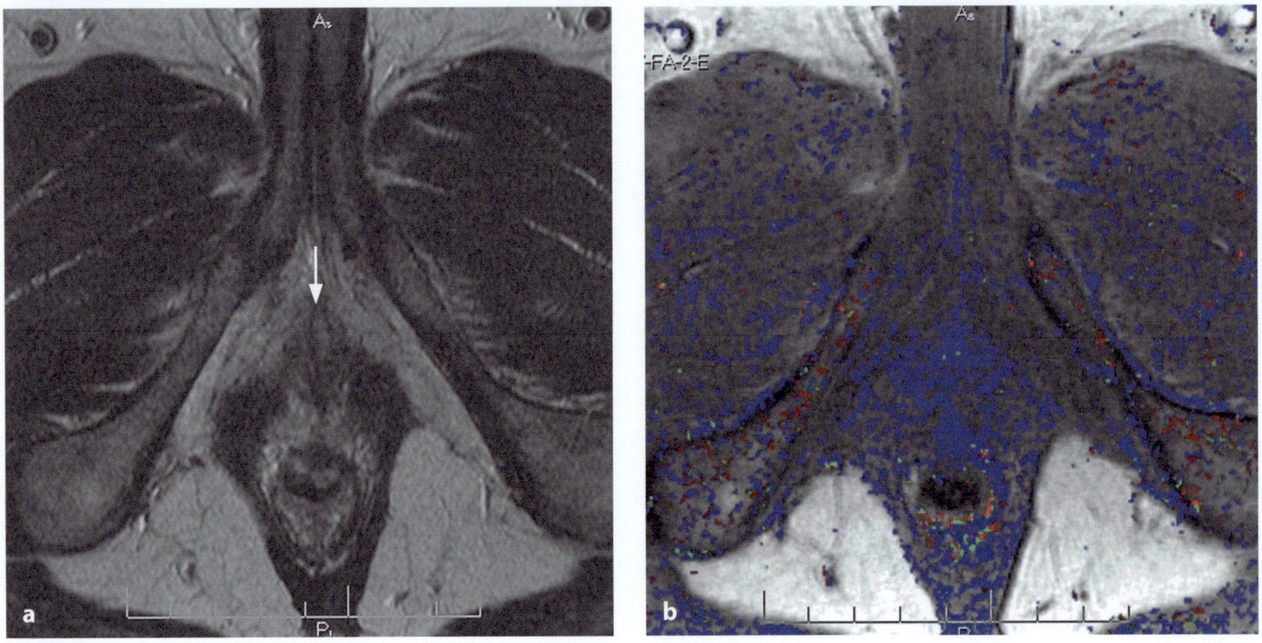

Fig. 9.3 a, b Normal apex

Fig. 9.3 c, d

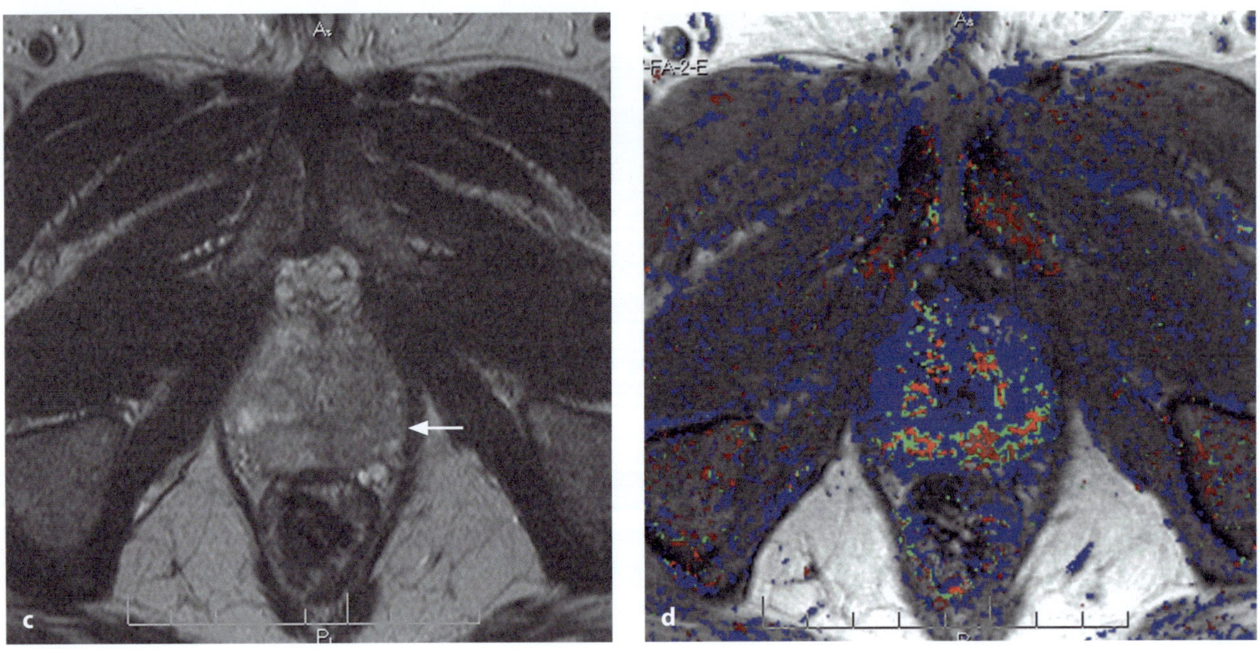

Fig. 9.3 c, d Left midgland Gleason 3

Fig. 9.3 e, f

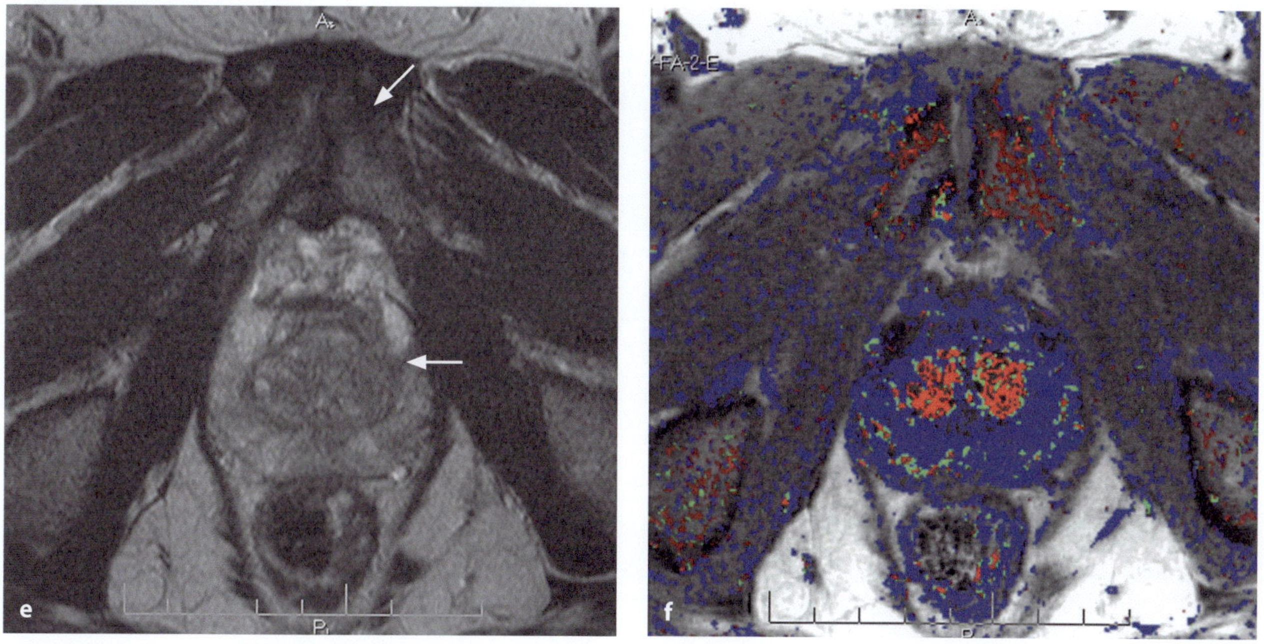

Fig. 9.3 e, f With central Gleason 4 and pubic bone mets

Fig. 9.3 g, h

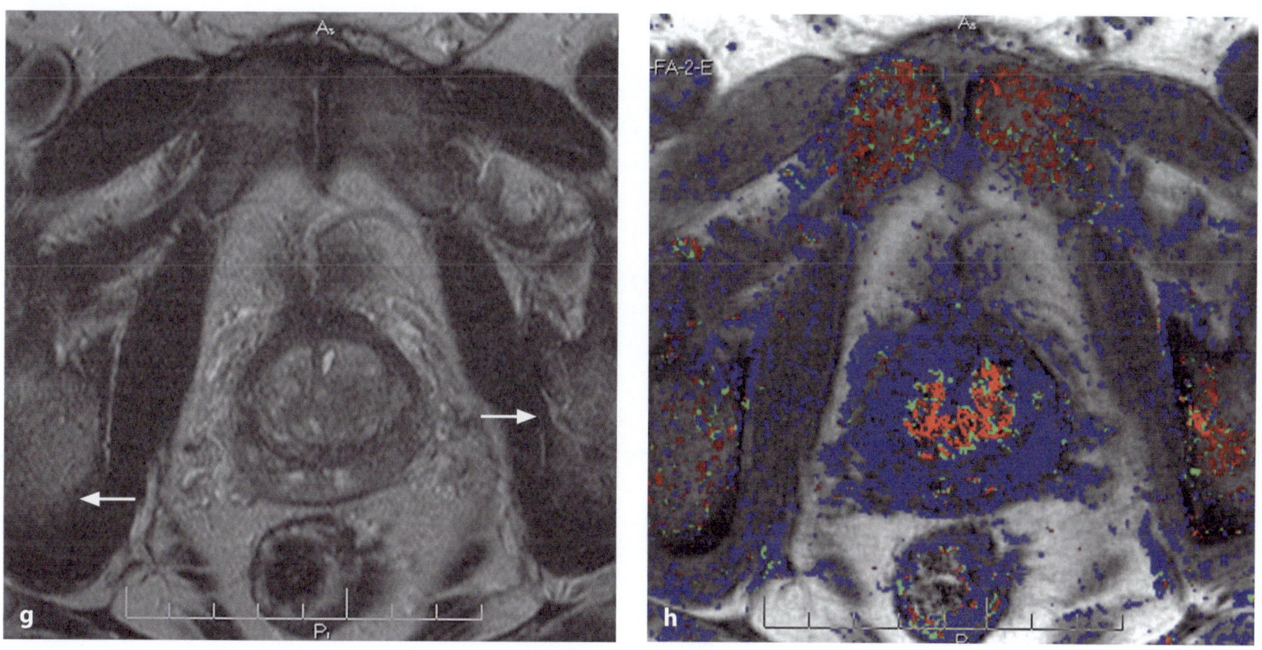

Fig. 9.3 g, h With bilateral acetabular and pubic symphysis metastases

Fig. 9.3 i, j

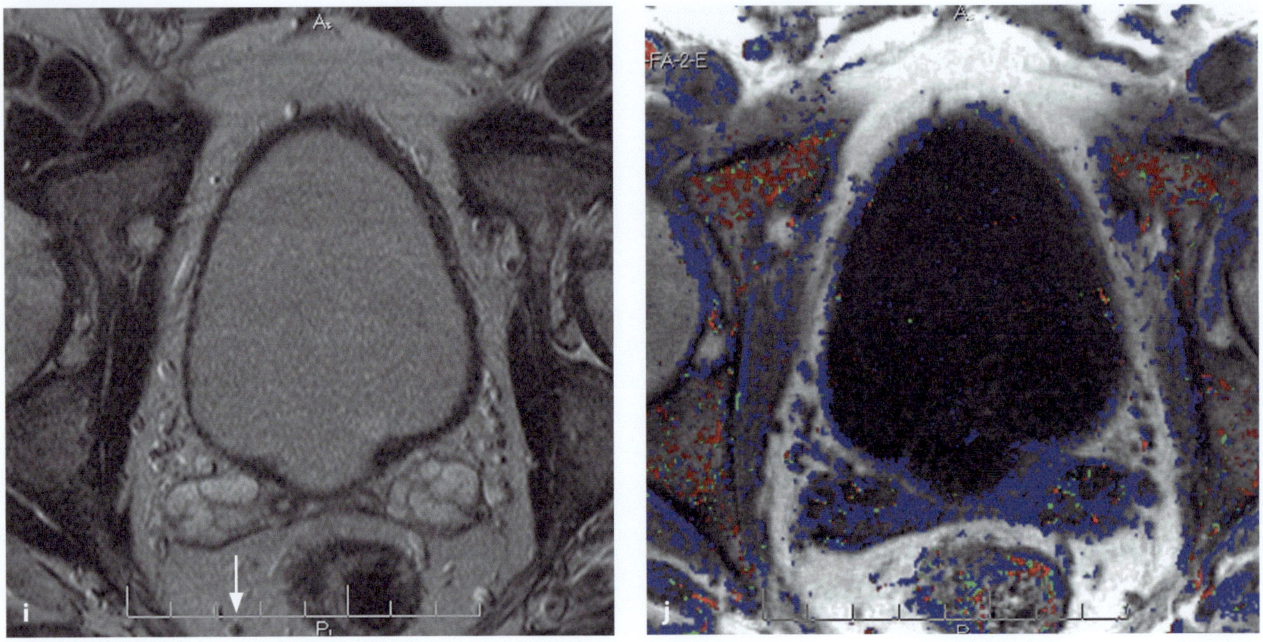

Fig. 9.3 i, j With right perirectal node and normal seminal vesicles

Fig. 9.4 a–h

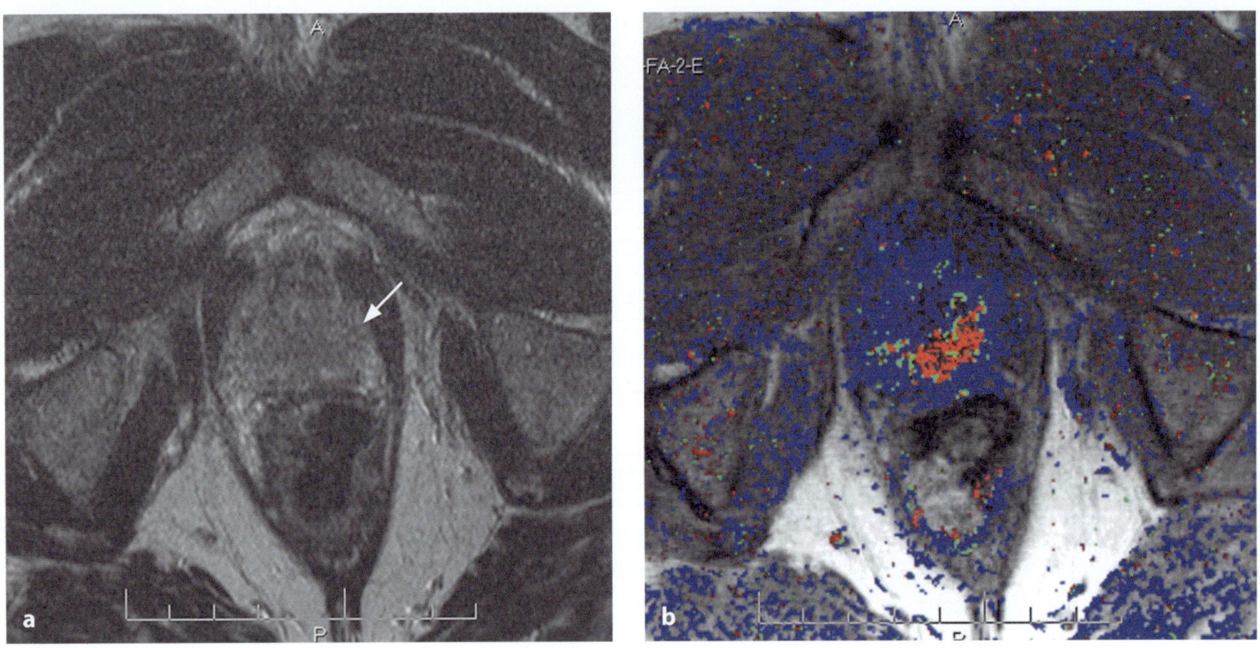

Fig. 9.4 a, b Apical focal left Gleason 4

Fig. 9.4 c, d

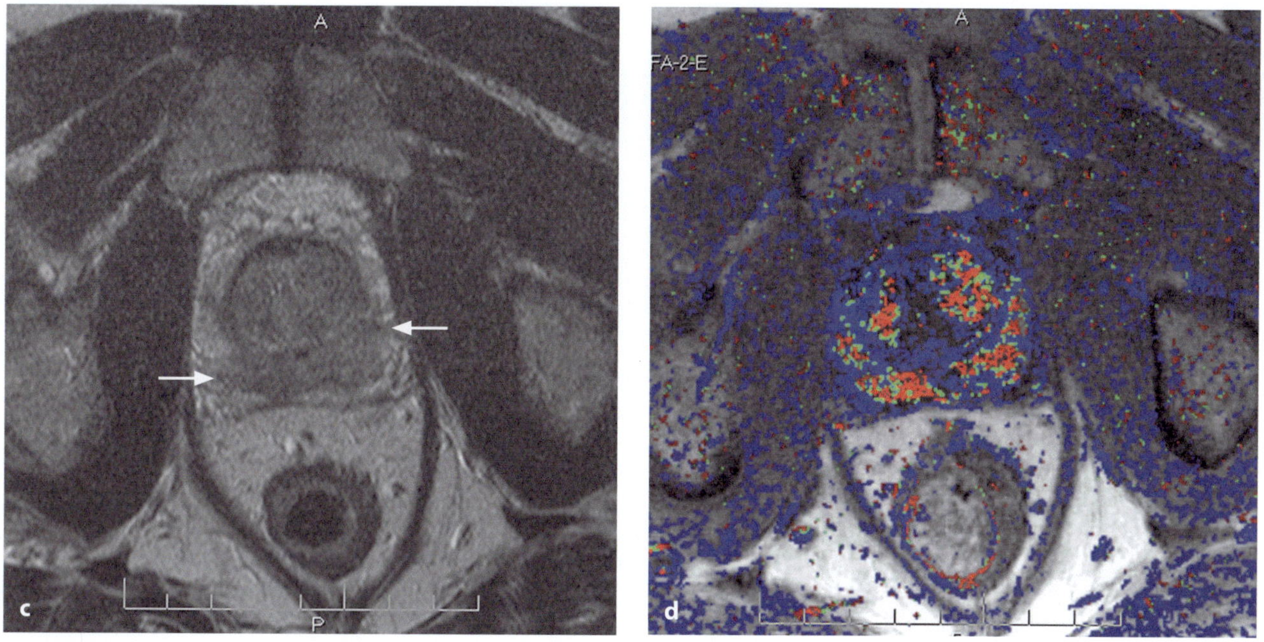

Fig. 9.4 c, d With extension into right and left midgland

Fig. 9.4 e, f

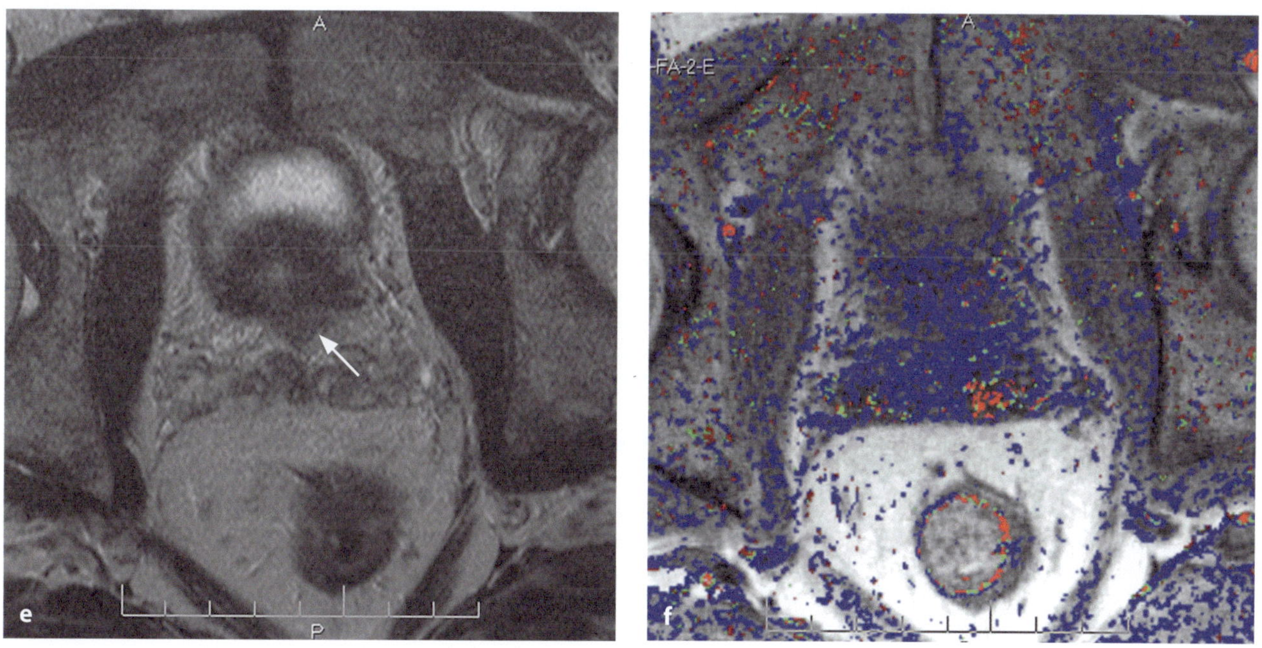

Fig. 9.4 e, f With extension into left posterior base

Fig. 9.4 g, h

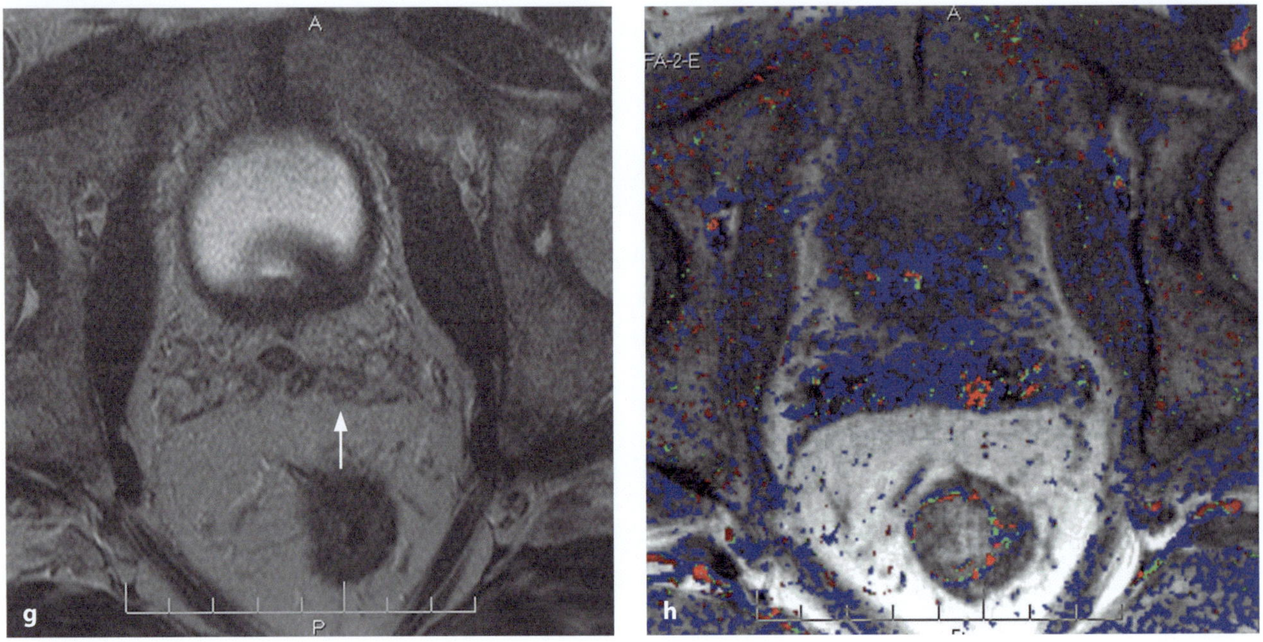

Fig. 9.4 g, h With invasion into left seminal vesicle

Fig. 9.5 a–d

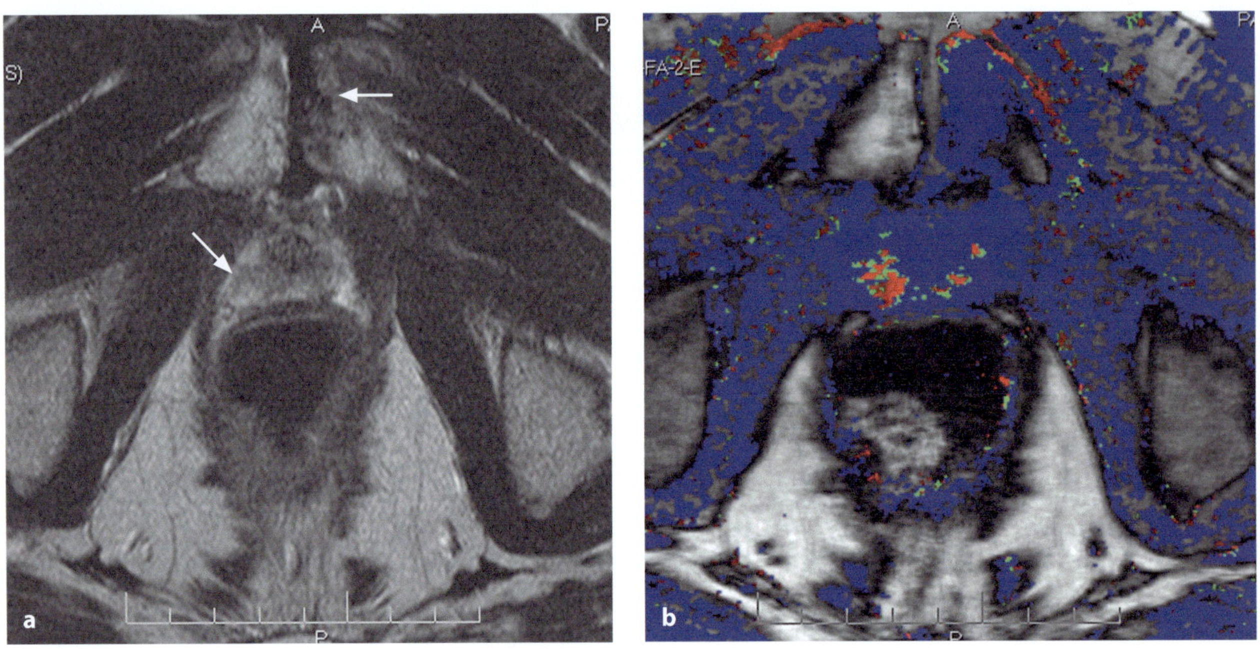

Fig. 9.5 a, b Right apical Gleason 4 (note left osteitis pubis)

Fig. 9.5 c, d

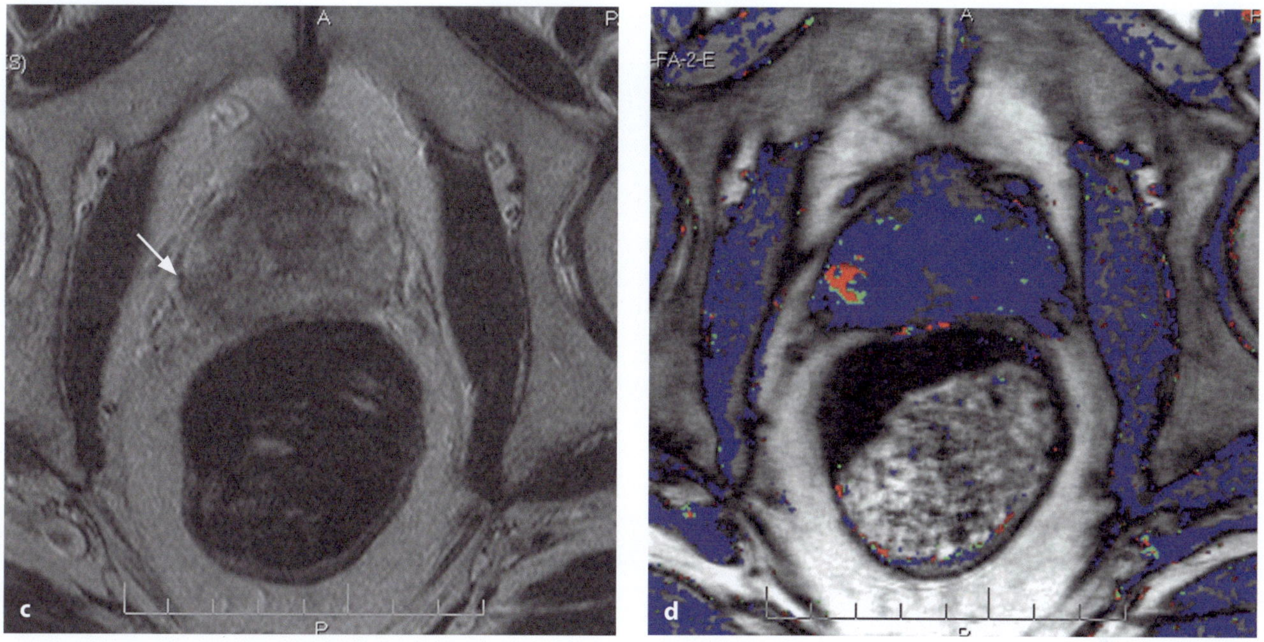

Fig. 9.5 c, d Right lateral midgland Gleason 3

Fig. 9.6 a–s

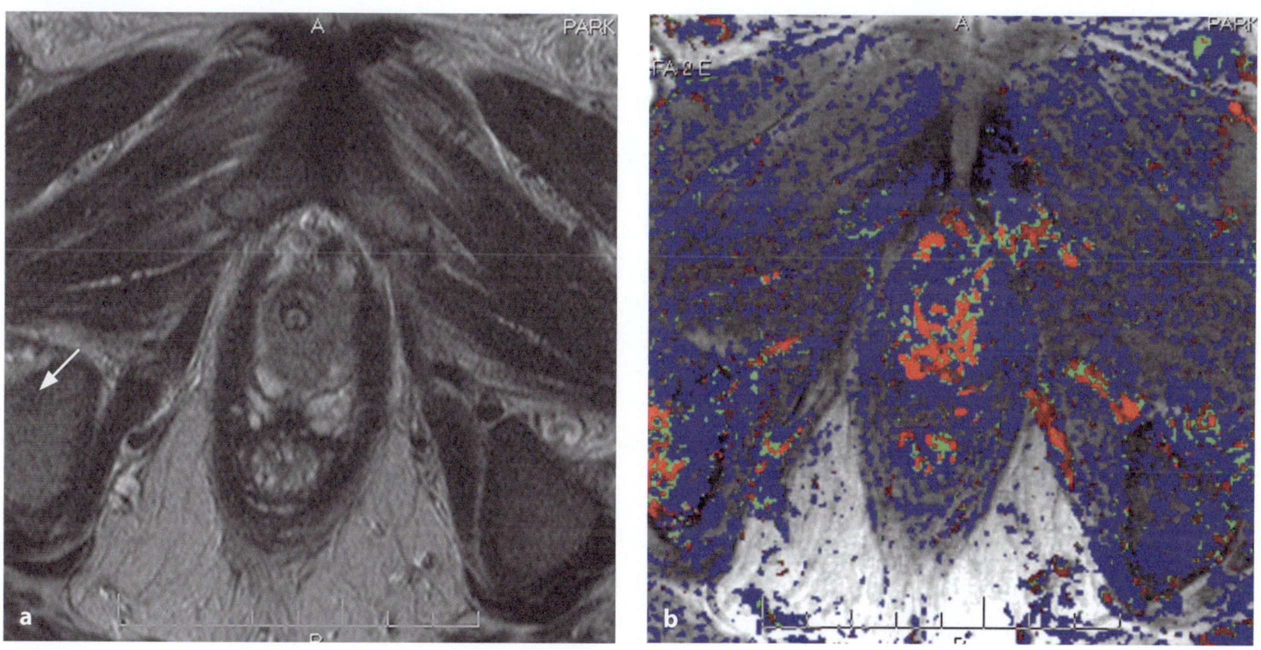

Fig. 9.6 a, b Apical Gleason 5 with right ischial tuberosity metastases (presenting symptom left leg edema/psa=291 ng/ml)

Fig. 9.6 c, d

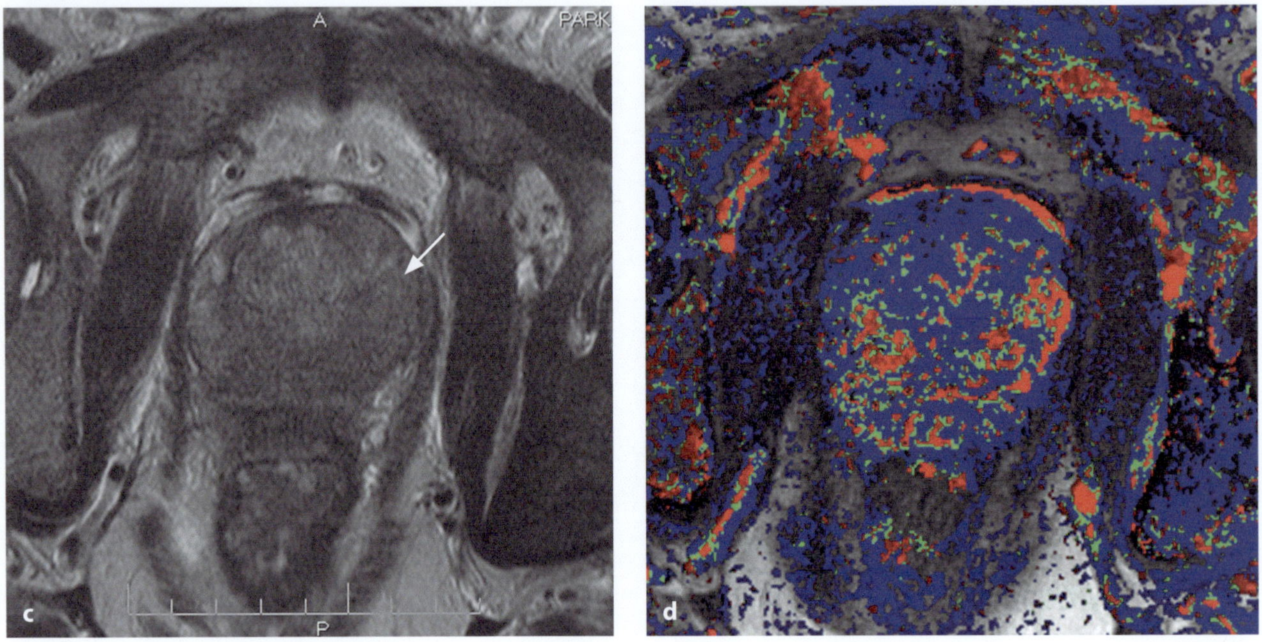

Fig. 9.6 c, d With midgland extension

Fig. 9.6 e, f

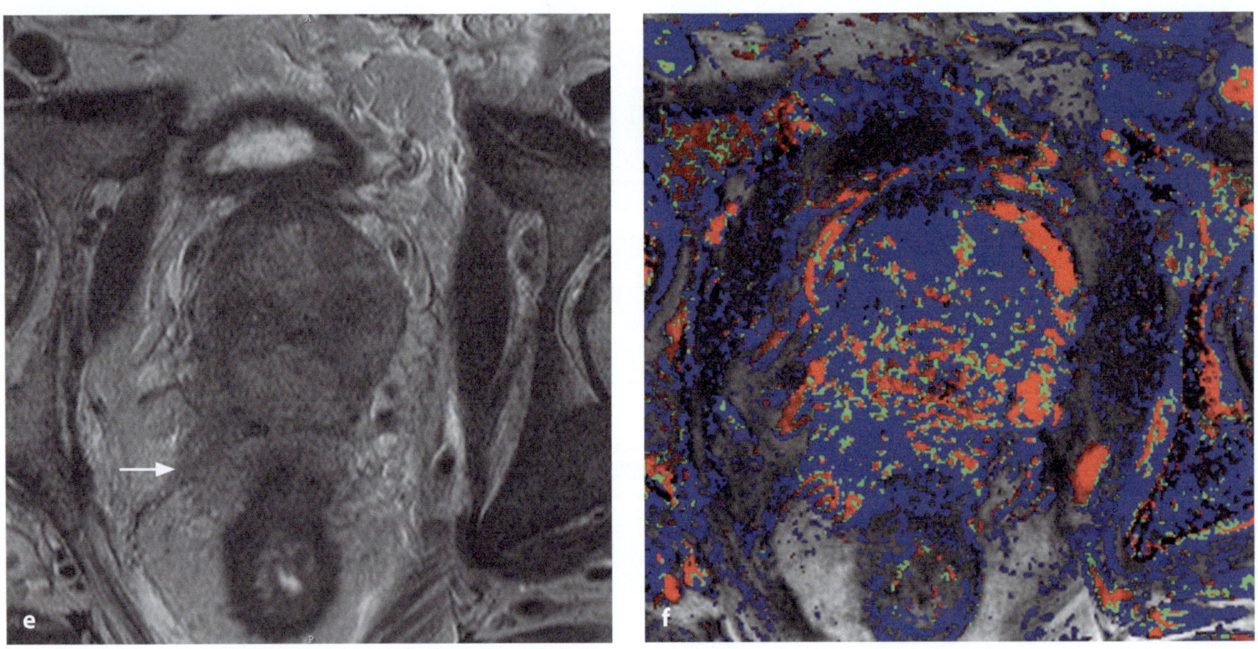

Fig. 9.6 e, f With right extracapsular extension

Fig. 9.6 g, h

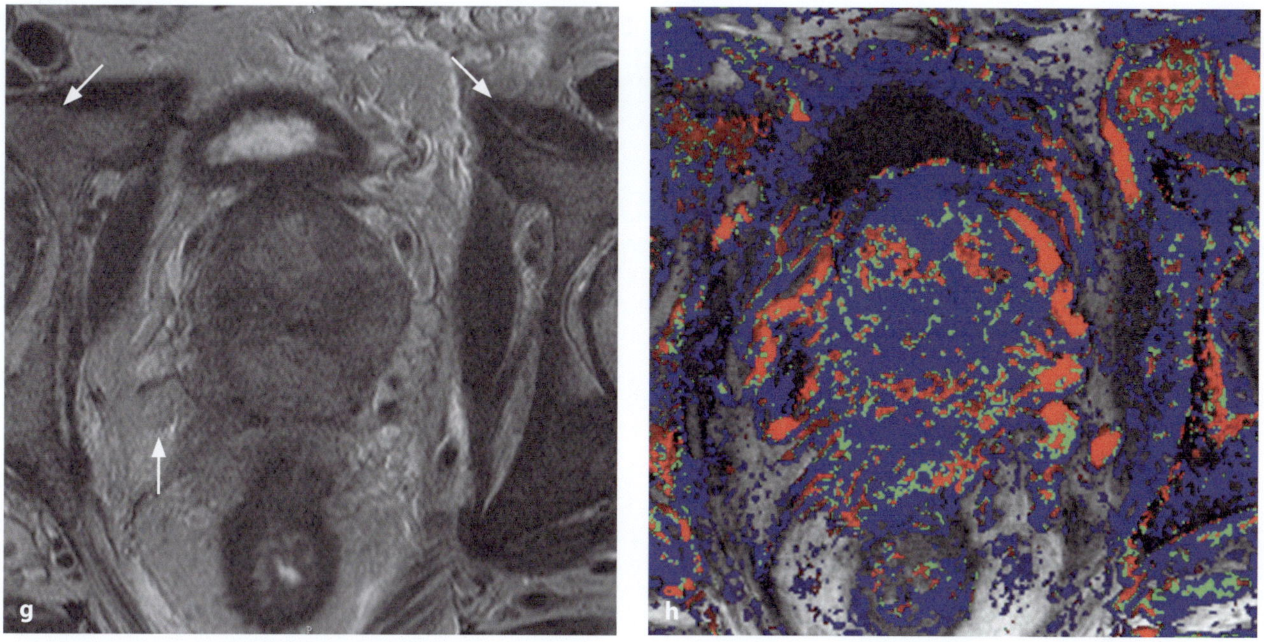

Fig. 9.6 g, h With boney mets and obturator adenopathy

Fig. 9.6 i, j

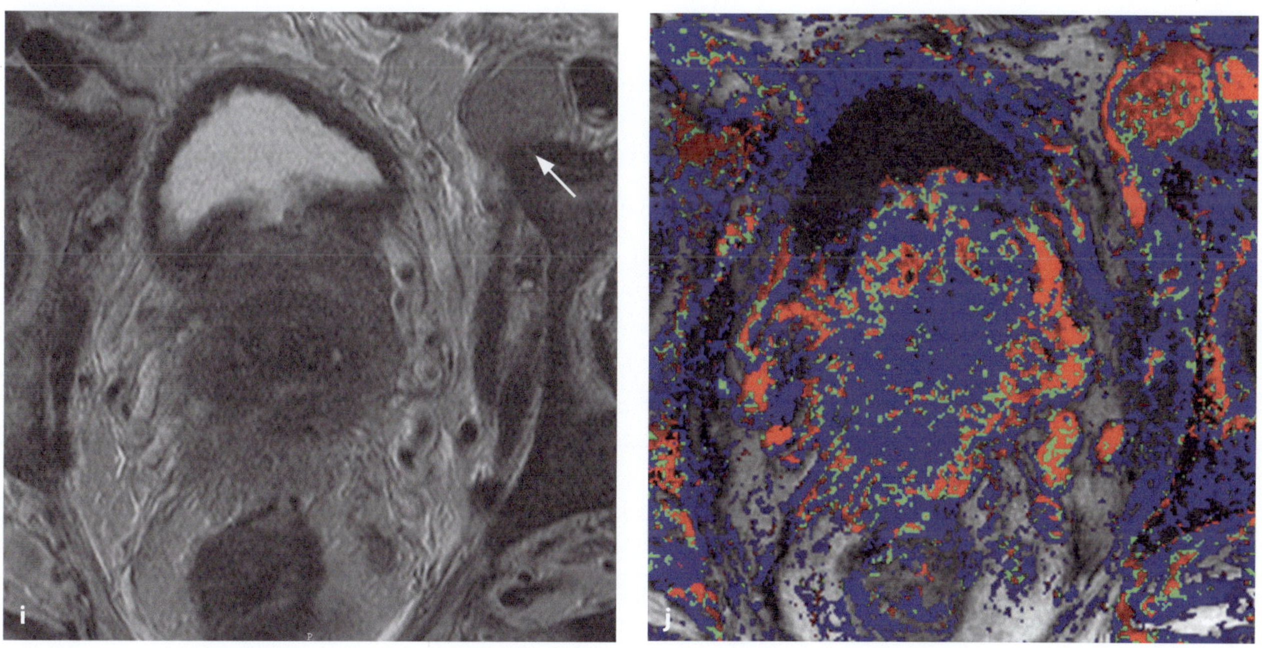

Fig. 9.6 i, j With left perirectal and pelvic side wall adenopathy

Fig. 9.6 k, l

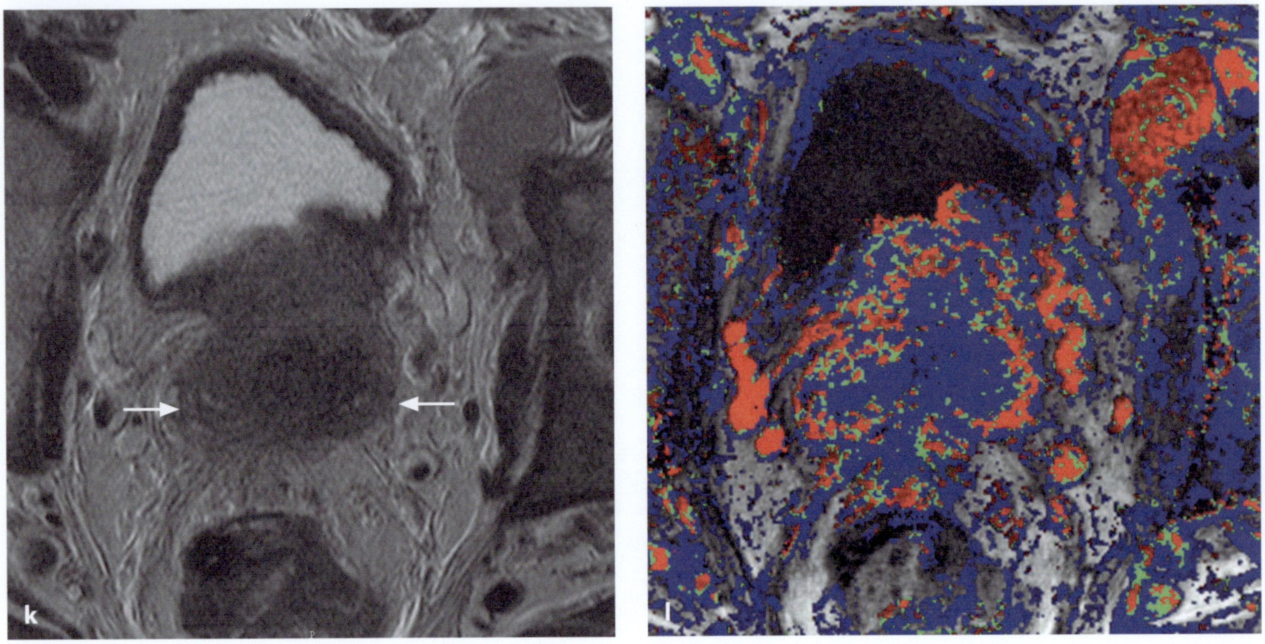

Fig. 9.6 k, l With seminal vesicle and bladder invasion

Fig. 9.6 m, n

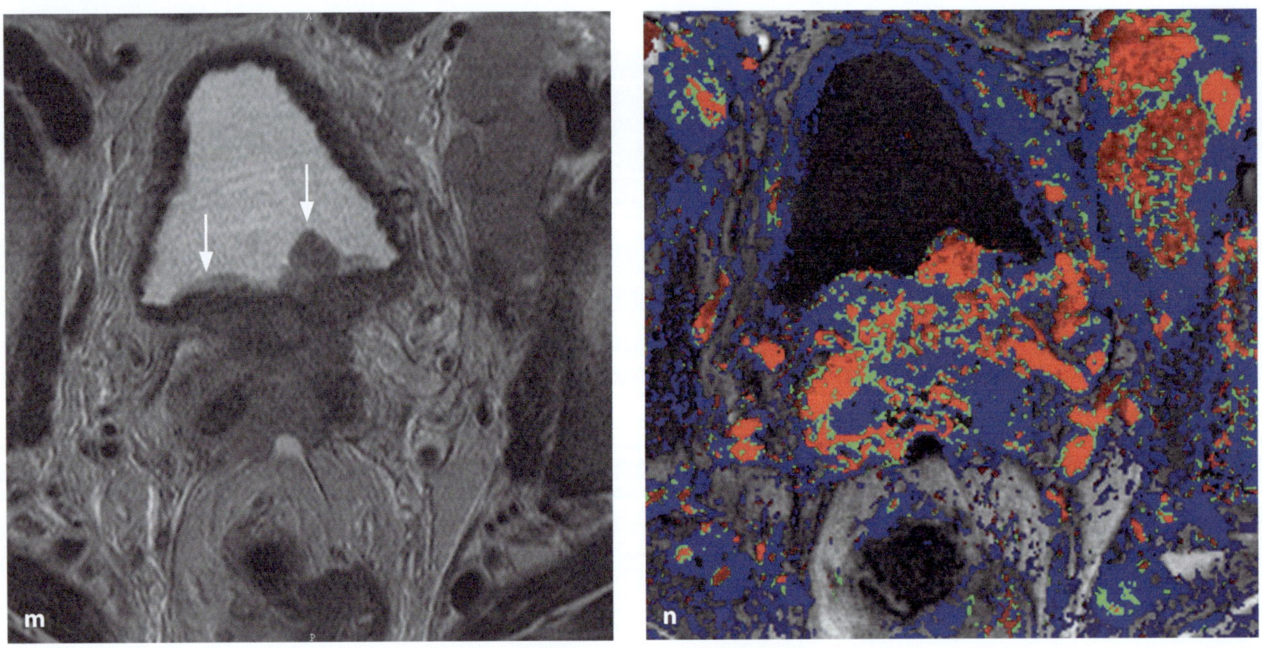

Fig. 9.6 m, n With small right/large left bladder base primary transitional cell carcinomas

Fig. 9.6 o, p

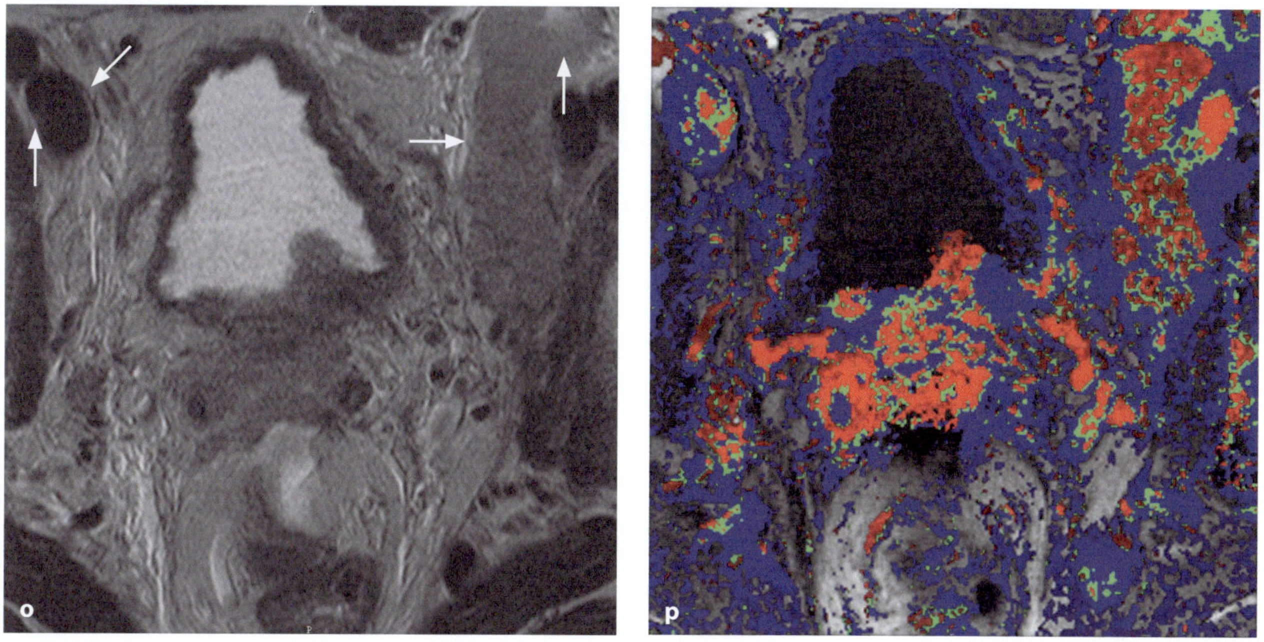

Fig. 9.6 o, p With massive external iliac adenopathy

Fig. 9.6 q, r

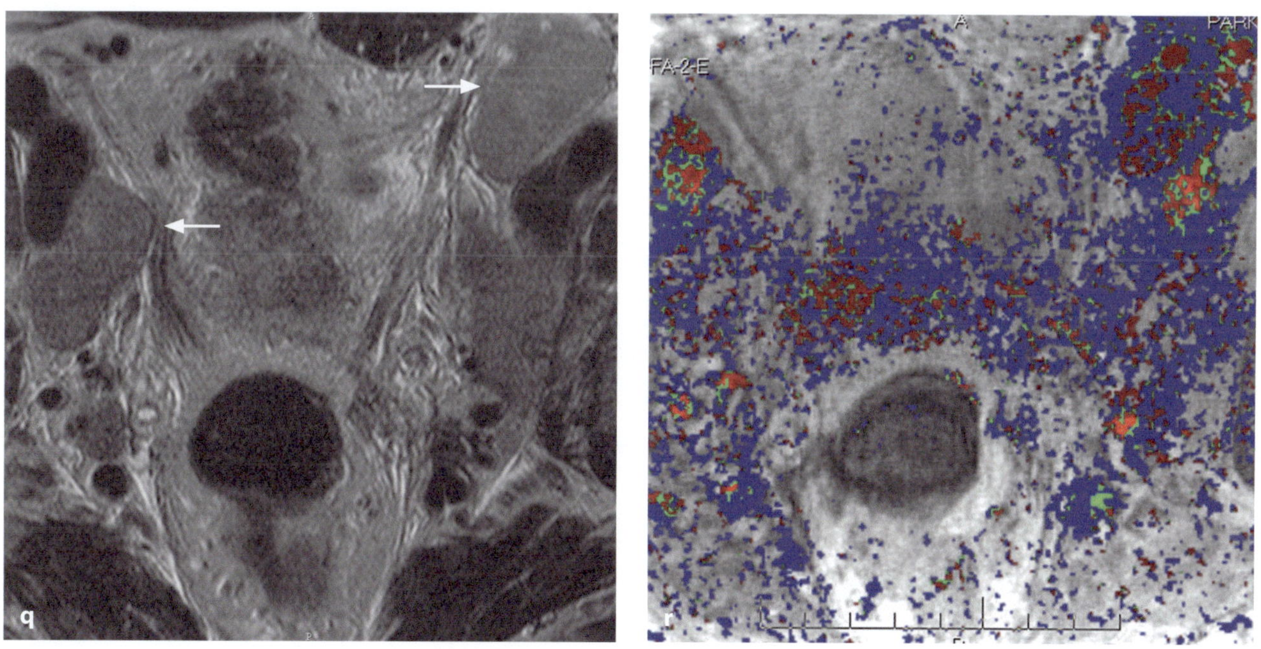

Fig. 9.6 q, r With bilateral external iliac adenopathy

Fig. 9.6 s

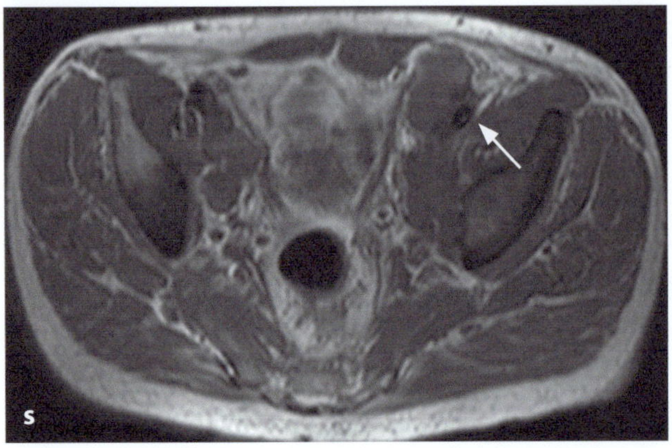

Fig. 9.6 s Left lymphedema due to metastatic transitional cell tumor with massive inguinal/femoral adenopathy (largest node 48mm) (image is T1 weighted large field of view of pelvis to show overview of extensive adenopathy)

Fig. 9.7 a–l

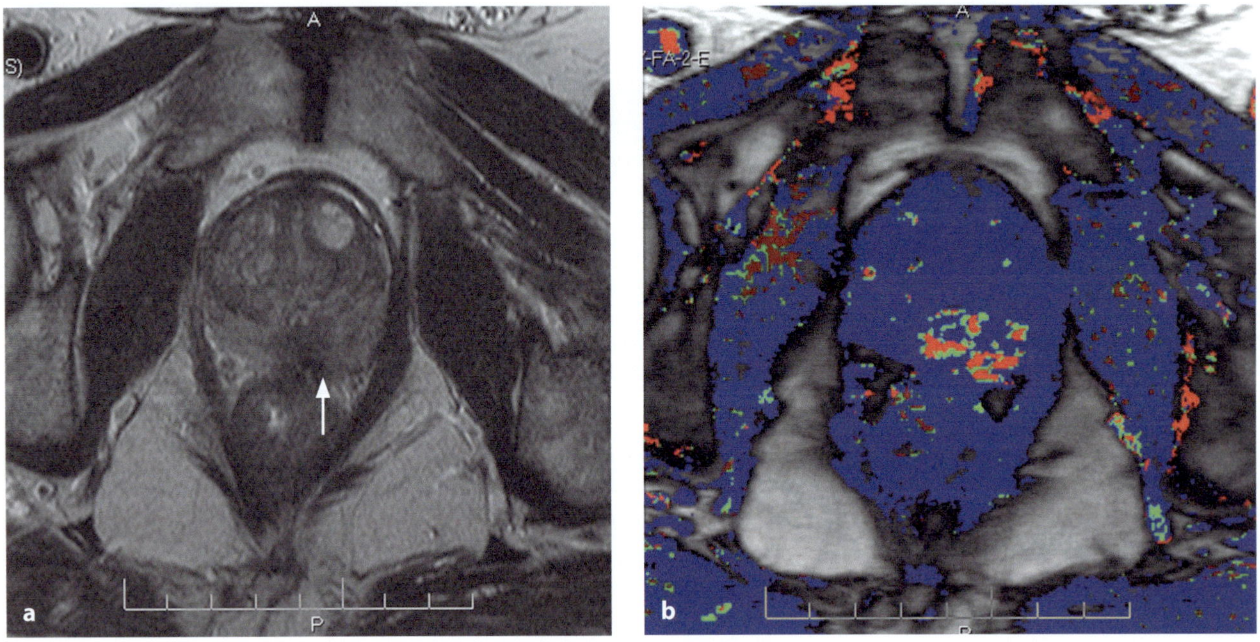

Fig. 9.7 a, b Midgland Gleason 5 with posterior extracapsular extension

Fig. 9.7 c, d

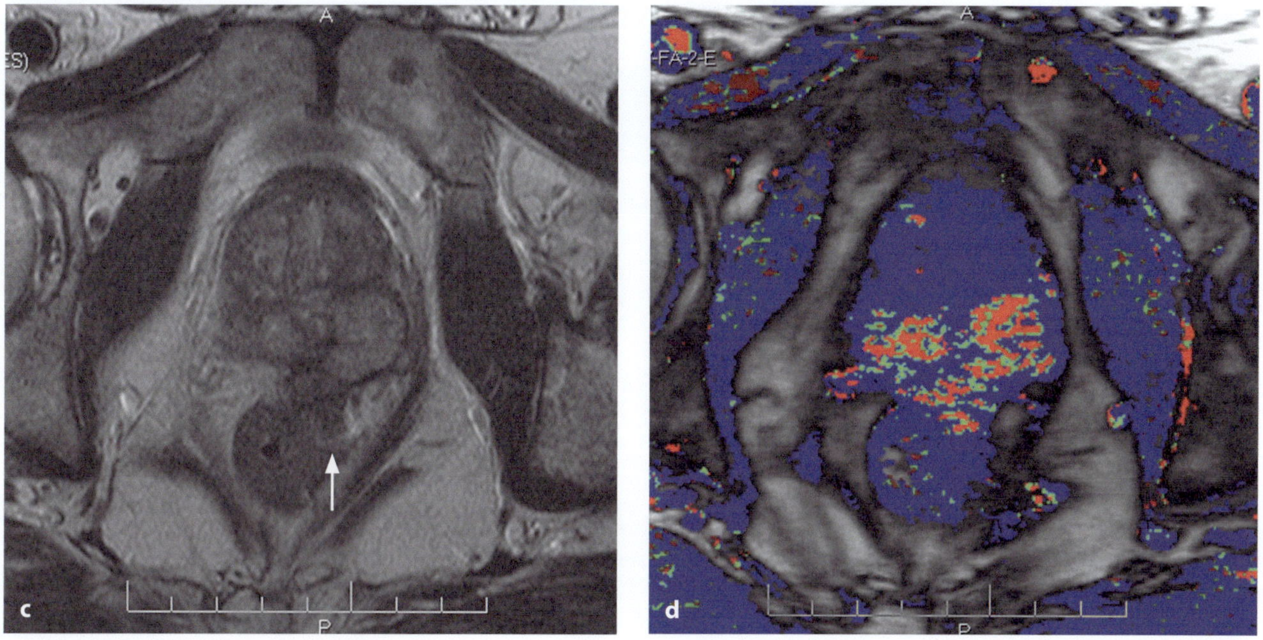

Fig. 9.7 c, d With invasion into rectum

Fig. 9.7 e, f

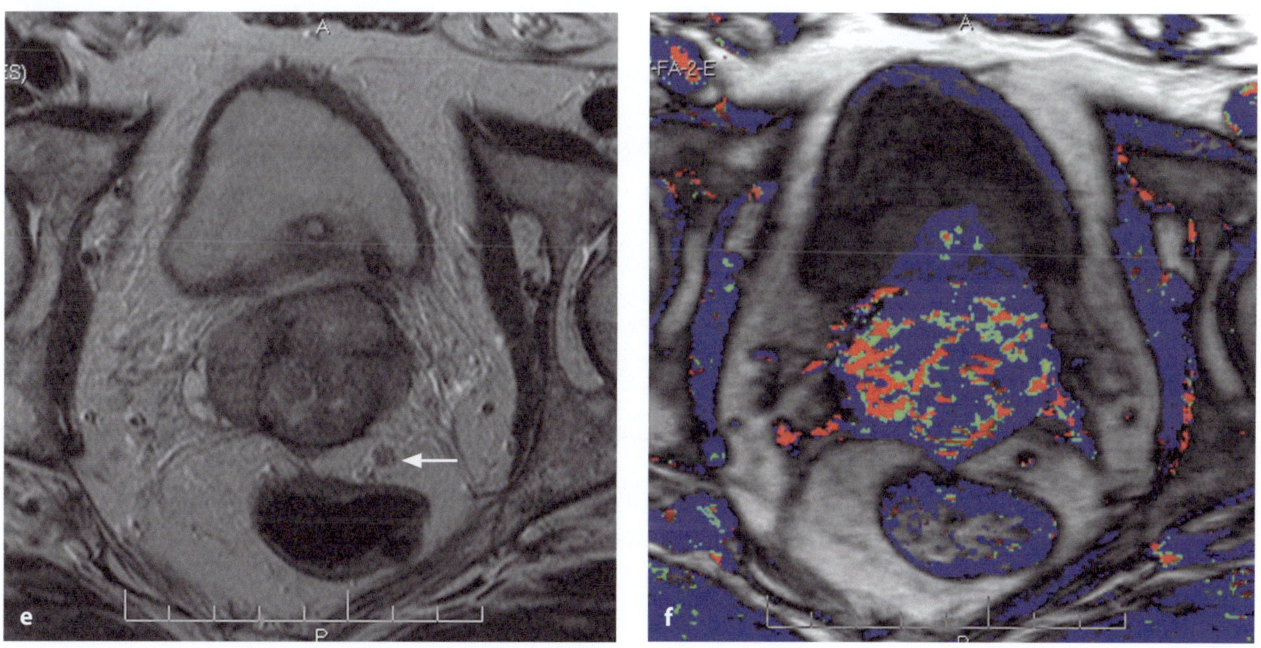

Fig. 9.7 e, f With seminal vesicle invasion and left perirectal node

Fig. 9.7 g, h

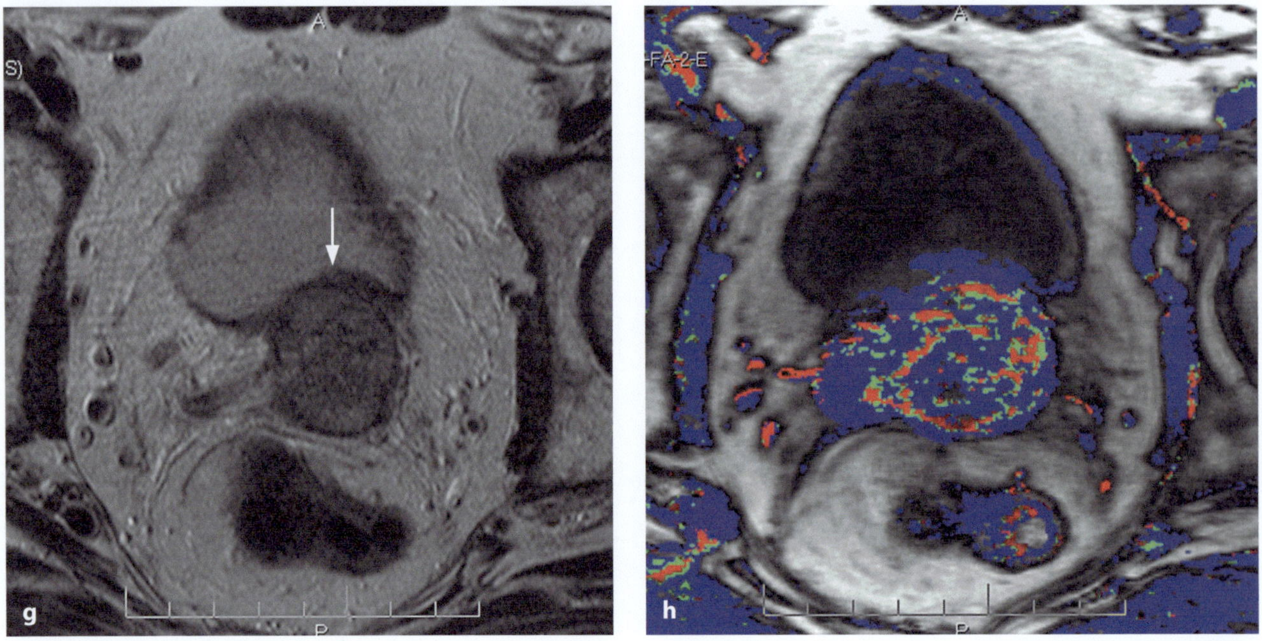

Fig. 9.7 g, h With bladder wall invasion

Fig. 9.7 i, j

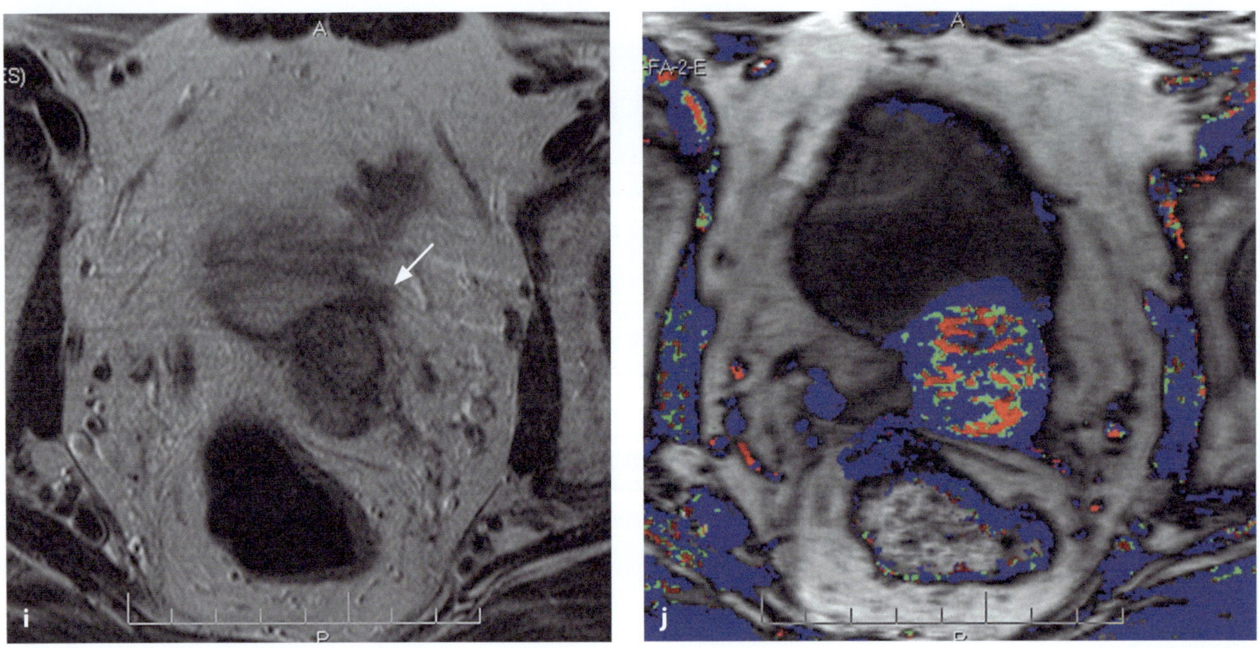

Fig. 9.7 i, j With bladder lumen invasion

Fig. 9.7 k, l

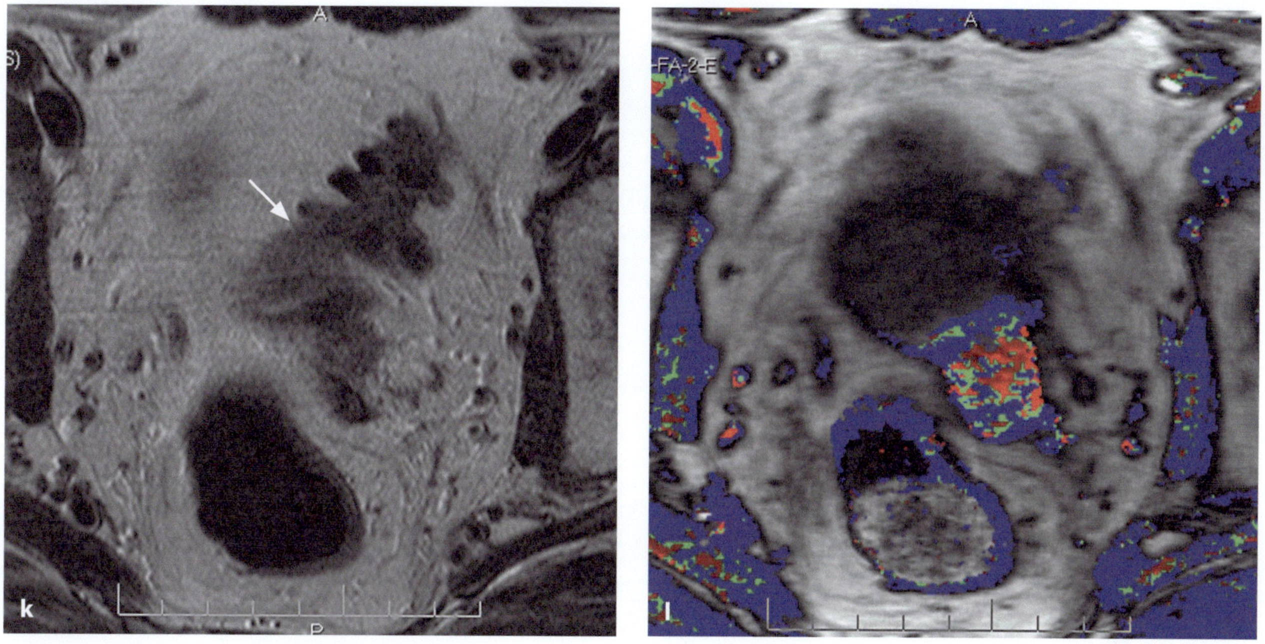

Fig. 9.7 k, l With distal sigmoid colon invasion

Fig. 9.8 a–n

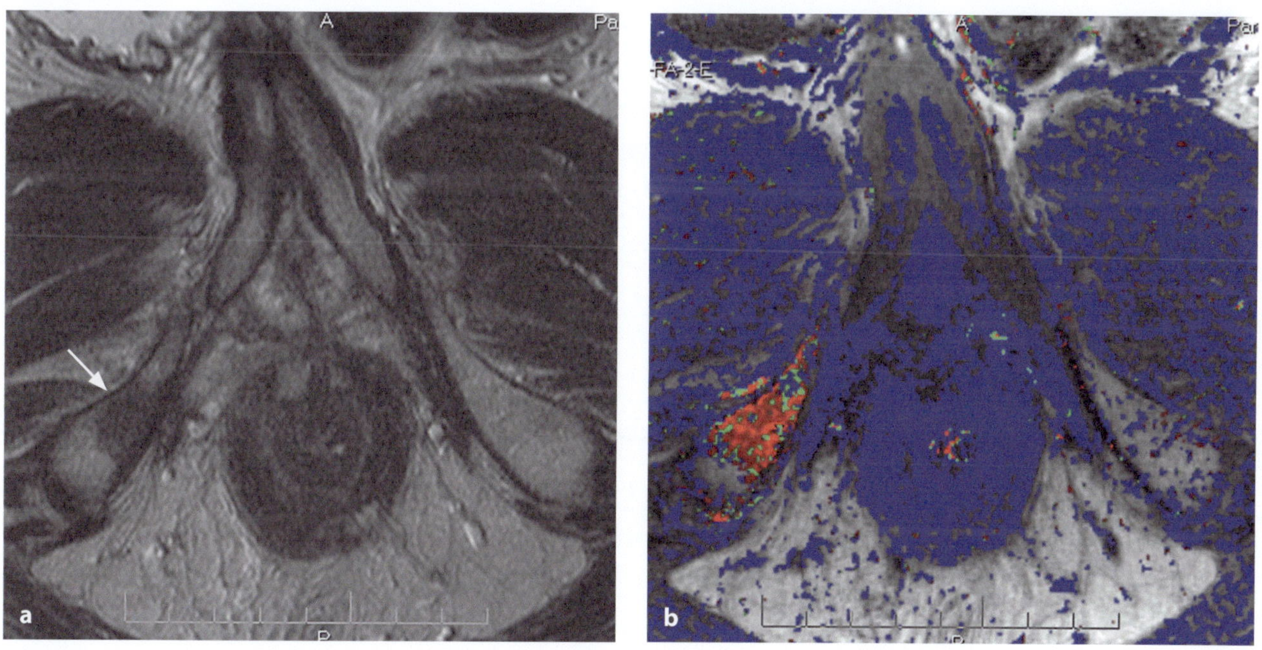

Fig. 9.8 a, b Gleason 5 with right inferior pubic ramus disease

Fig. 9.8 c, d

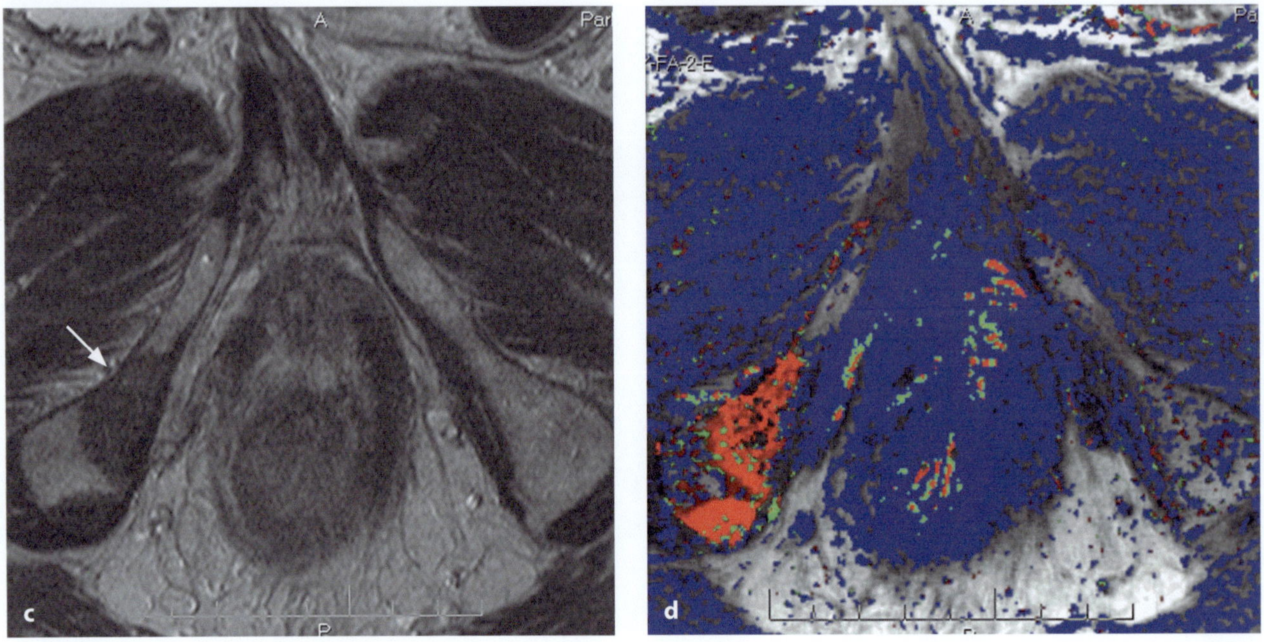

Fig. 9.8 c, d With right ischial tuberosity metastases

Fig. 9.8 e, f

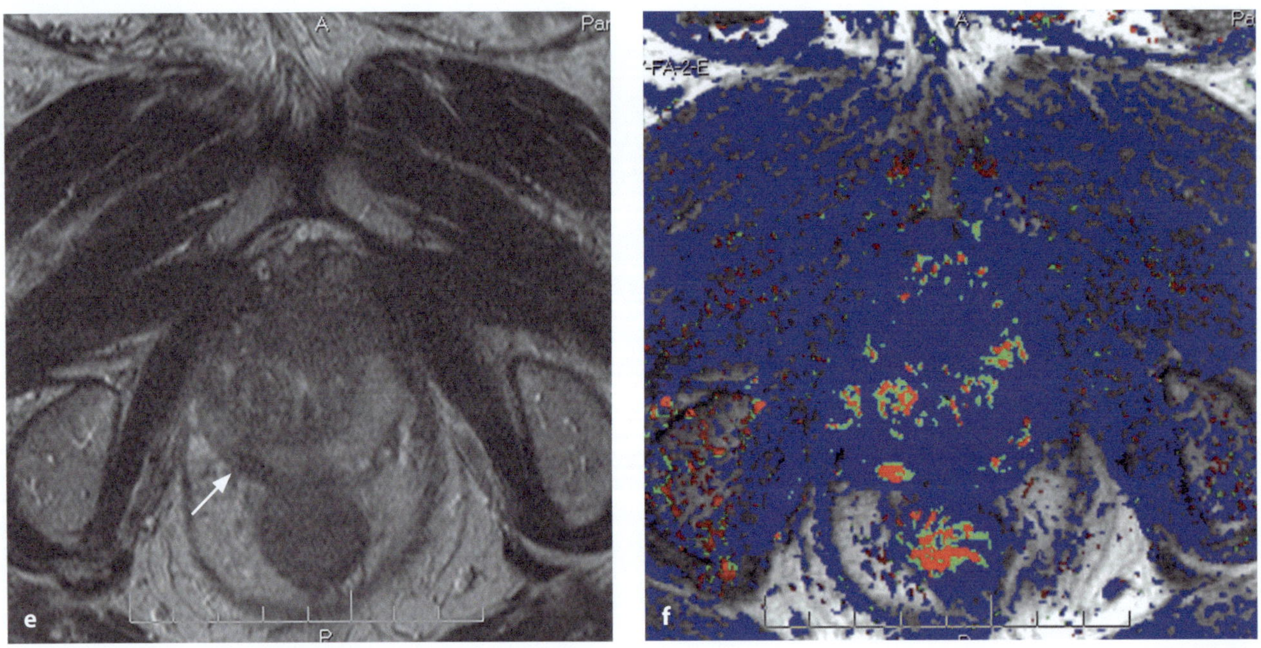

Fig. 9.8 e, f With right midgland posterior lesion

Fig. 9.8 g, h

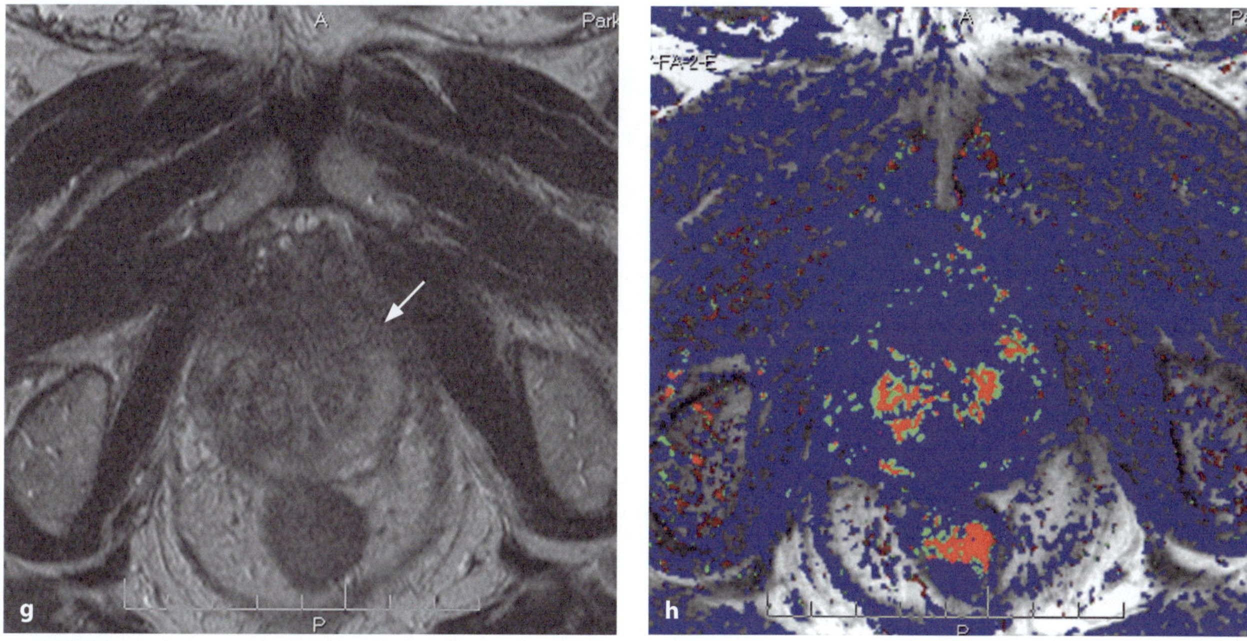

Fig. 9.8 g, h With left anterior base lesion

Fig. 9.8 i, j

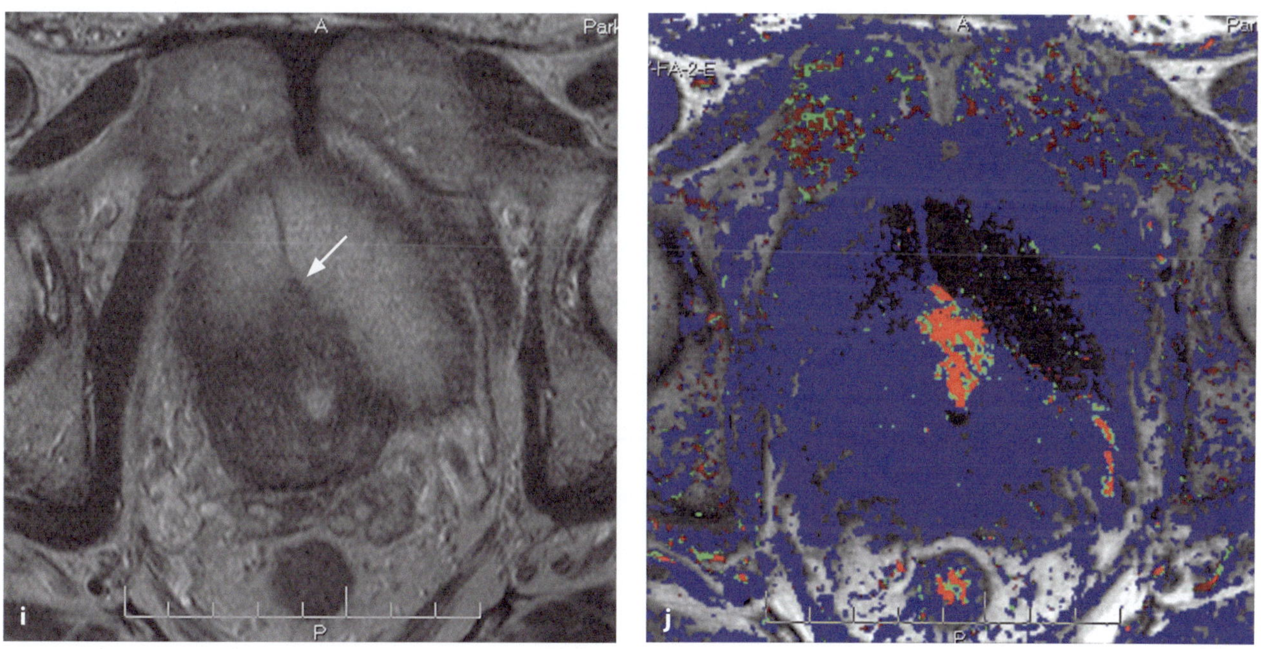

Fig. 9.8 i, j With base lesion invading bladder

Fig. 9.8 k, l

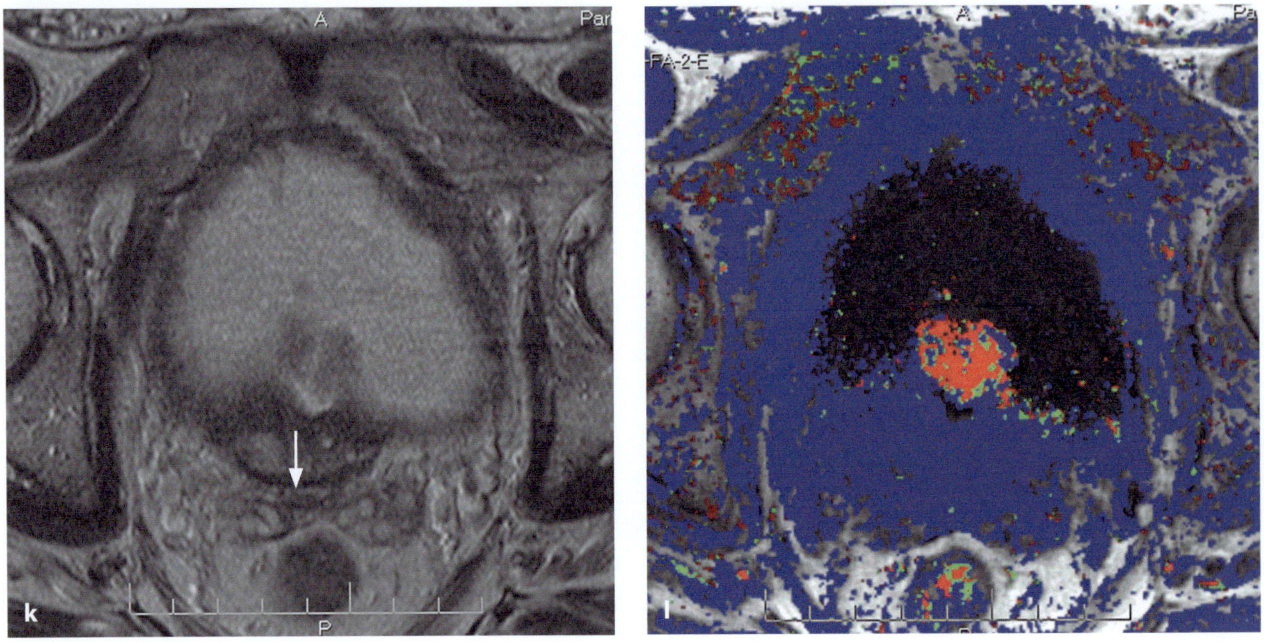

Fig. 9.8 k, l With seminal vesicle central invasion

Fig. 9.8 m, n

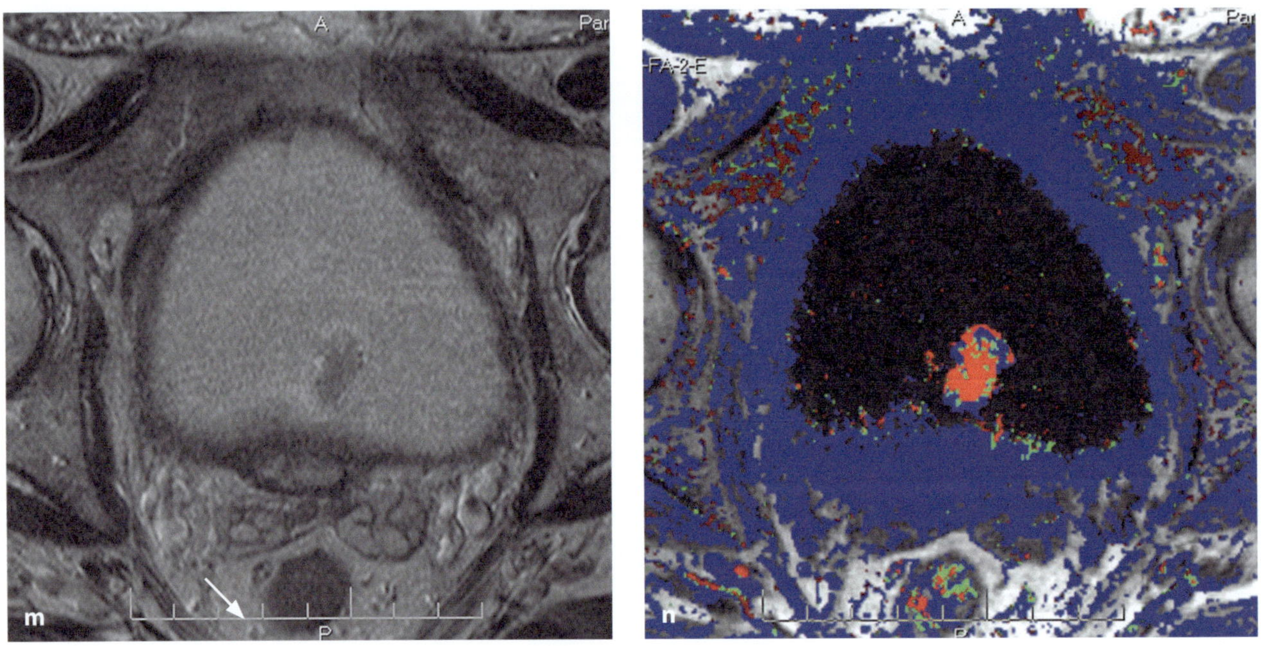

Fig. 9.8 m, n With right perirectal adenopathy and polypoid bladder mass

Fig. 9.9 a–j

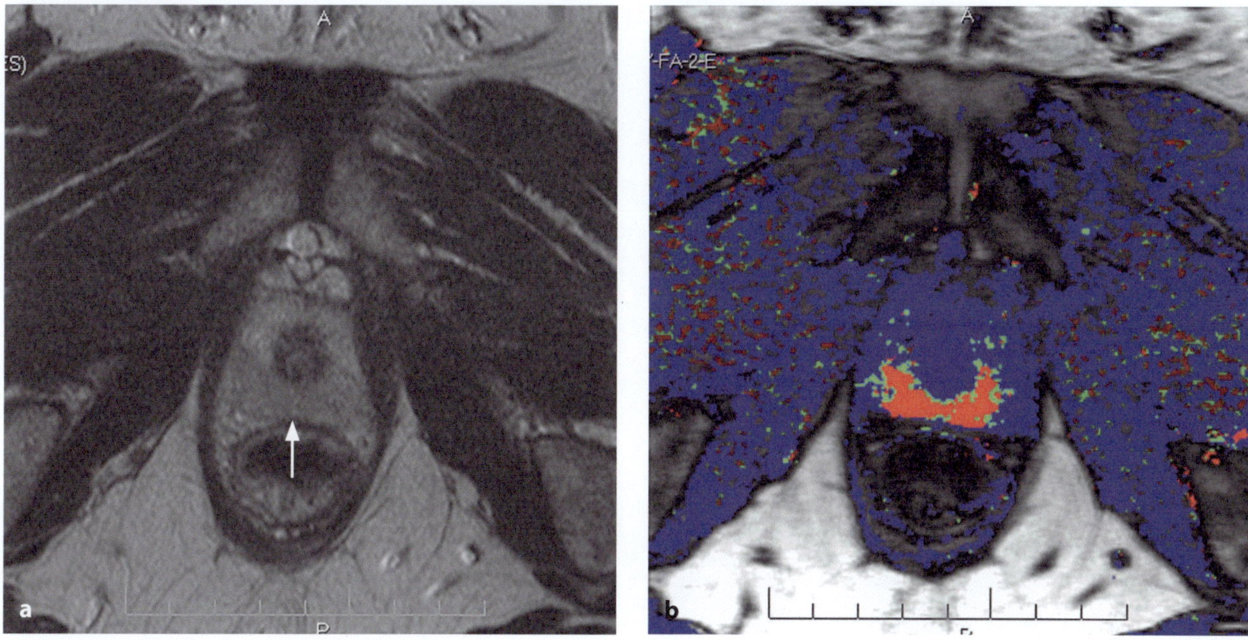

Fig. 9.9 a, b Gleason 4 with symmetric apical disease simulating inflammation

Fig. 9.9 c, d

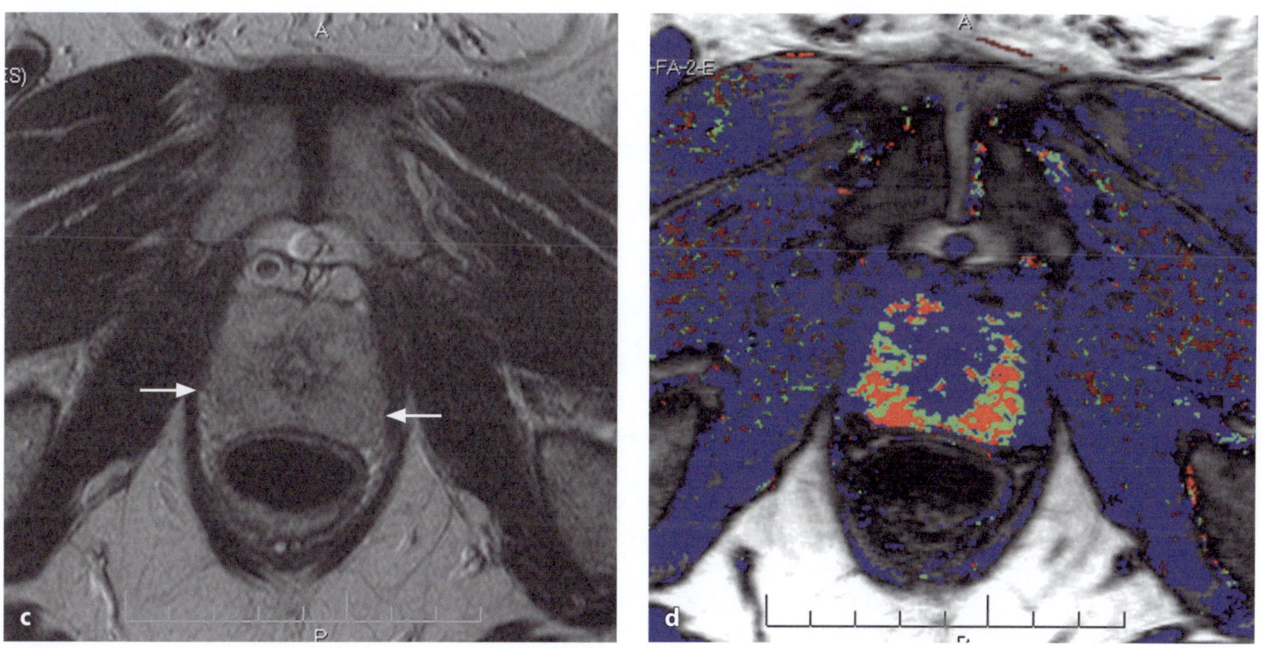

Fig. 9.9 c, d Symmetric distal midgland disease

Fig. 9.9 e, f

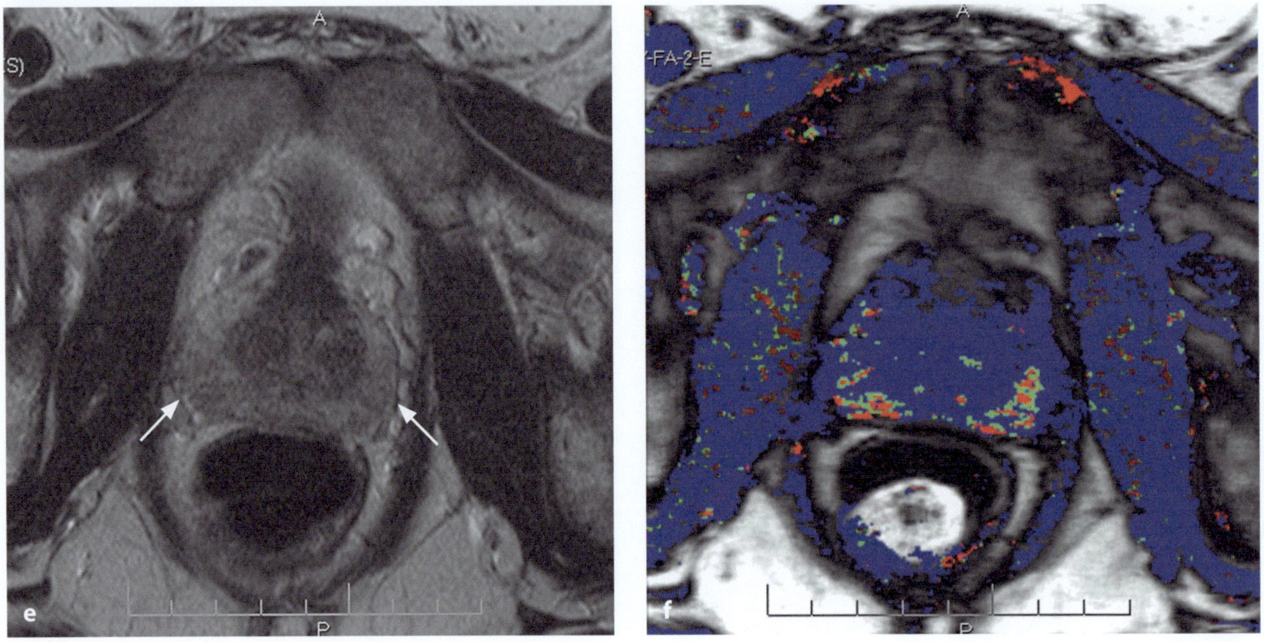

Fig. 9.9 e, f Symmetric proximal midgland disease

Fig. 9.9 g, h

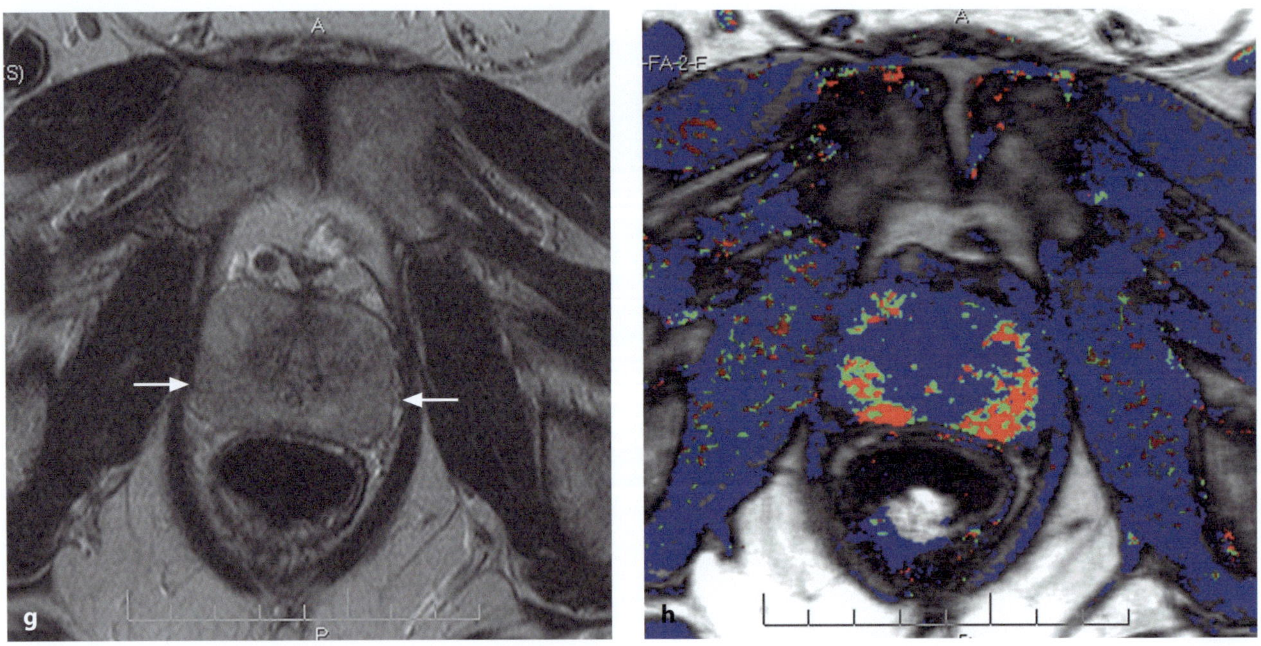

Fig. 9.9 g, h Symmetric base disease

Fig. 9.9 i, j

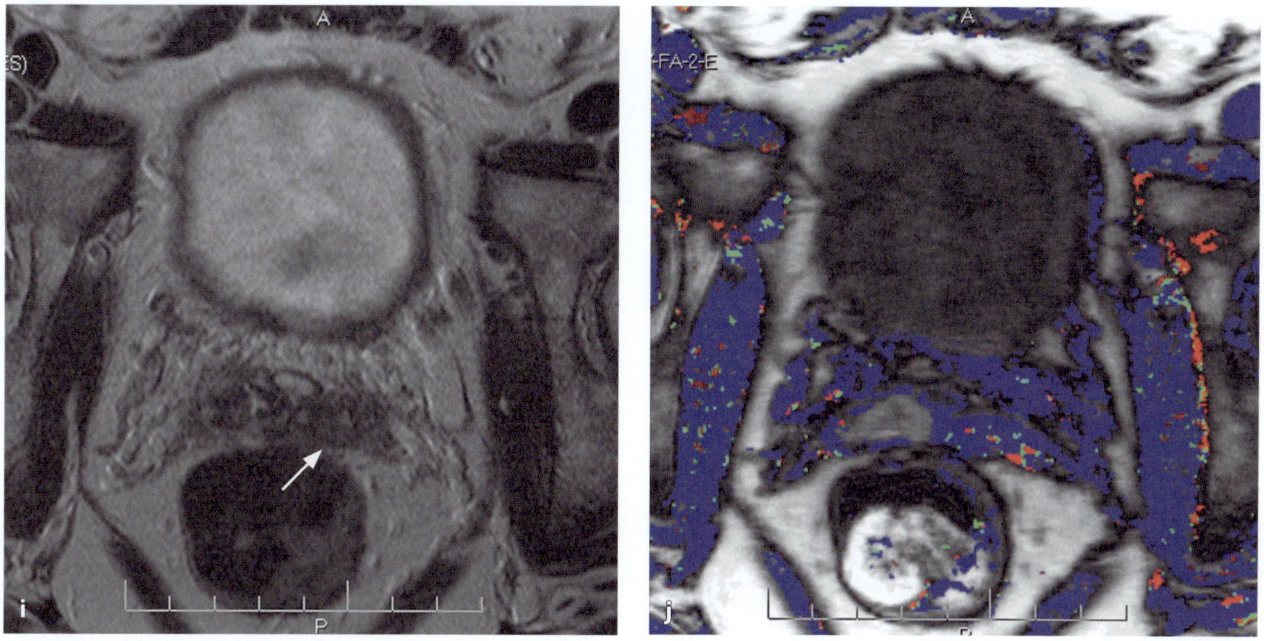

Fig. 9.9 i, j Asymmetric seminal vesicle invasion on left

Fig. 9.10 a–h

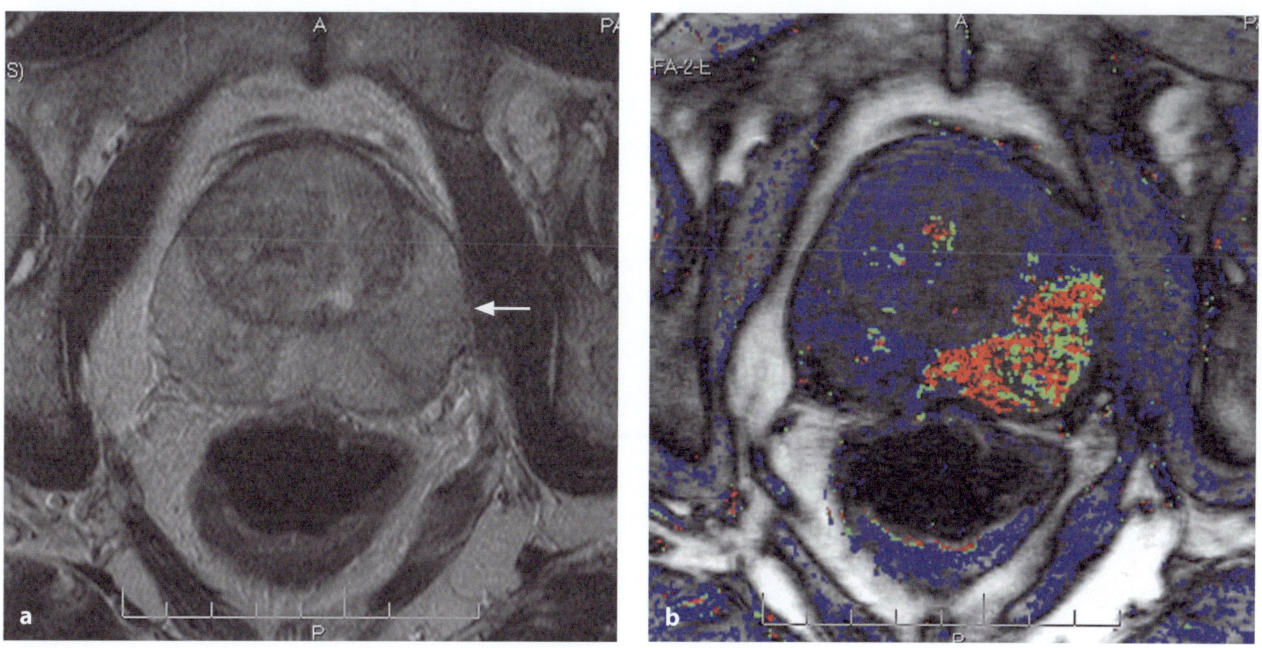

Fig. 9.10 a, b Left midgland Gleason 4 with lateral extracapsular erosion

Fig. 9.10 c, d

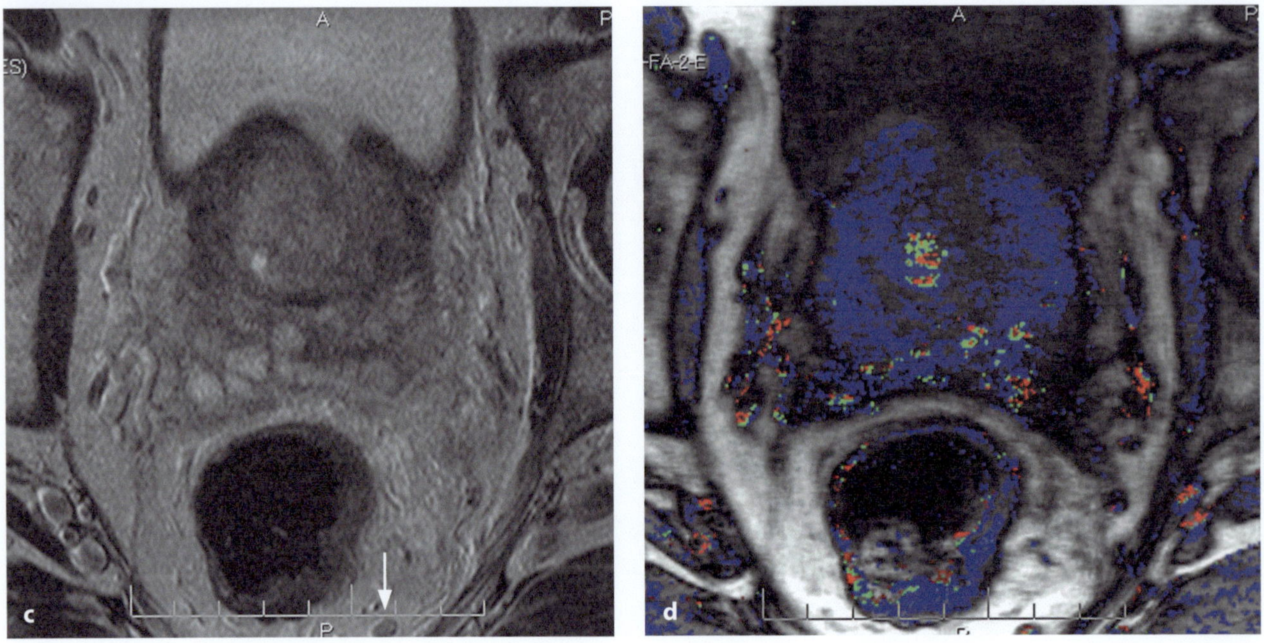

Fig. 9.10 c, d With vascular left perirectal node

Fig. 9.10 e, f

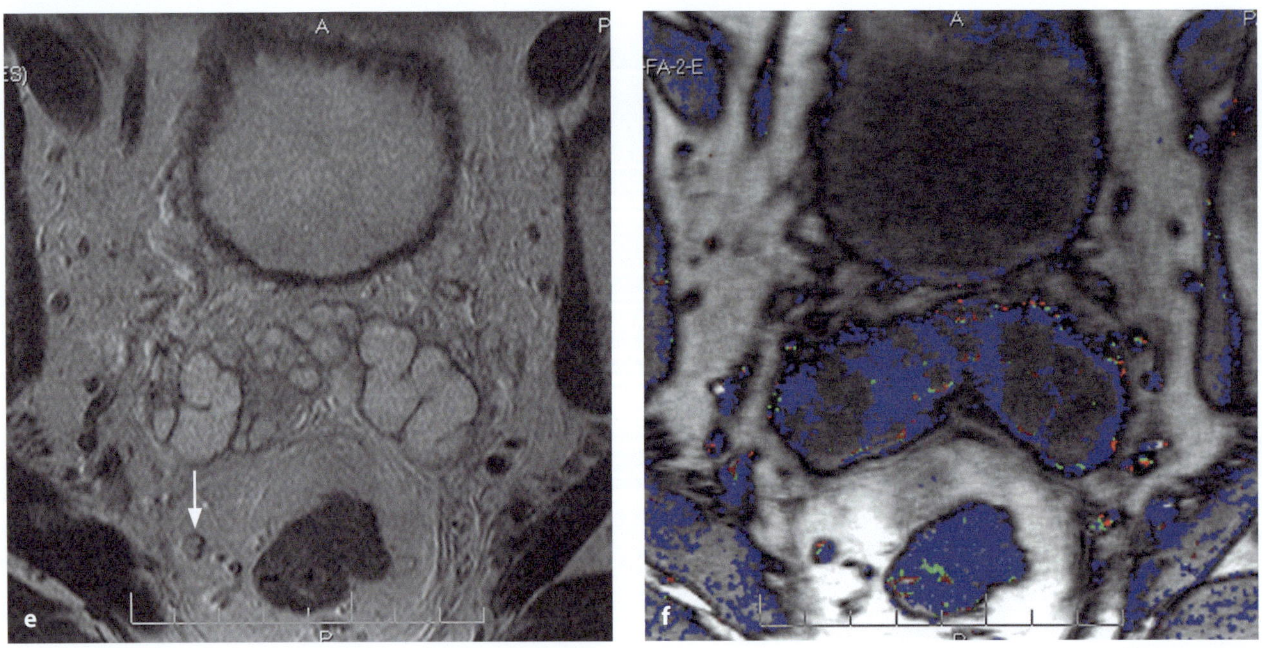

Fig. 9.10 e, f With vascular bilateral perirectal nodes

Fig. 9.10 g, h

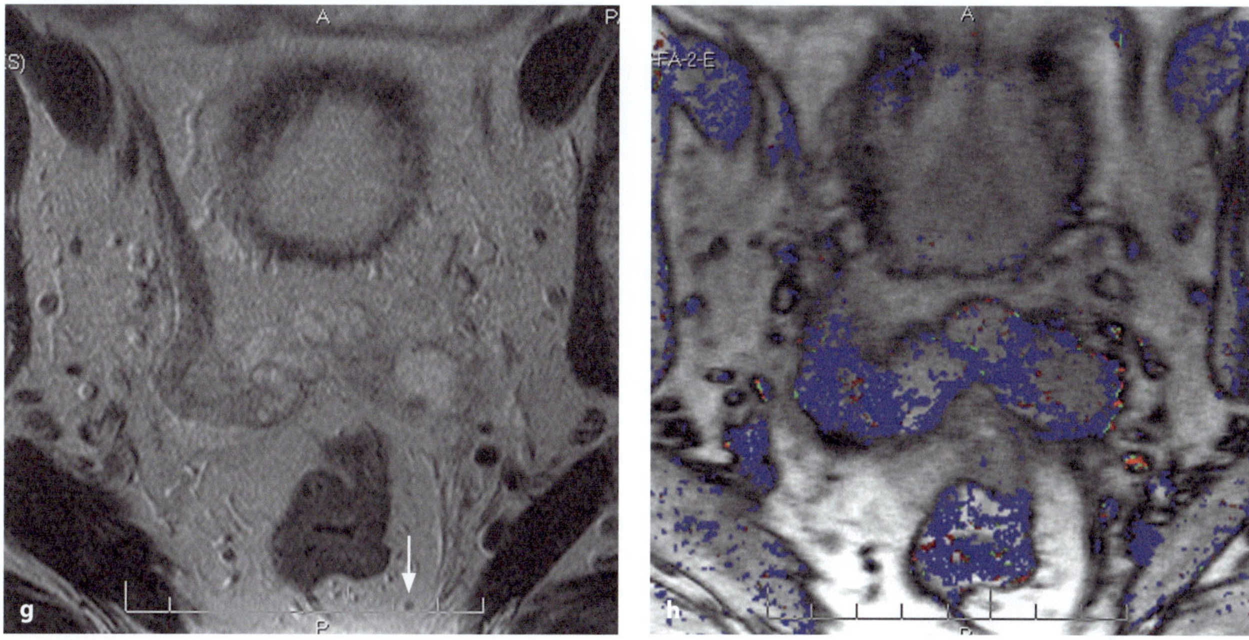

Fig. 9.10 g, h With avascular left perirectal 3 mm node

Fig. 9.11 a–h

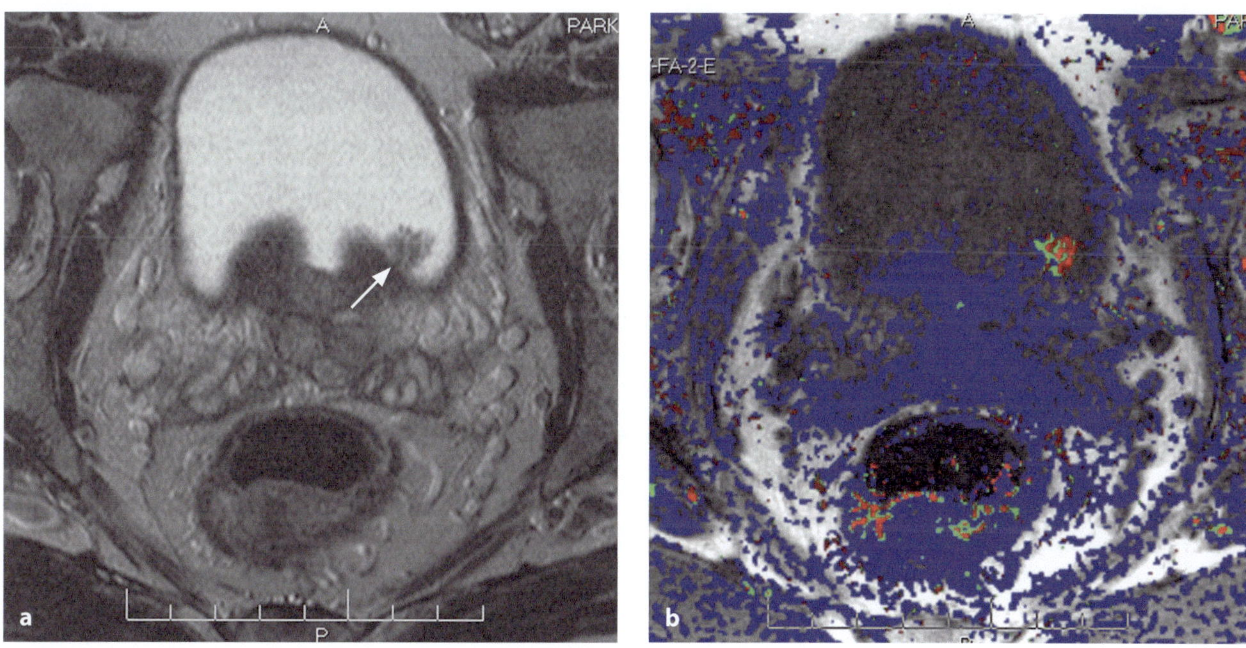

Fig. 9.11 a, b Left bladder mass incidentally discovered

Fig. 9.11 c, d

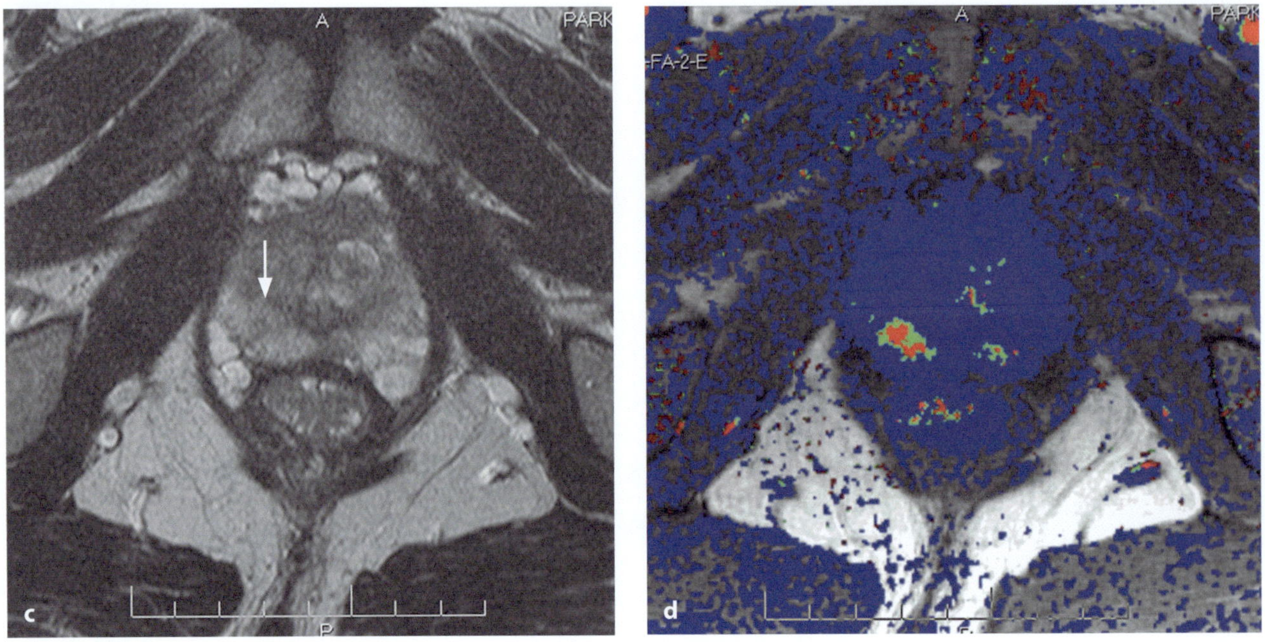

Fig. 9.11 c, d With right midgland Gleason 4

Fig. 9.11 e, f

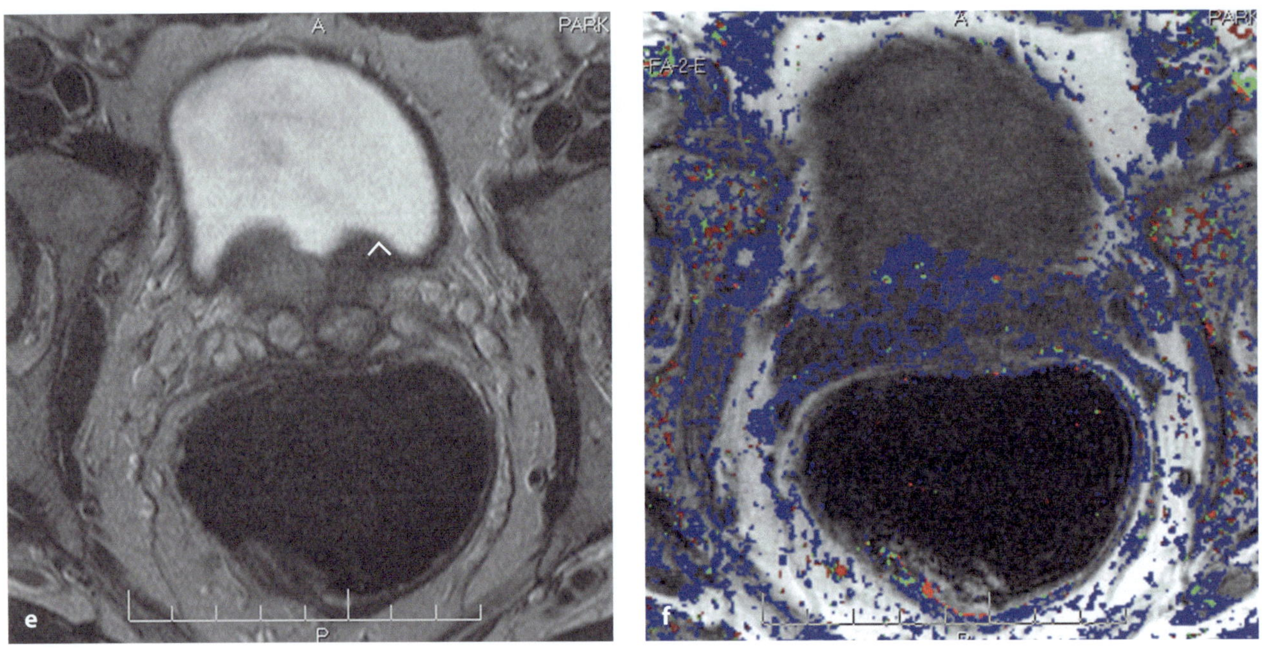

Fig. 9.11 e, f 8 month followup-high grade transitional cell tumor removed

Fig. 9.11 g, h

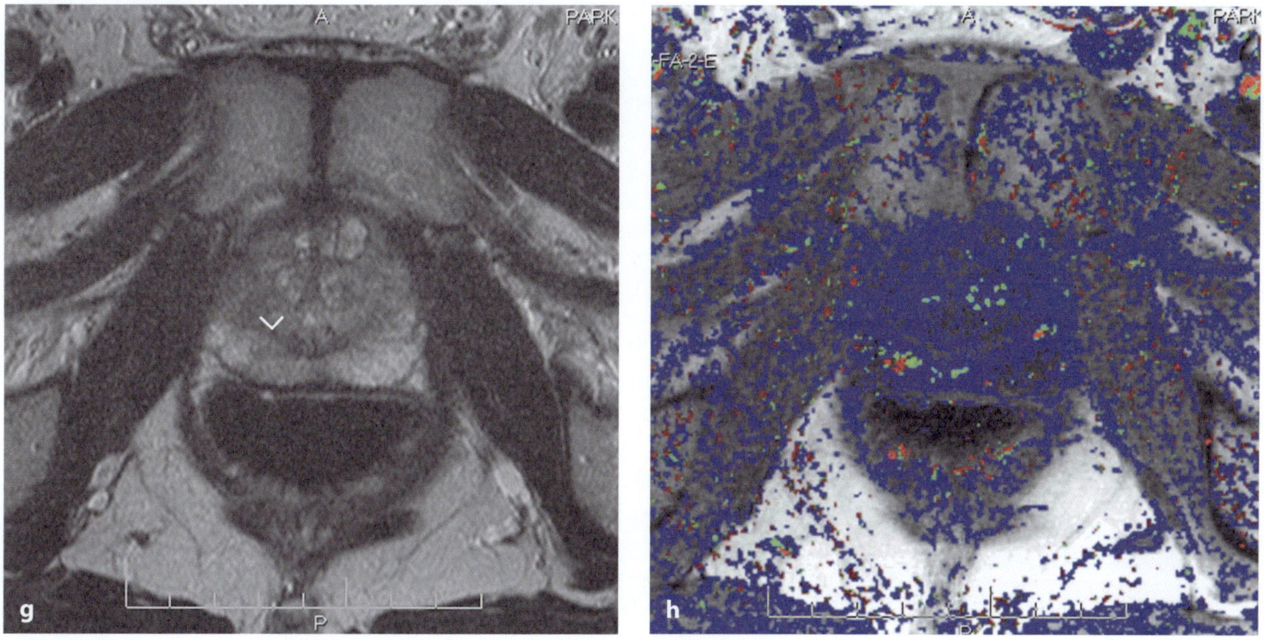

Fig. 9.11 g, h Antioxidant treatments reduce midgland prostate lesion

Fig. 9.12 a–h

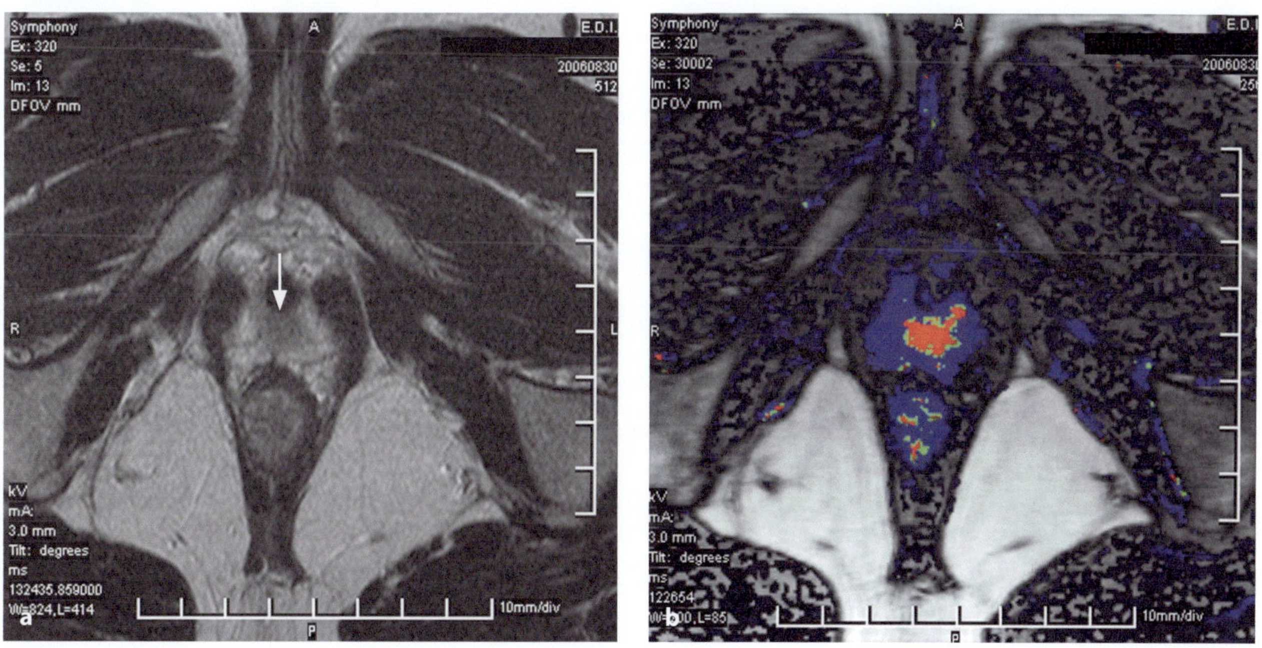

Fig. 9.12 a, b Gleason 4 with central apical disease

Fig. 9.12 c, d

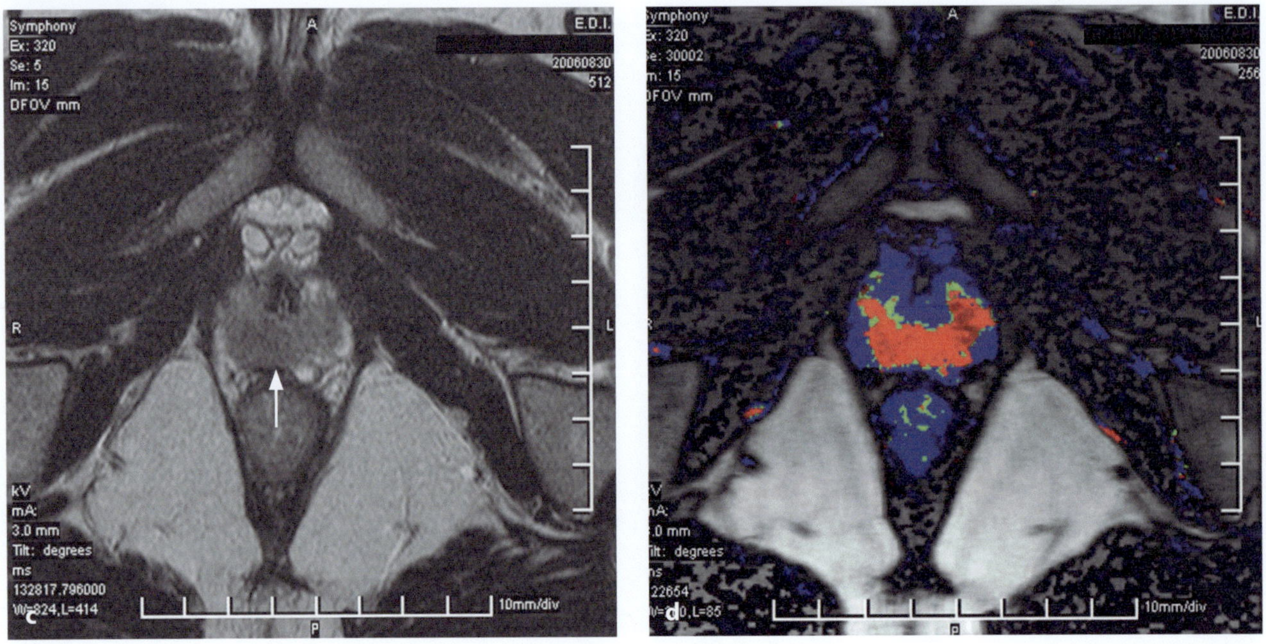

Fig. 9.12 c, d With central midgland extension

Fig. 9.12 e, f

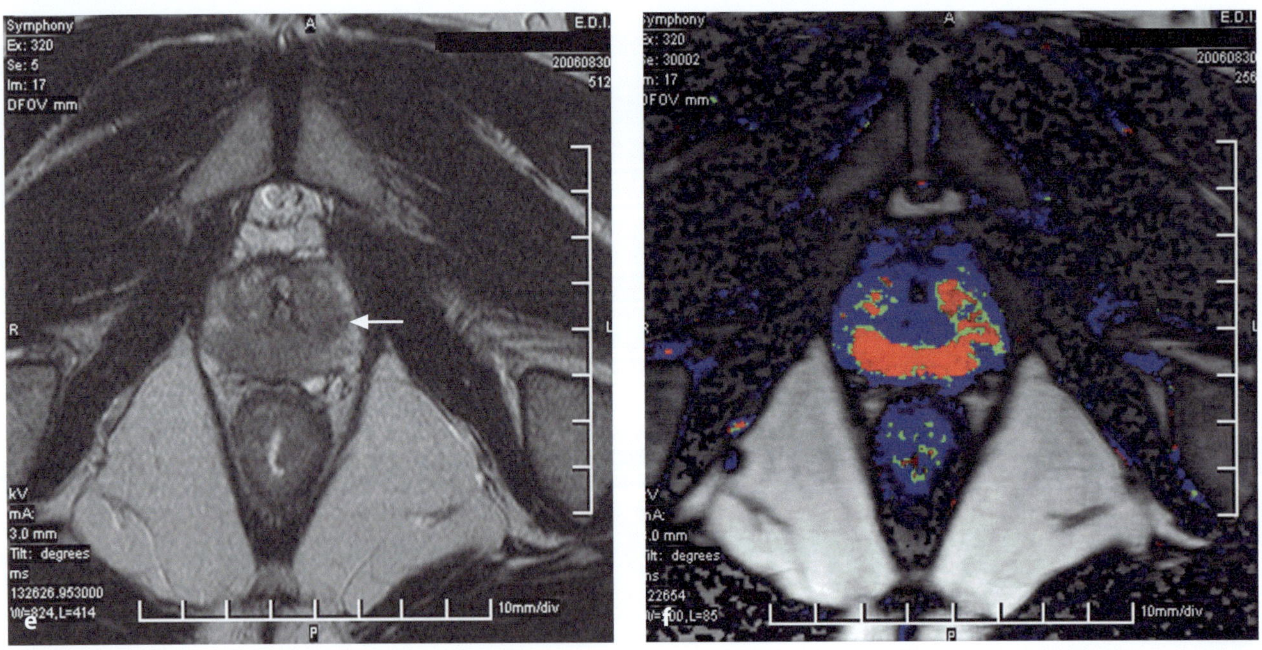

Fig. 9.12 e, f With peripheral midgland extension

Fig. 9.12 g, h

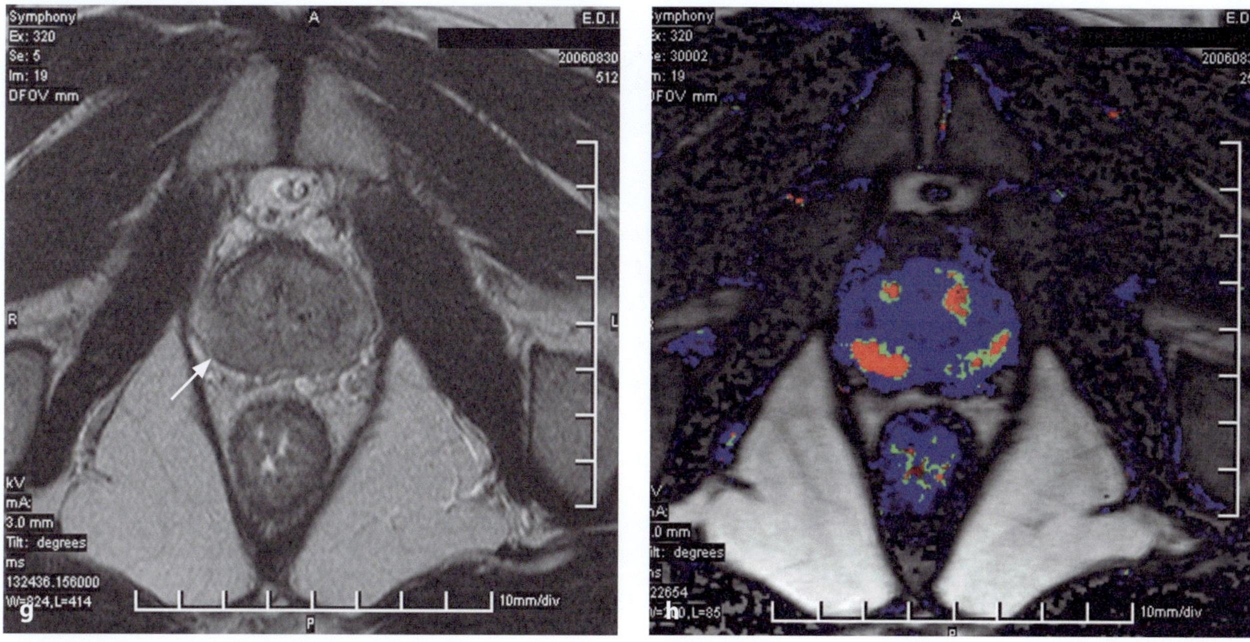

Fig. 9.12 g, h With peripheral base extension

Fig. 9.13 a–h

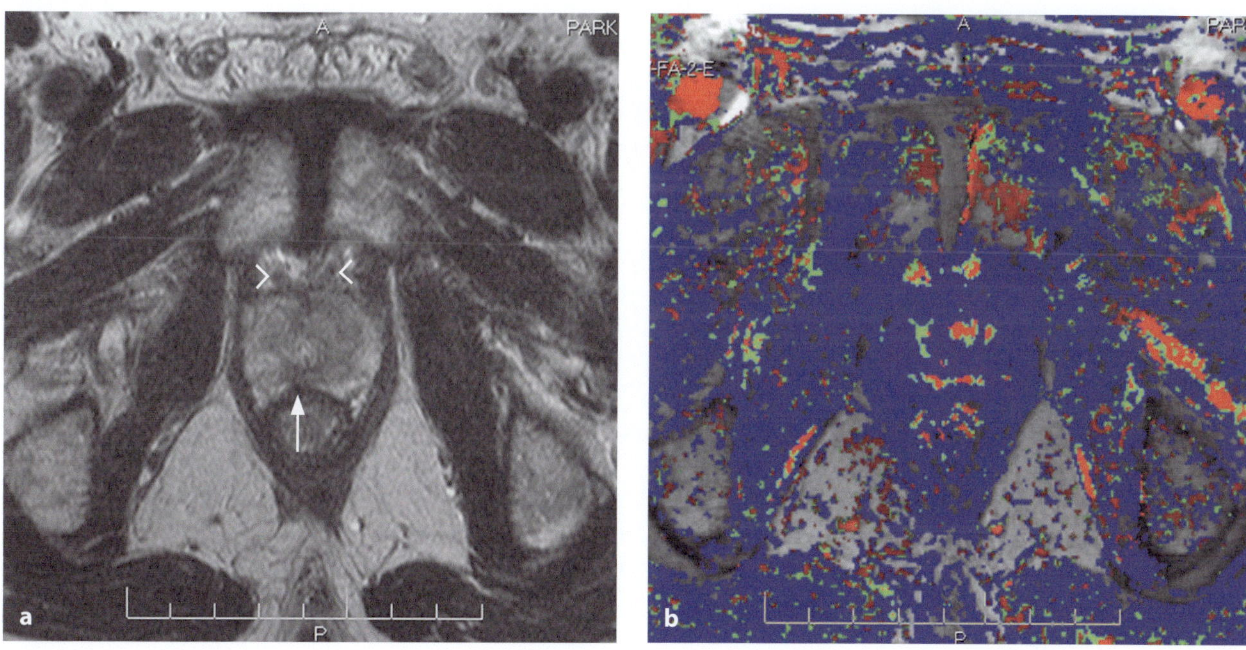

Fig. 9.13 a, b Apical posterior Gleason 4-note anterior veins

Fig. 9.13 c, d

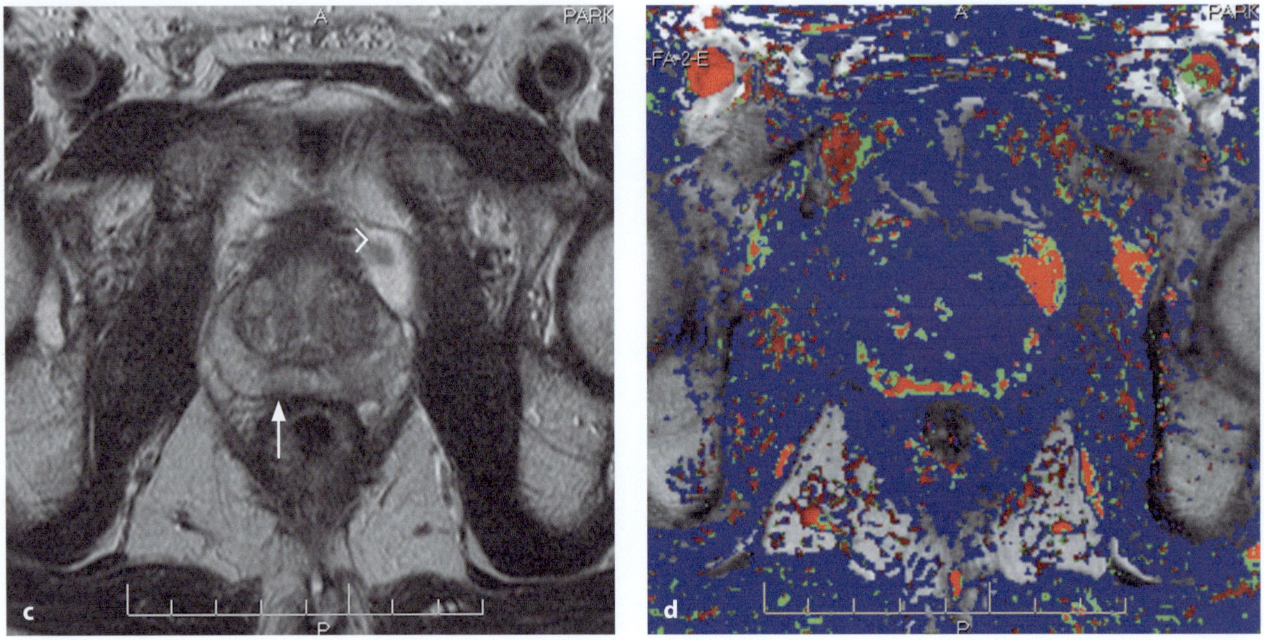

Fig. 9.13 c, d With midgland posterior Gleason 3 with peripheral veins

Fig. 9.13 e, f

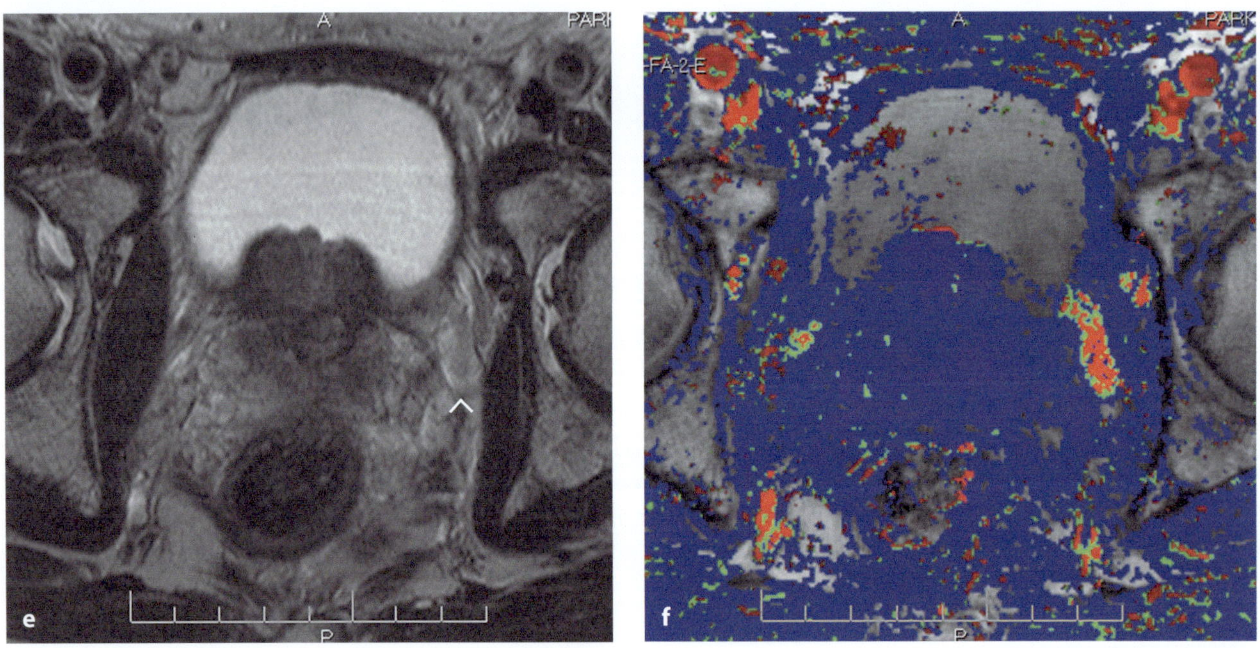

Fig. 9.13 e, f With normal base with peripheral venous dilation

Fig. 9.13 g, h

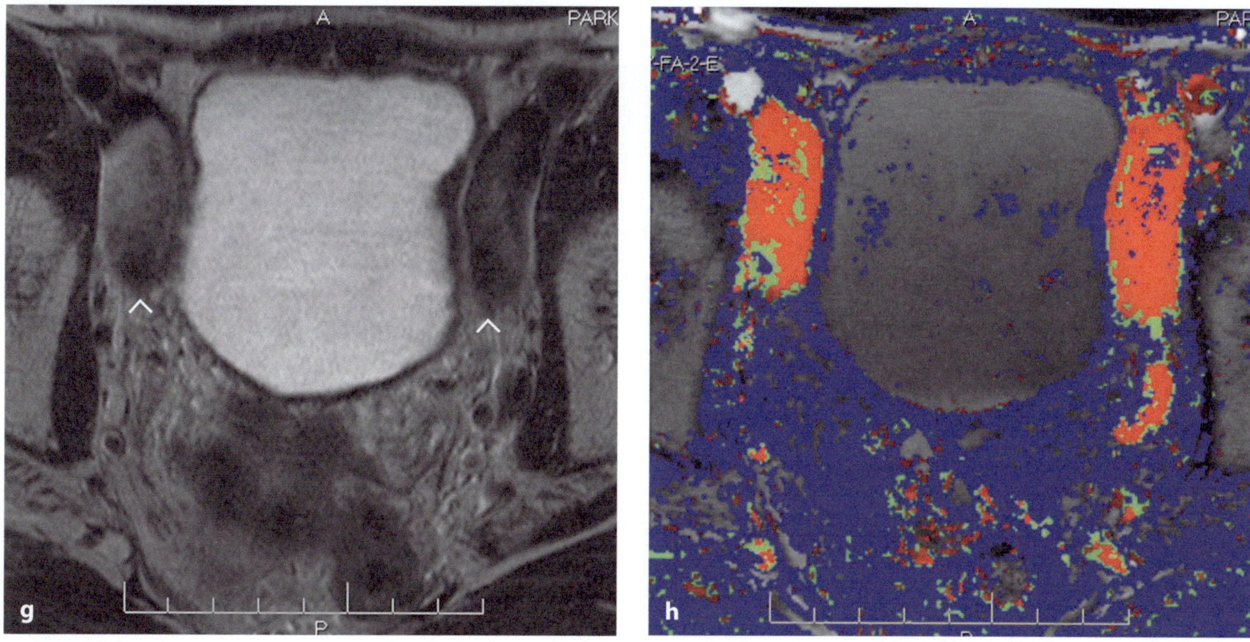

Fig. 9.13 g, h With massive perivesical obturator venous dilation

Fig. 9.14 a–j

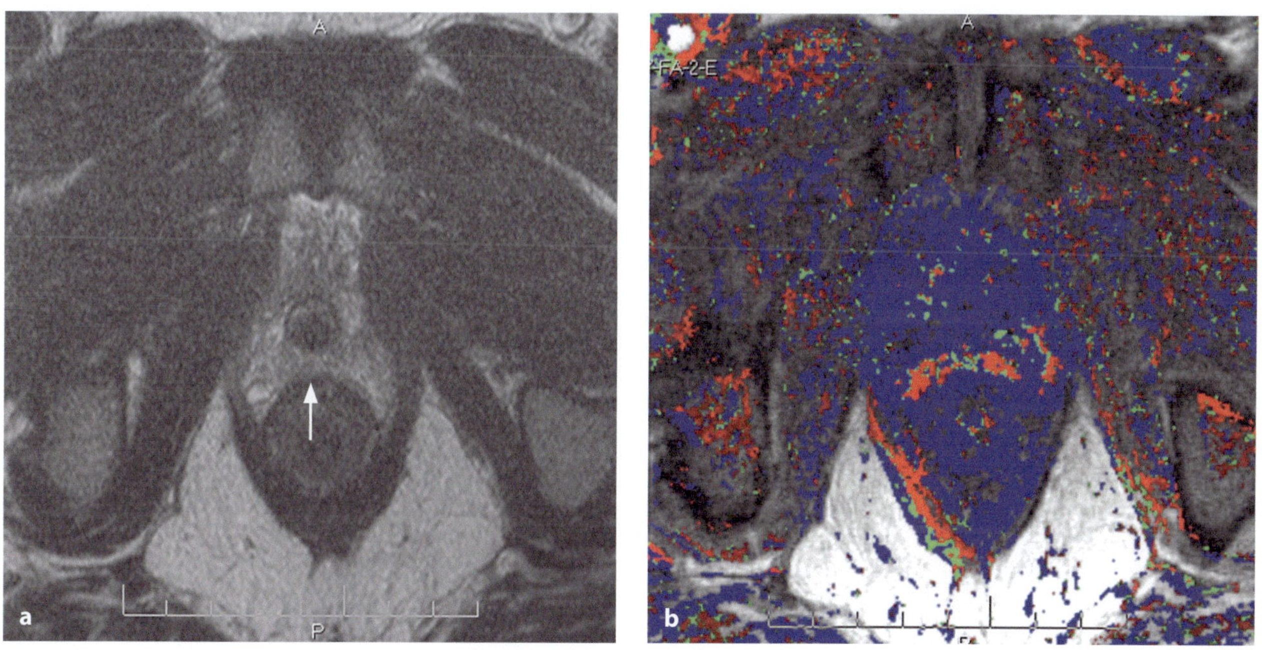

Fig. 9.14 a, b Gleason 5 with posterior apex tumor

Fig. 9.14 c, d

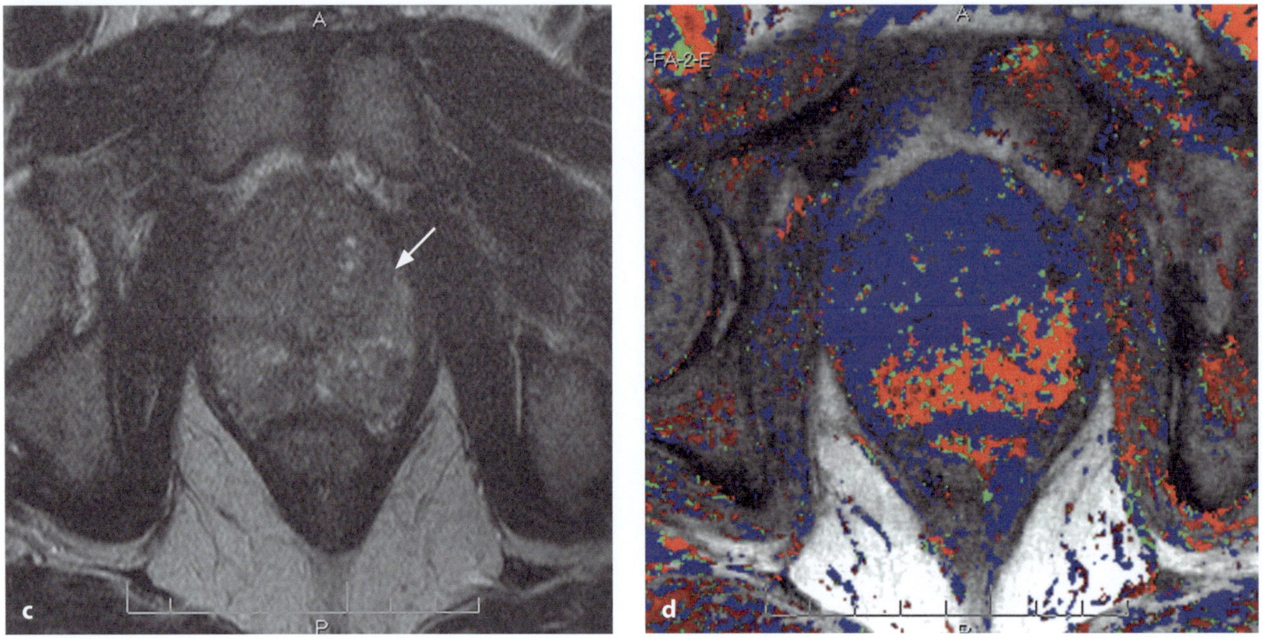

Fig. 9.14 c, d With extension into midgland

Fig. 9.14 e, f

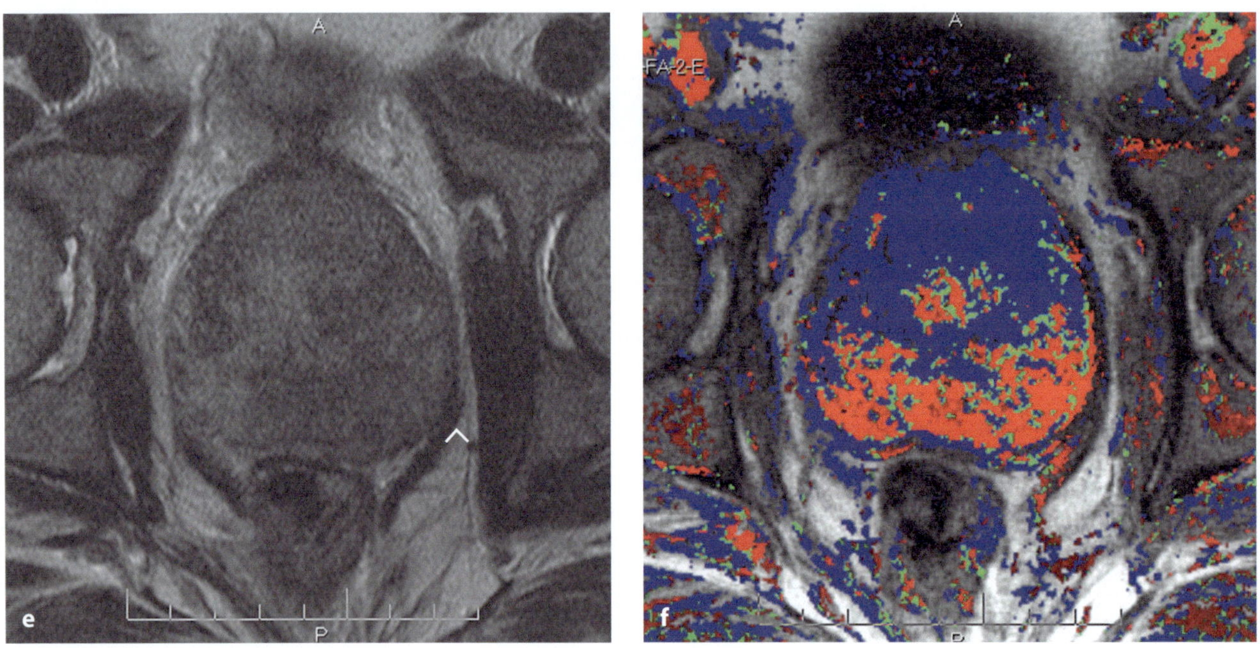

Fig. 9.14 e, f With left capsular bulging

Fig. 9.14 g, h

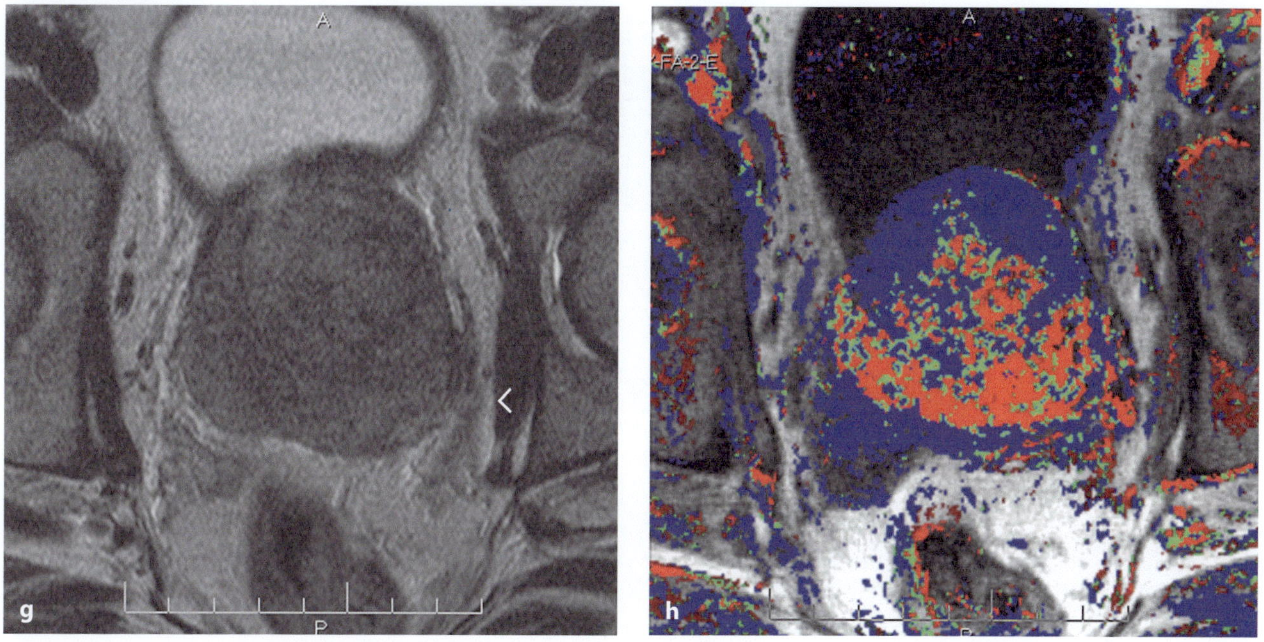

Fig. 9.14 g, h With extension into base and extracapsular tumor

Fig. 9.14 i, j

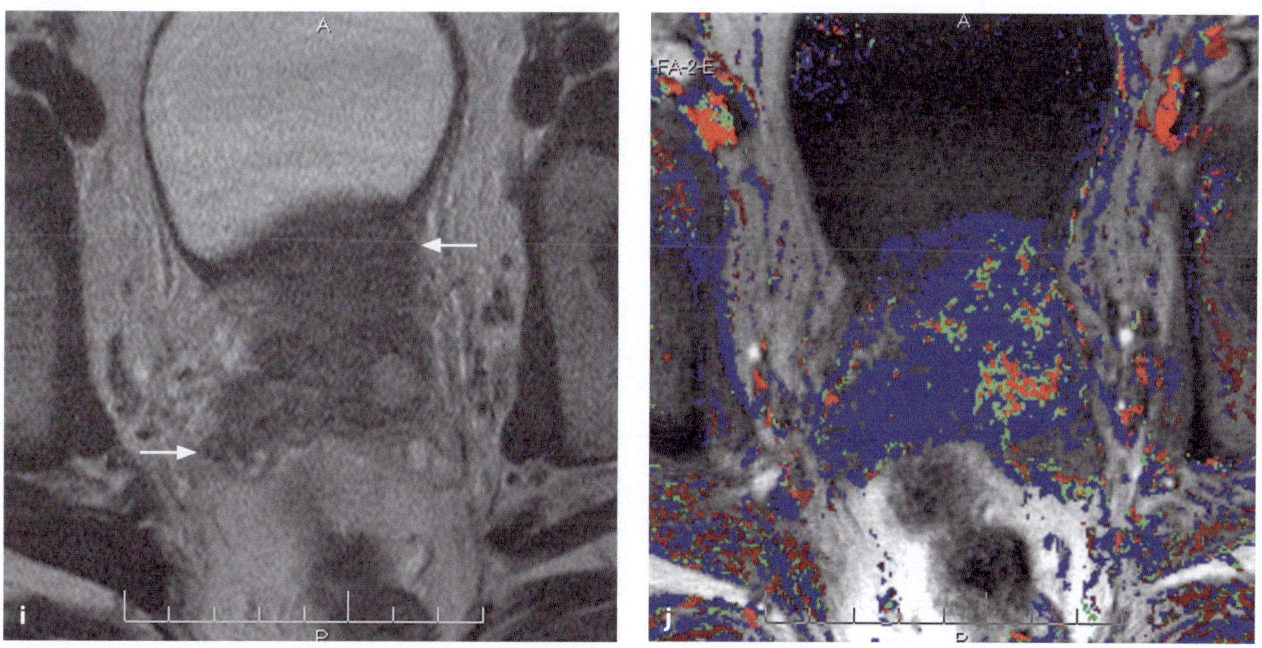

Fig. 9.14 i, j With extension into both seminal vesicles and posterior bladder

Fig. 9.15 a, b

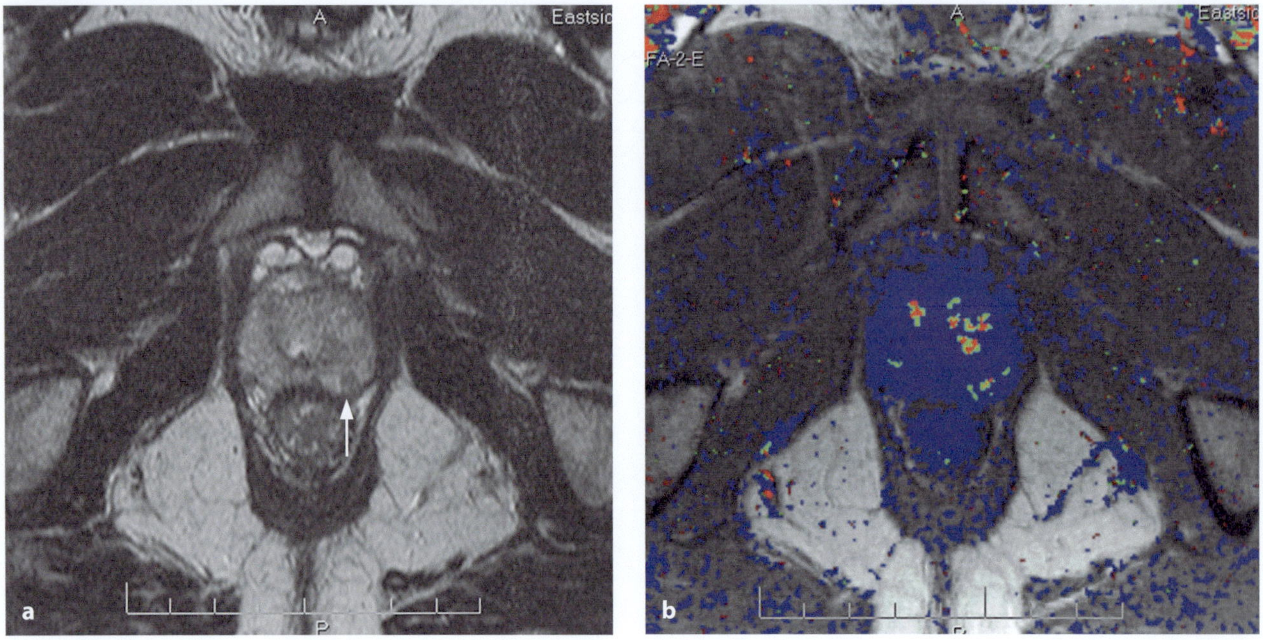

Fig. 9.15 a, b 4 mm left apical posterior Gleason 5

Fig. 9.15 c, d

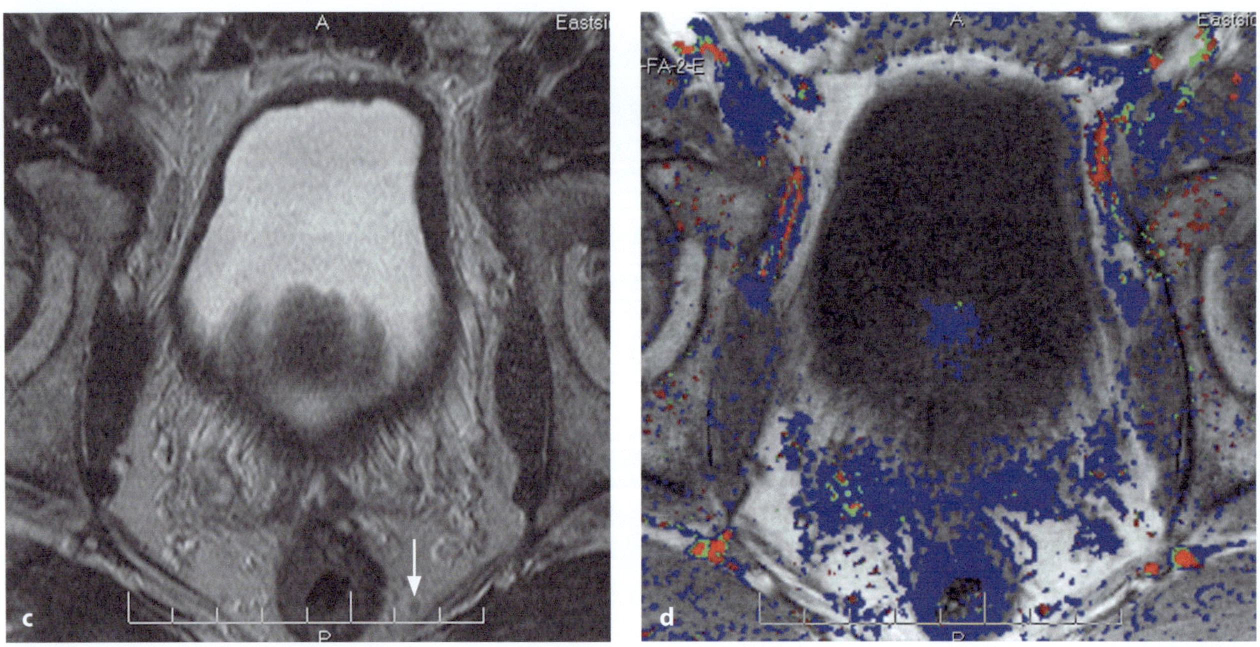

Fig. 9.15 c, d With left perirectal vascular node

Fig. 9.15 e, f

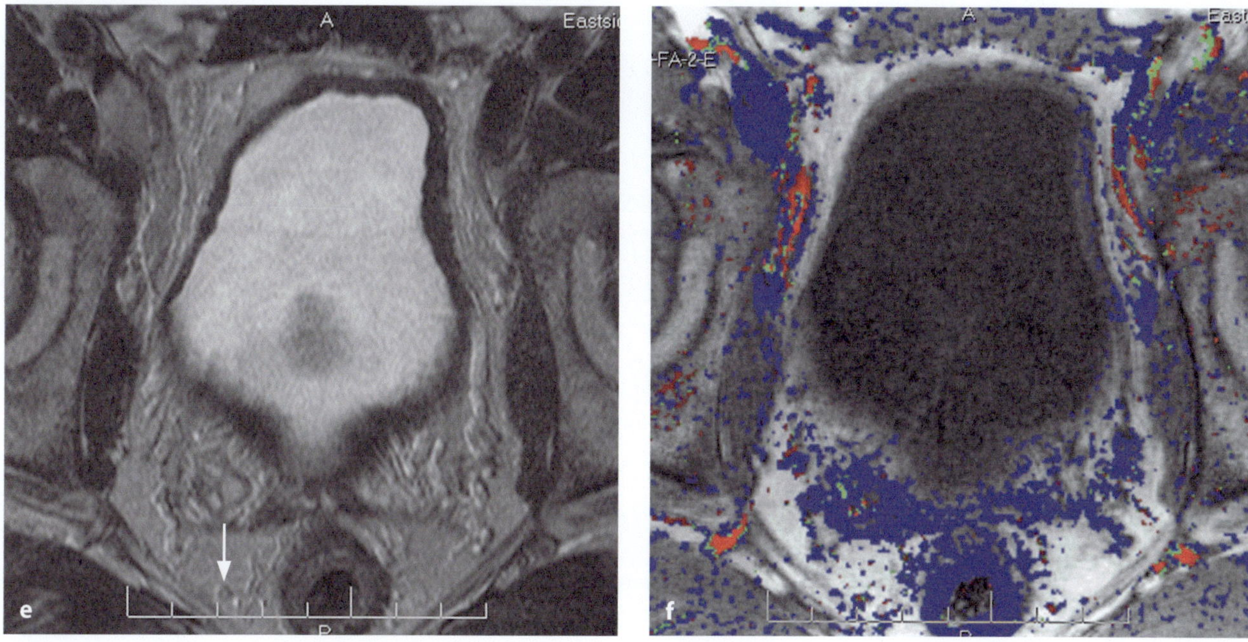

Fig. 9.15 e, f With 3 mm right perirectal vascular node

Fig. 9.15 g, h

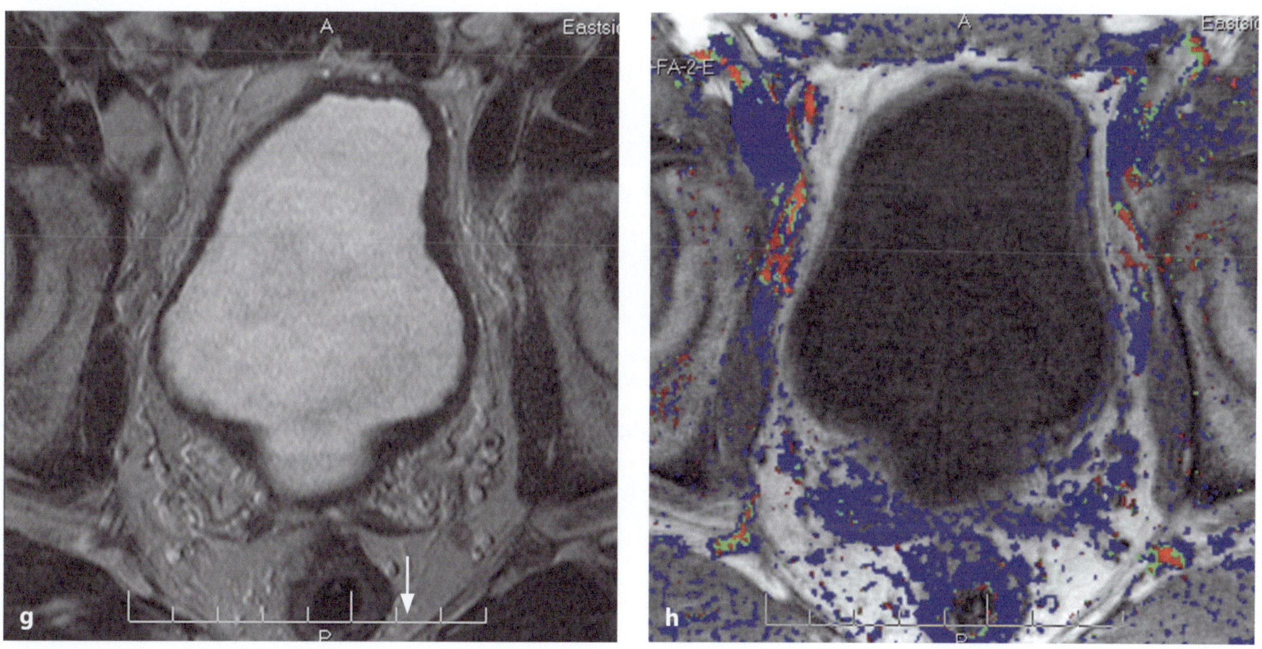

Fig. 9.15 g, h With left perirectal vascular node

Fig. 9.15 i, j

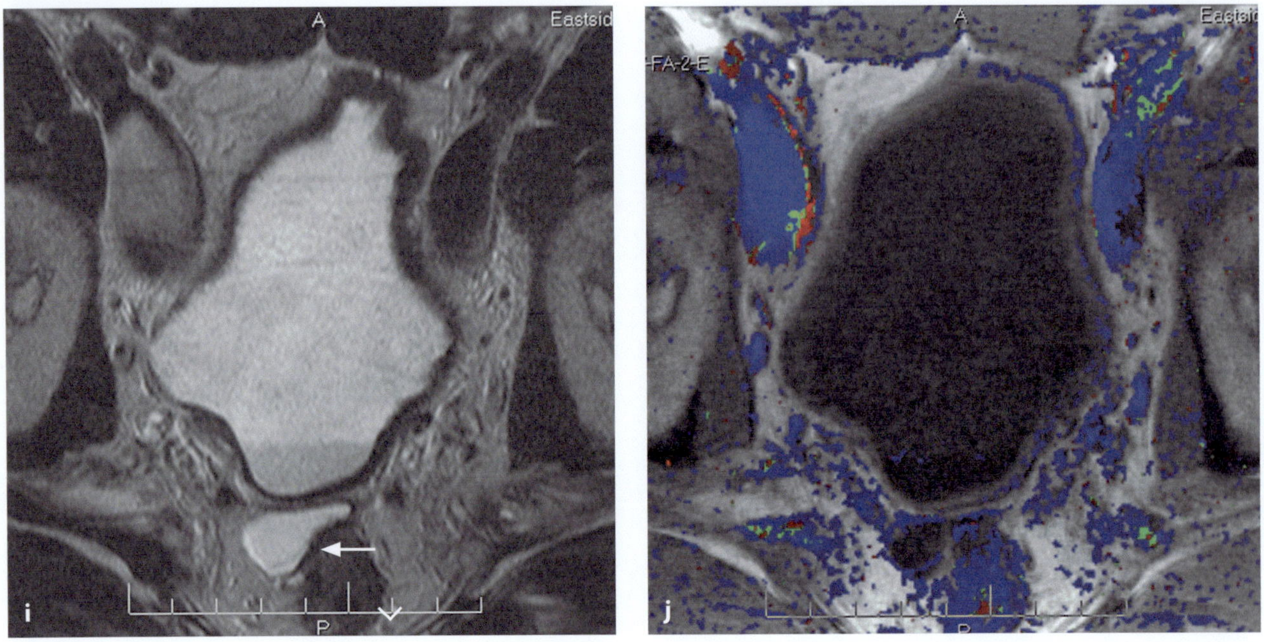

Fig. 9.15 i, j With ascites and left perirectal vascular node

Fig. 9.16 a–h

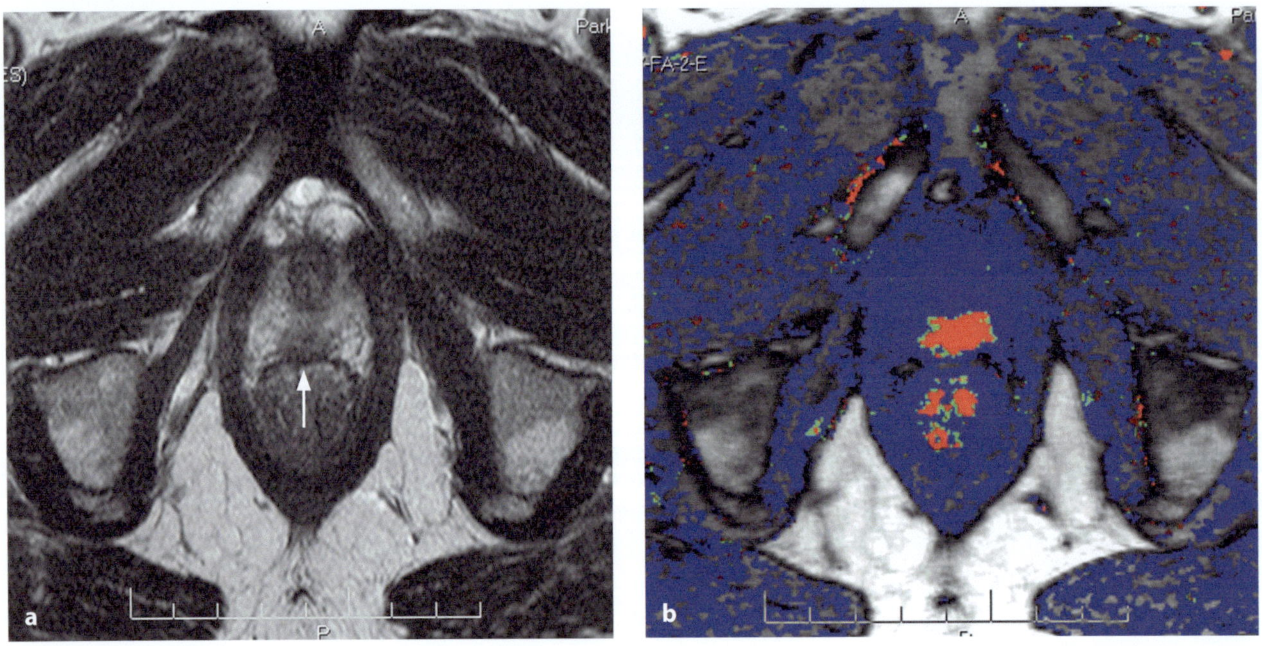

Fig. 9.16 a, b Gleason 5 apex-focal posterior lesion

Fig. 9.16 c, d

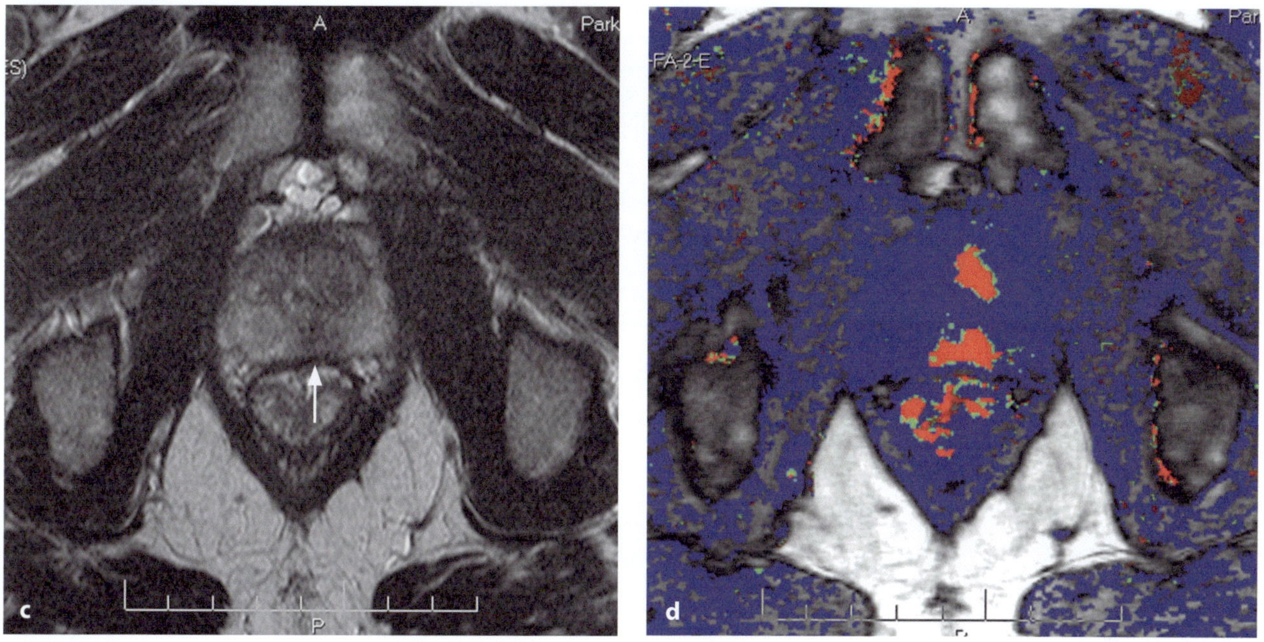

Fig. 9.16 c, d With extension to midgland-focal lesion

Fig. 9.16 e, f

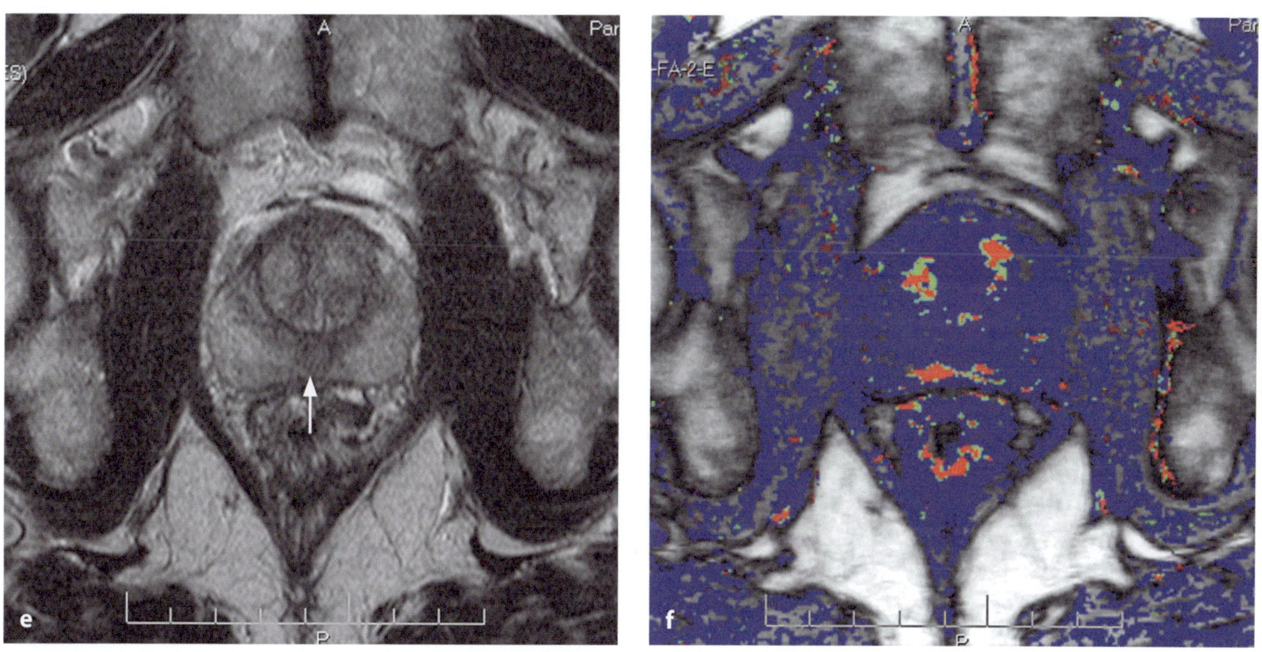

Fig. 9.16 e, f With Gleason 4 in proximal midgland-focal lesion

Fig. 9.16 g, h

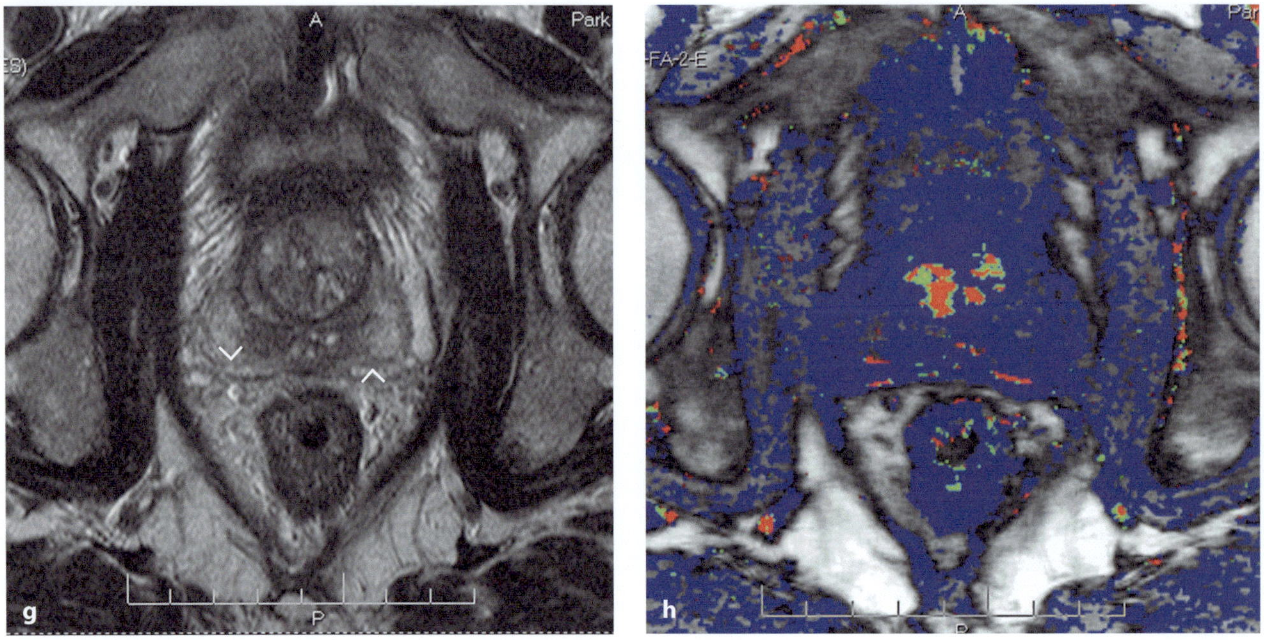

Fig. 9.16 g, h With Gleason 3 in both bases as linear lesions

Fig. 9.17 a, b

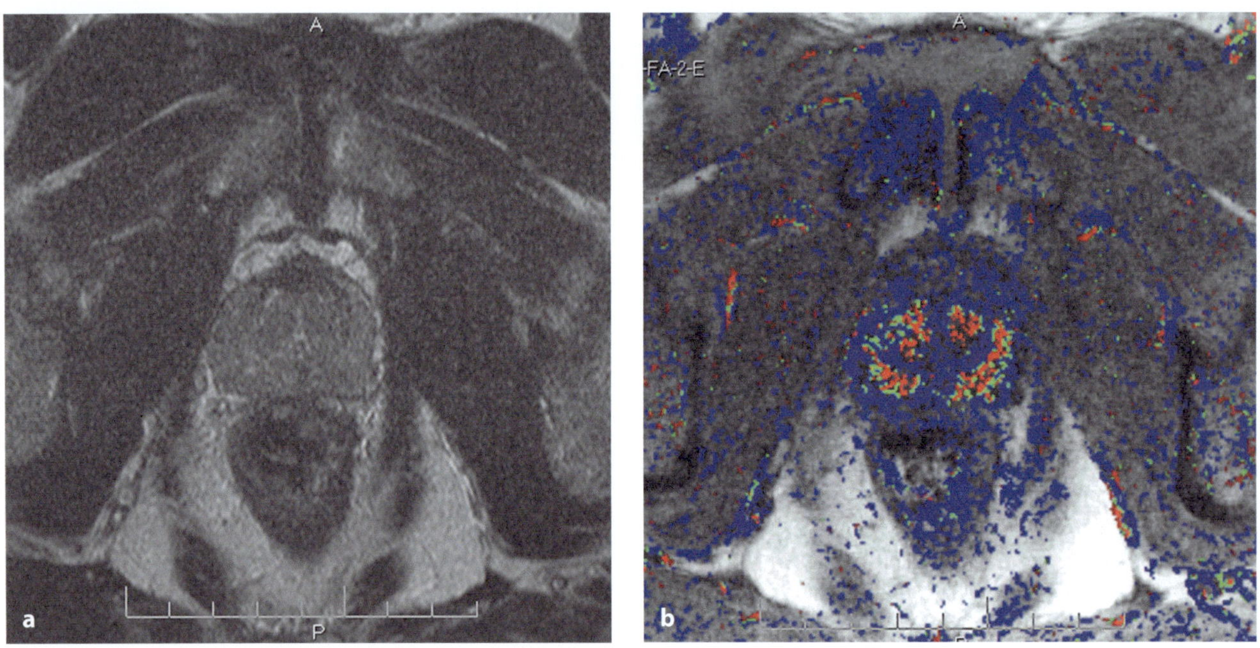

Fig. 9.17 a, b Post radiation prostatitis-T2 weighted low signal and symmetric migland flows

Fig. 9.18 a–j

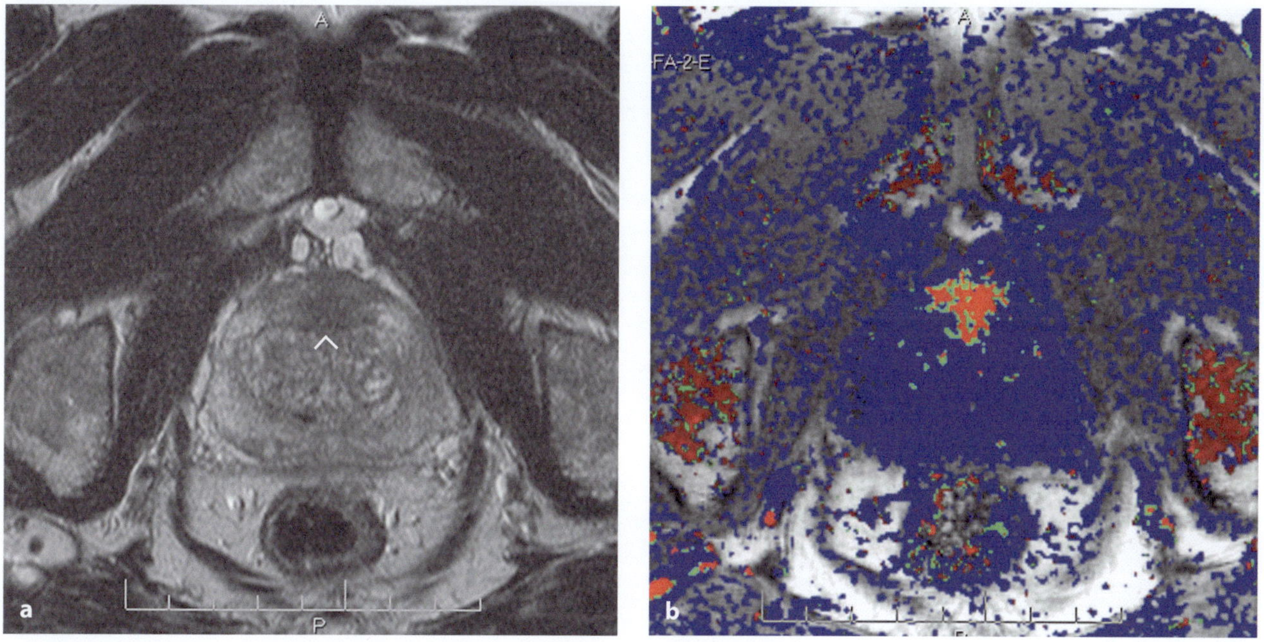

Fig. 9.18 a, b Ab small anterior Gleason 5 with extensive bone disease

Fig. 9.18 c, d

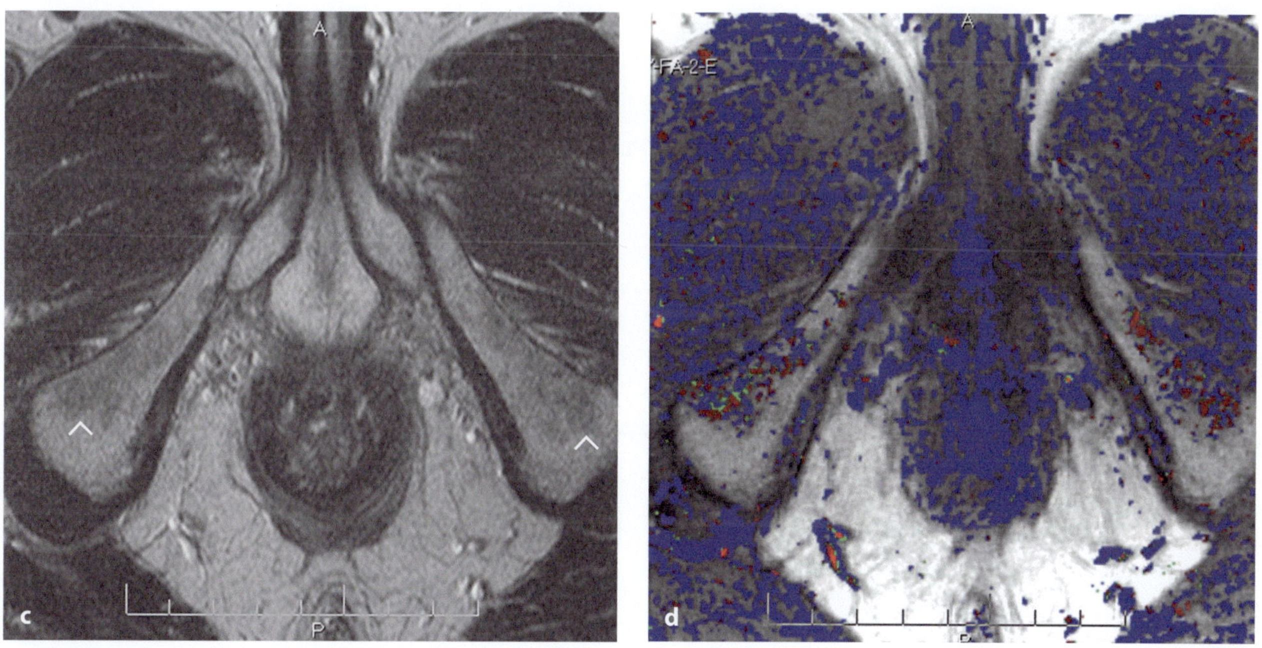

Fig. 9.18 c, d To right and left inferior pubic rami

Fig. 9.18 e, f

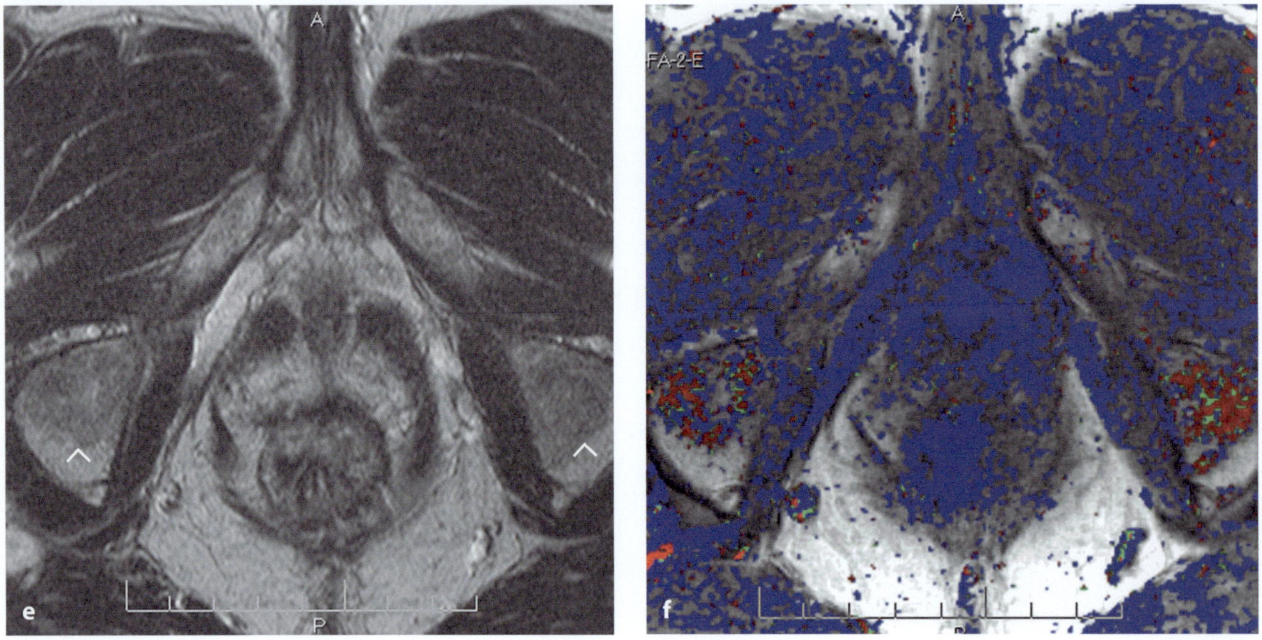

Fig. 9.18 e, f To right and left ischial tuberosity

Fig. 9.18 g, h

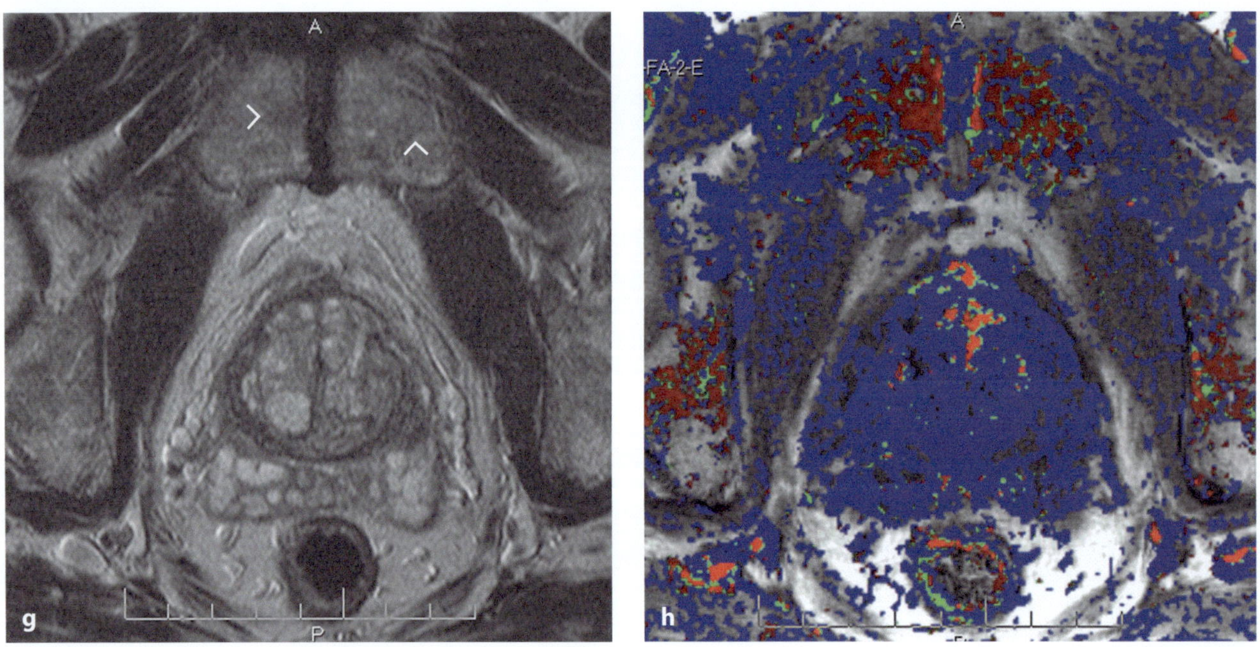

Fig. 9.18 g, h To right and left pubis symphysis

Fig. 9.18 i, j

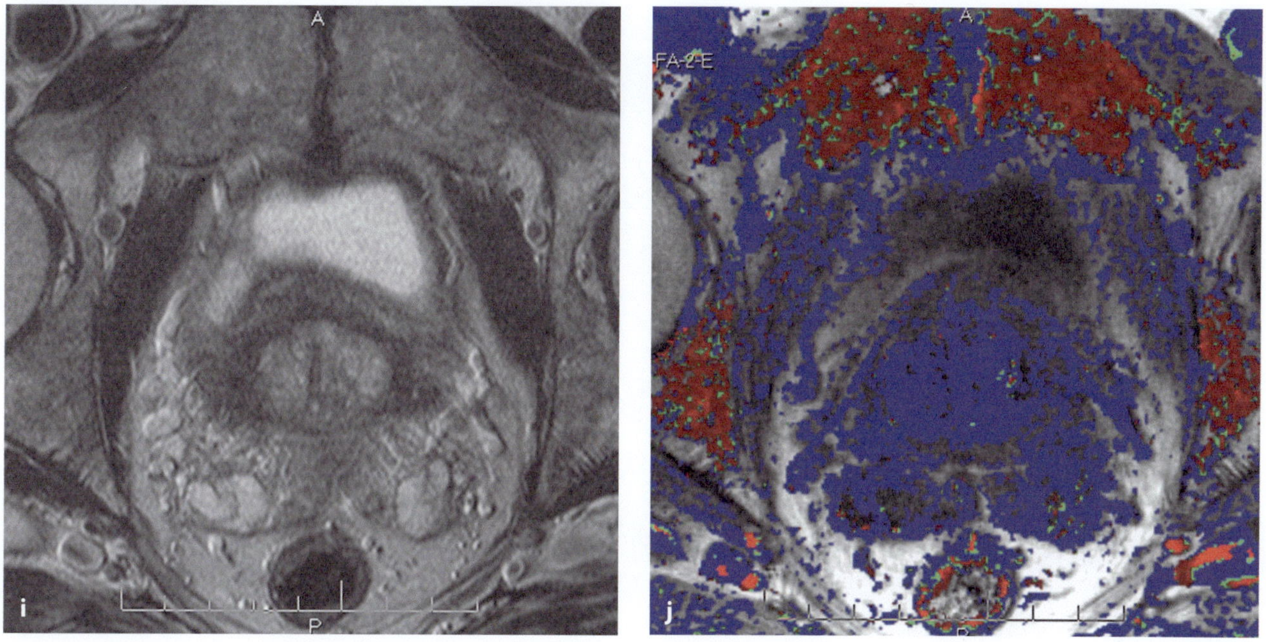

Fig. 9.18 i, j To post acetabuli and both pubic symphysis

Fig. 9.19 a–p

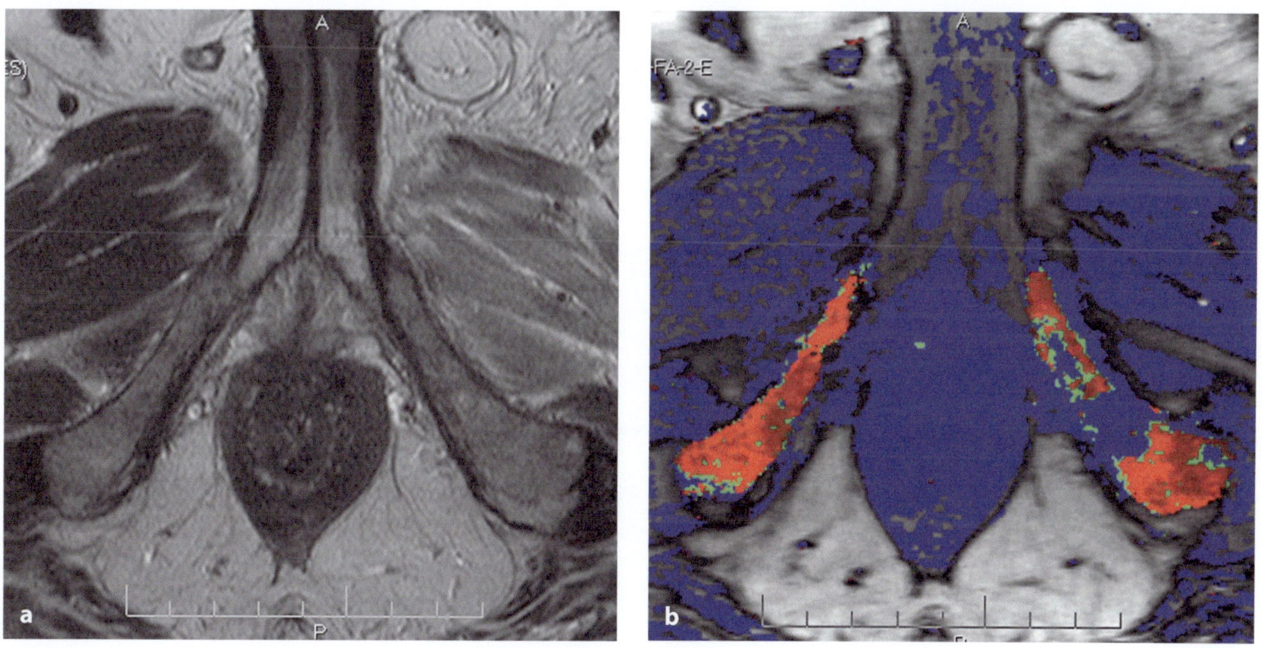

Fig. 9.19 a, b Anterior Gleason 5 with inferior pubic rami metastases

Fig. 9.19 c, d

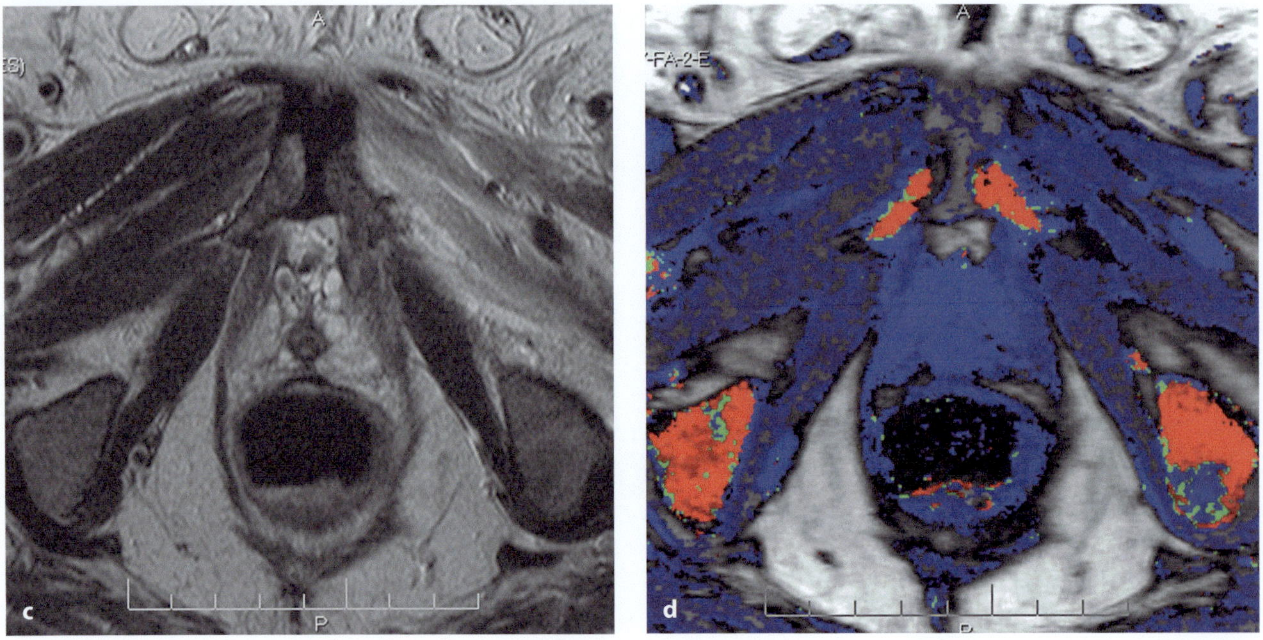

Fig. 9.19 c, d With bilateral ischial tuberosity and inferior pubic sypmhysis metatases

Fig. 9.19 e, f

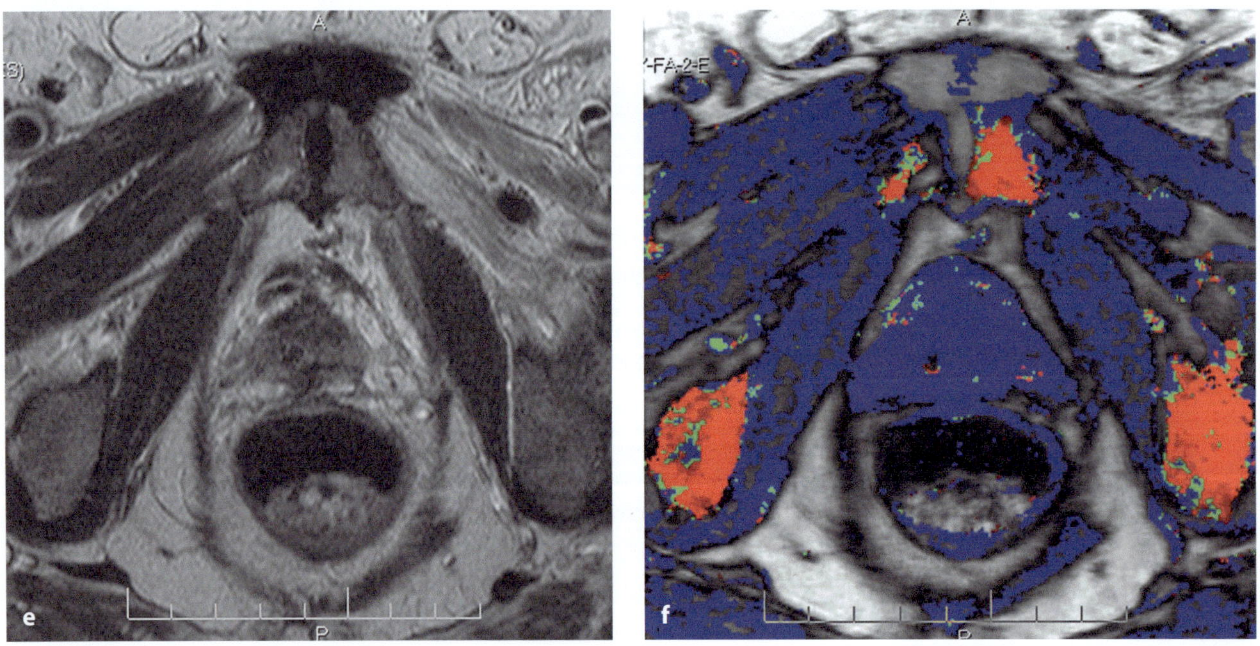

Fig. 9.19 e, f With inferior acetabular metastases

Fig. 9.19 g, h

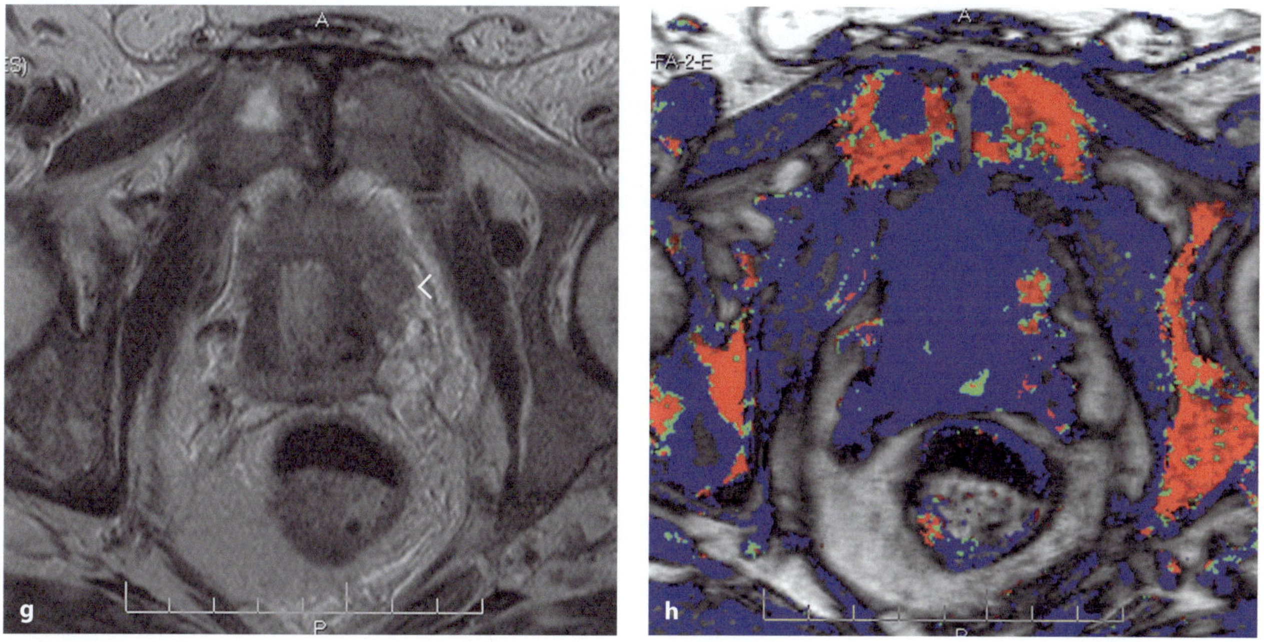

Fig. 9.19 g, h With mid acetabular metastases and left midgland extracapsular erosion

Fig. 9.19 i, j

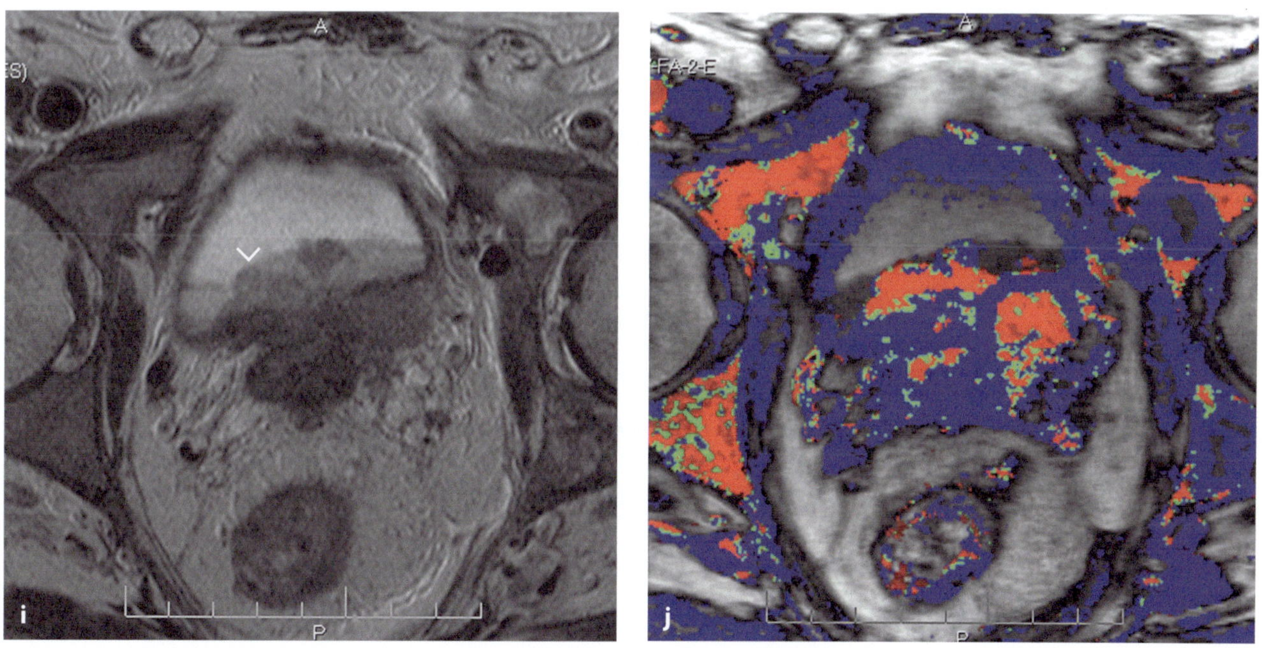

Fig. 9.19 i, j With superior acetabular metastases and anterior bladder wall invasion

Fig. 9.19 k, l

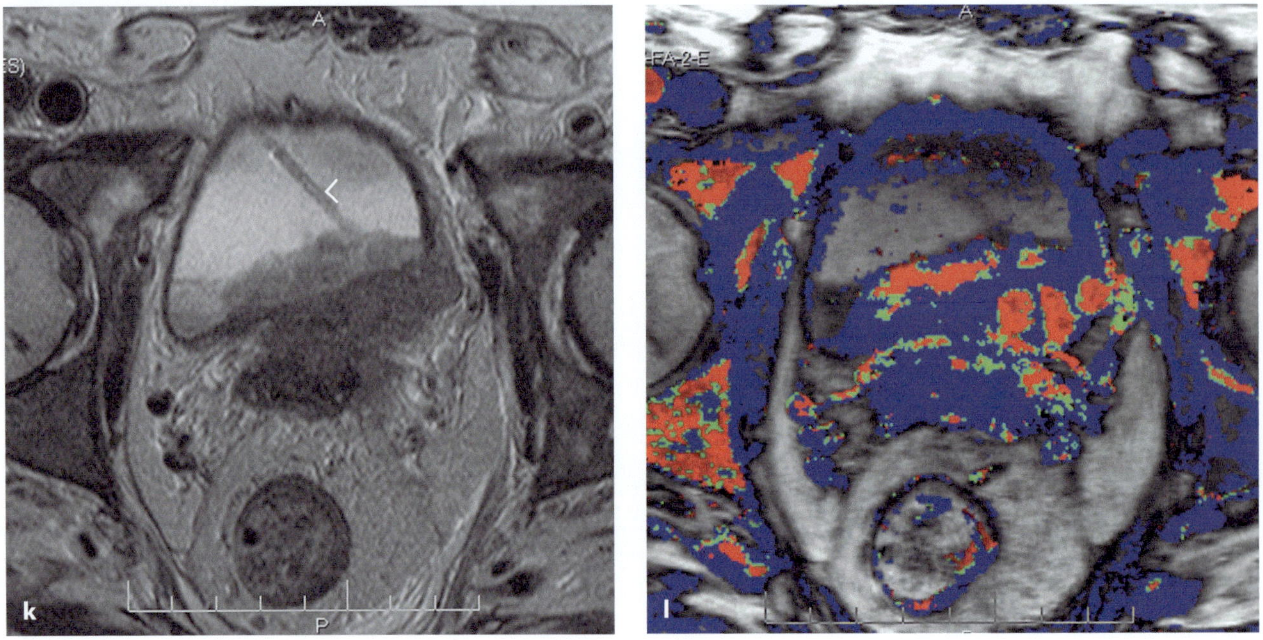

Fig. 9.19 k, l With bladder catheter and right perirectal avascular node

Fig. 9.19 m, n

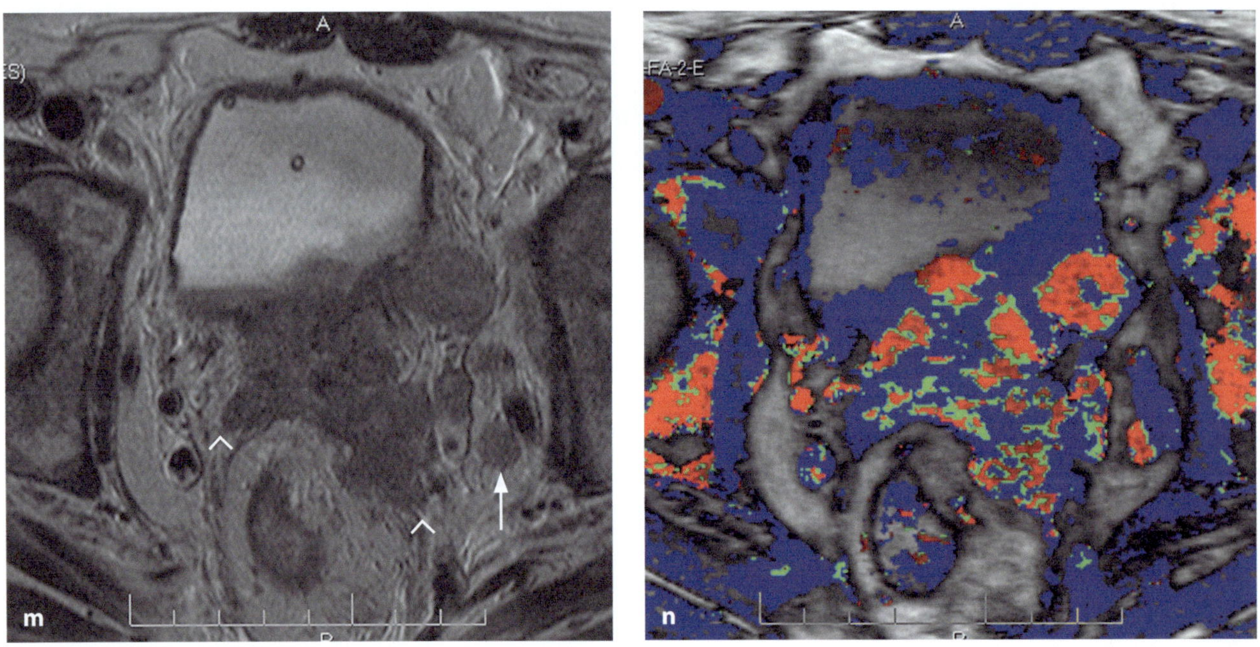

Fig. 9.19 m, n With seminal vesical invasion and left obturator nodes

Fig. 9.19 o, p

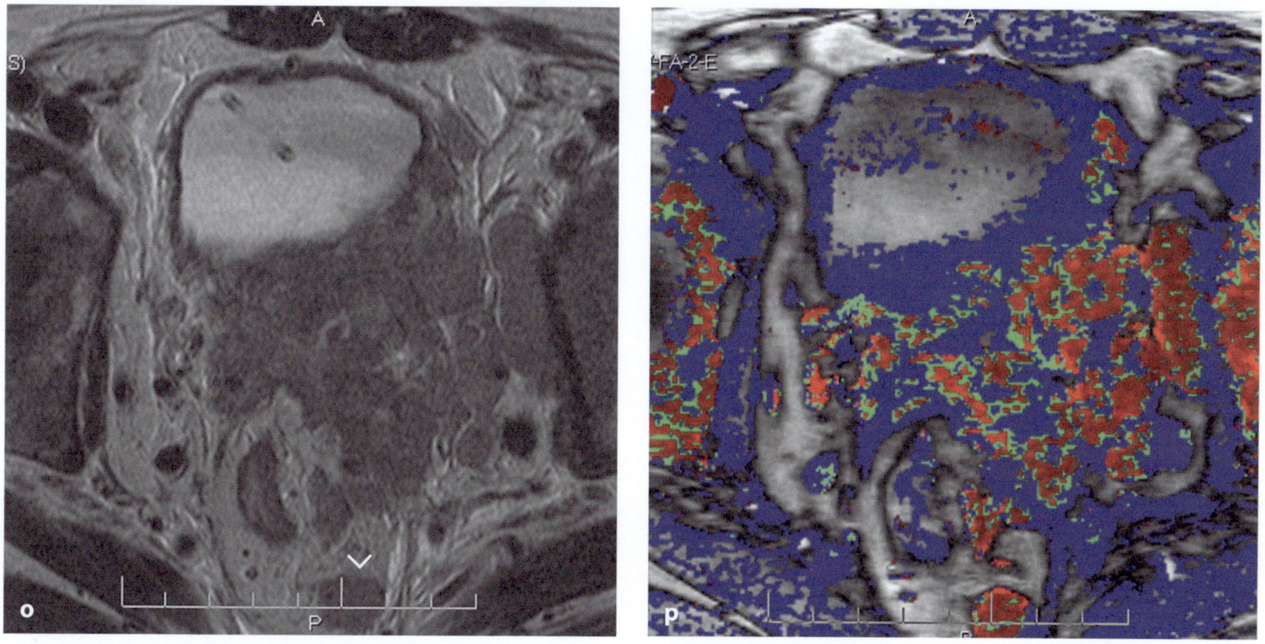

Fig. 9.19 o, p With iliac boney metastases and large left perirectal node

Fig. 9.20 a–j

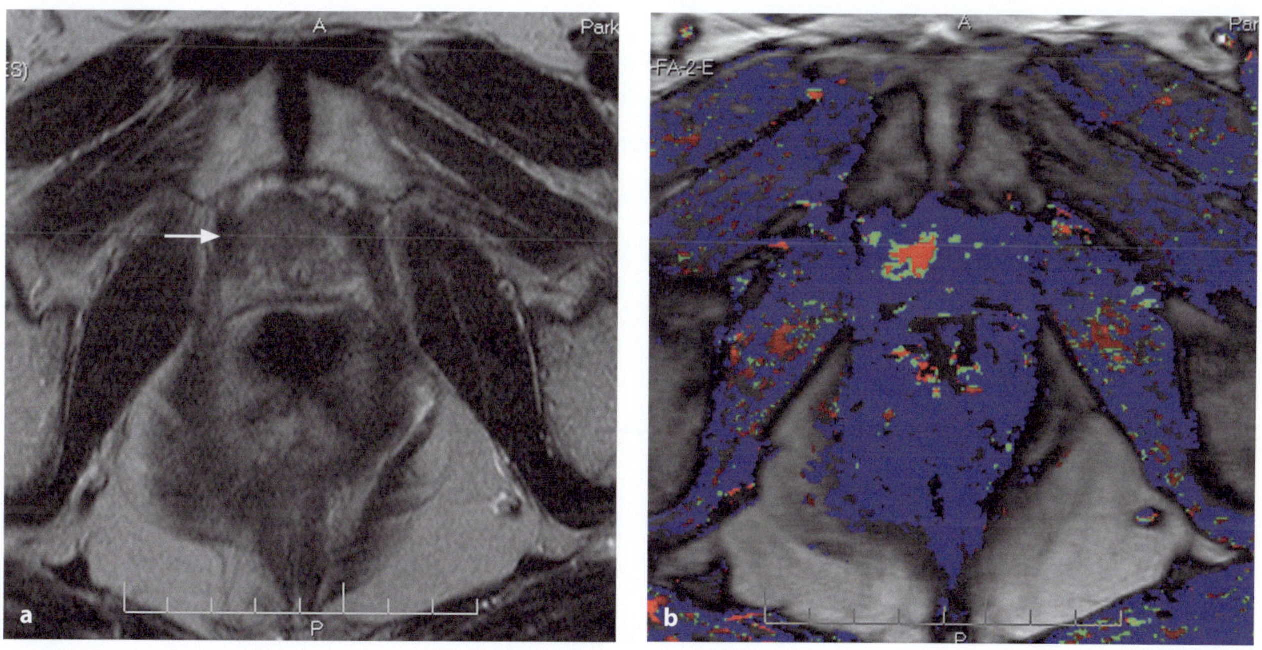

Fig. 9.20 a, b Apical Gleason 5 focal mass with right extracapsular extension

Fig. 9.20 c, d

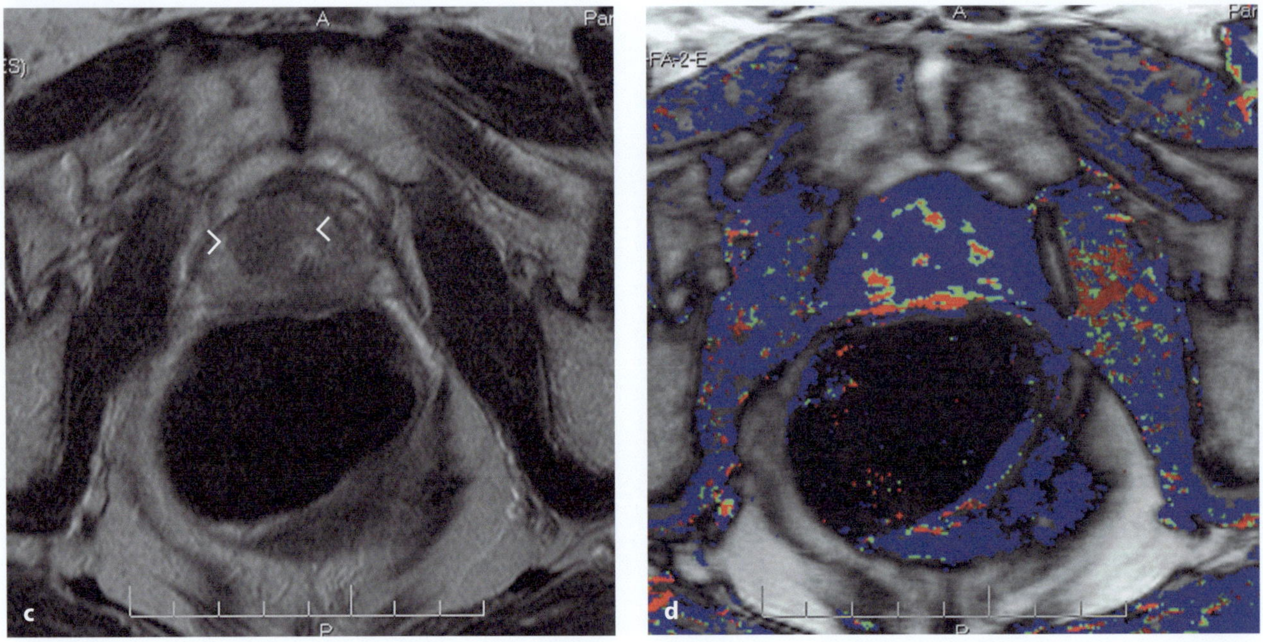

Fig. 9.20 c, d With midgland central zone Gleason 4 tumor-note dark and irregular right central region on T2 weighted scan as compared with mottled higher signal on contralateral side and circumferential vascularity surrounding periphery of right central mass. Also present are posterior Gleason 3 and right lateral Gleason 3 tumors.

Fig. 9.20 e, f

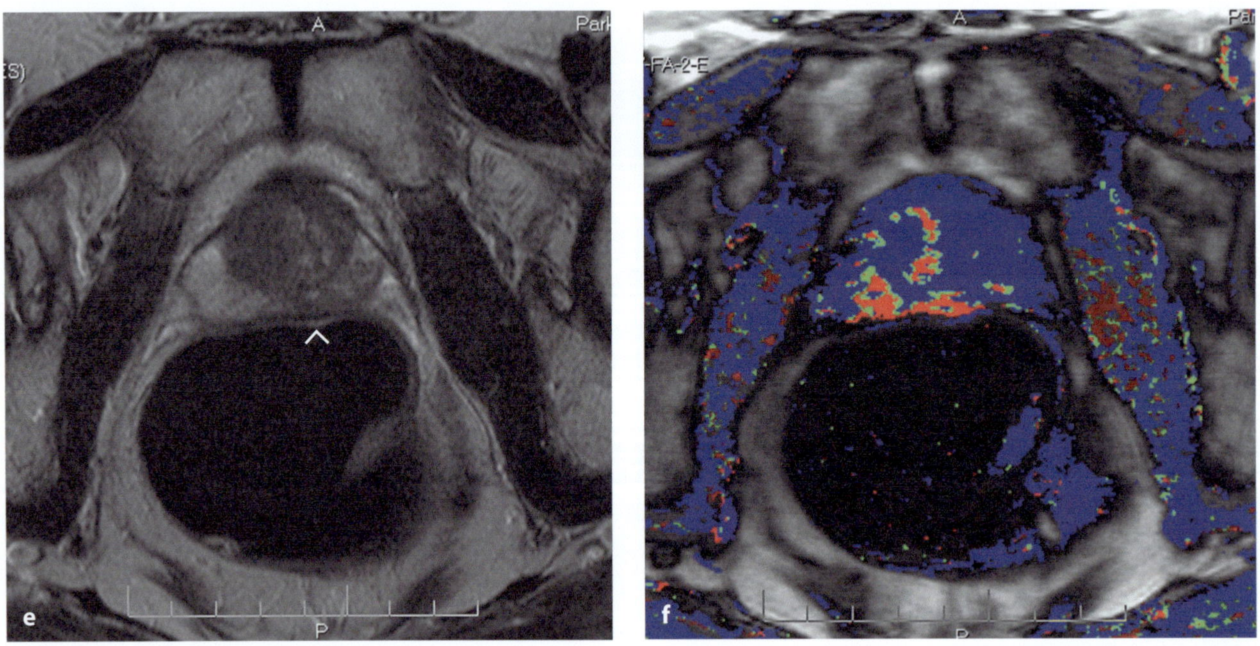

Fig. 9.20 e, f With left paramedian midgland Gleason 3 bulging capsule posteriorly

Fig. 9.20 g, h

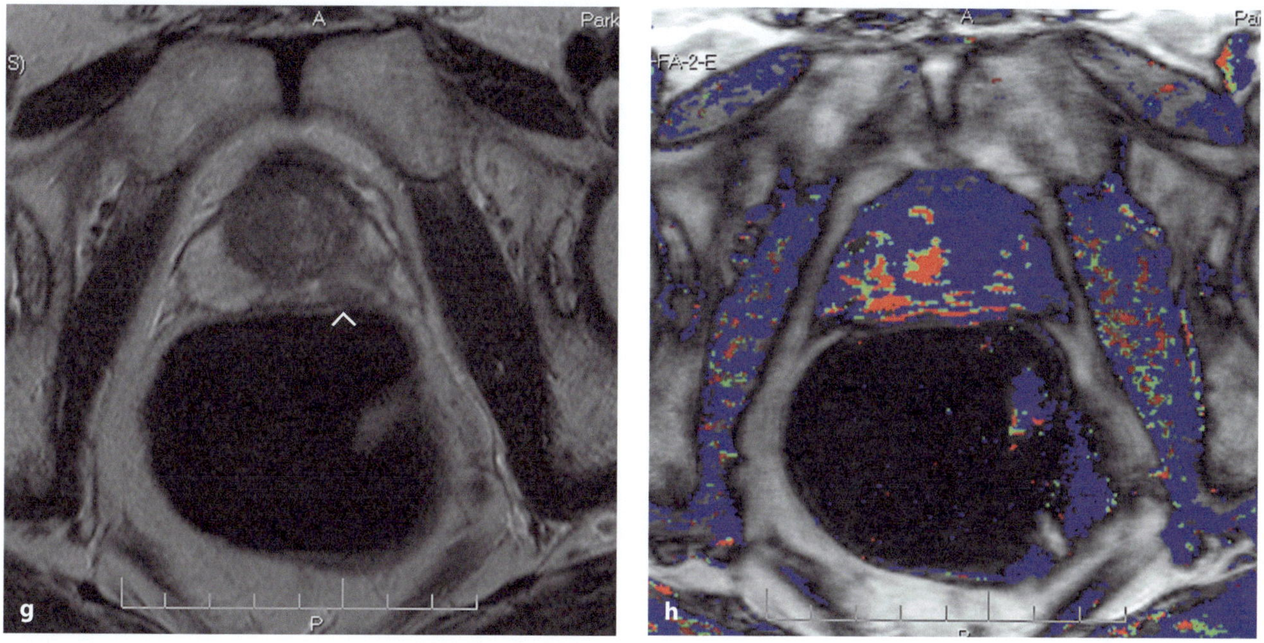

Fig. 9.20 g, h Left lateral and posterior capsular erosion

Fig. 9.20 i, j

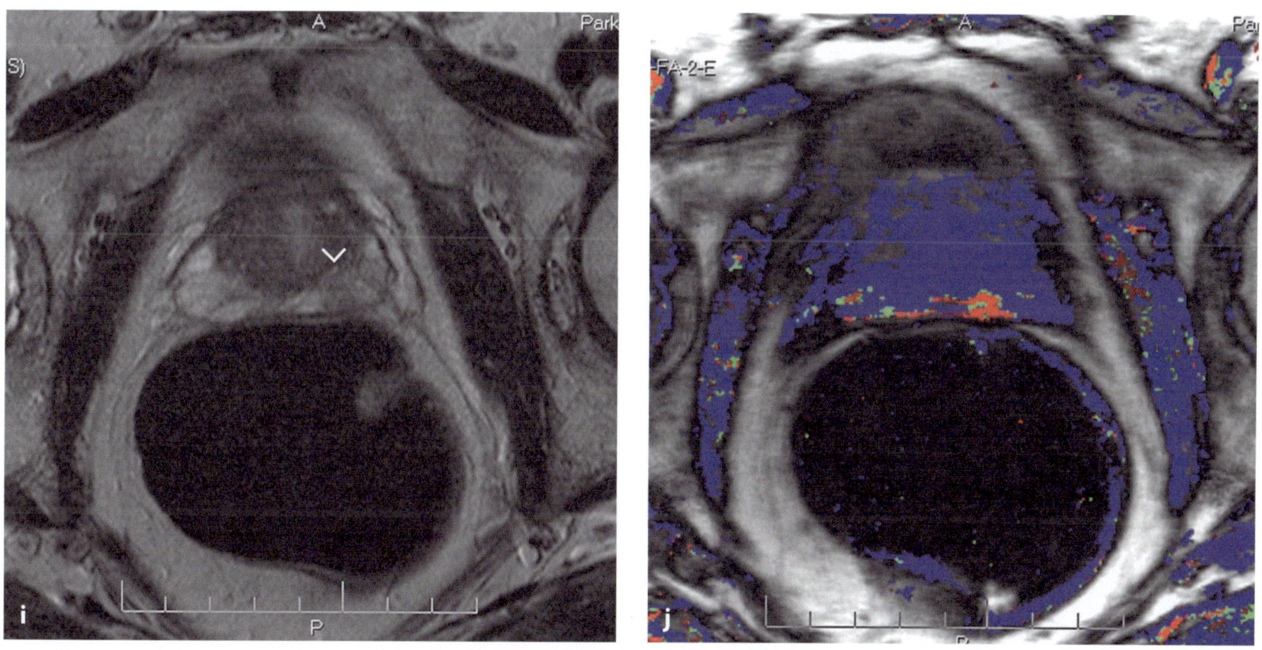

Fig. 9.20 i, j With focal left posterior base Gleason 4 tumor-note increased vascularity to central gland tumor

Chapter

Advanced Imaging Techniques

10

Bladder tumors are well imaged as intraluminal masses. Wall invasion may be noted and vascularity assessed. Staging is possible with DCE-MRI including vascular preoperative mapping. The presence of a bladder cancer requires renal pelvis and ureteral imaging to rule out "drop metastases"

Fig. 10.1 a, b

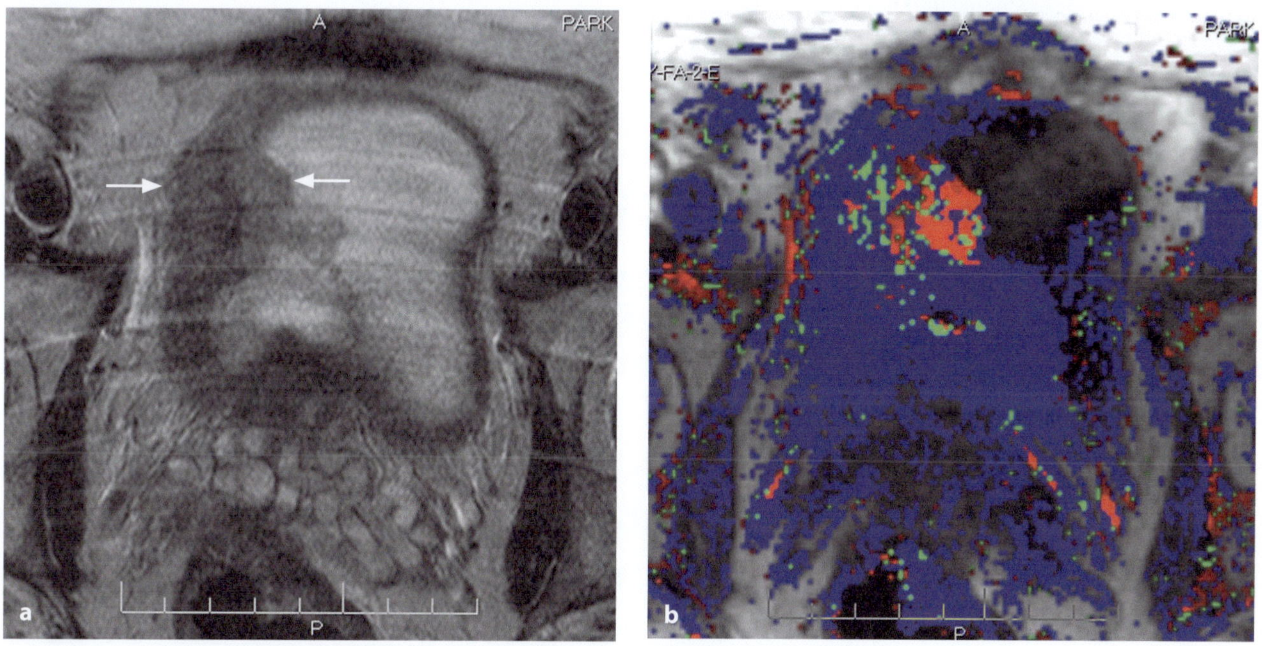

Fig. 10.1 a, b Bladder transitional cell carcinoma with right bladder wall thickening

Fig. 10.1 c, d

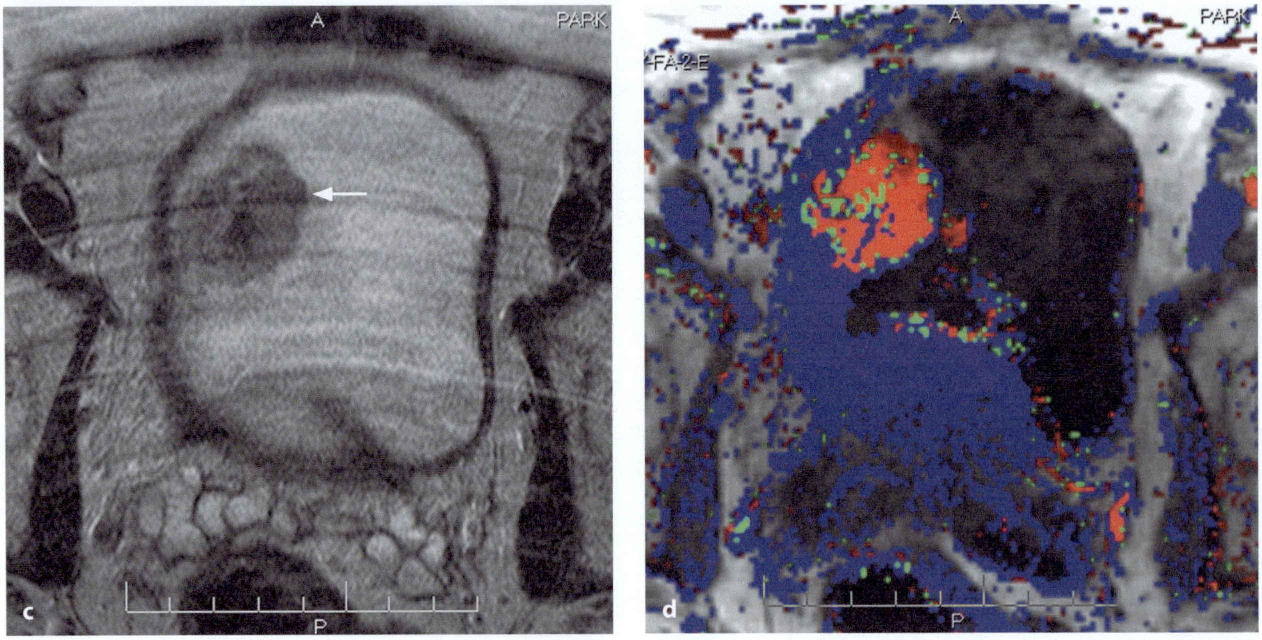

Fig. 10.1 c, d Extending into lumen as polypoid right tumor mass

Fig. 10.2 a–d

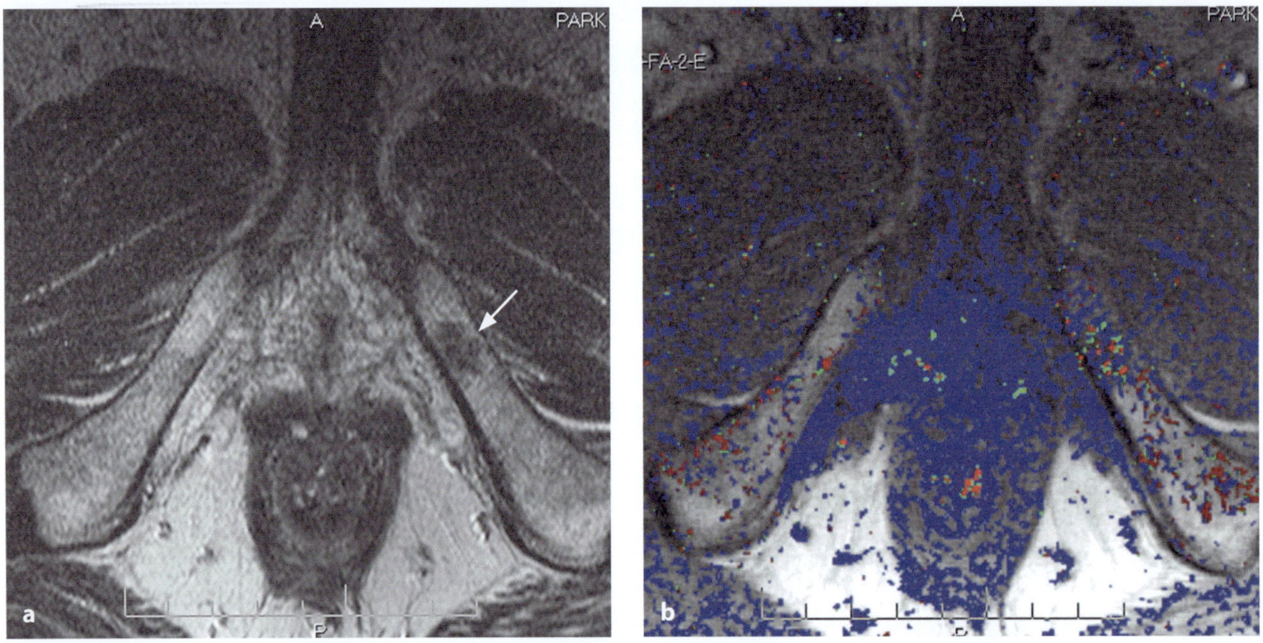

Fig. 10.2 Primary TCC of prostate and bladder Rare sub types of prostate cancer include: small cell carcinoma, transitional cell carcinoma (TCC), ductal carcinoma and carcinosarcoma with neuroendocrine variations a, b Right apical carcinoma with left inferior pubic ramus metastases

Fig. 10.2 c, d

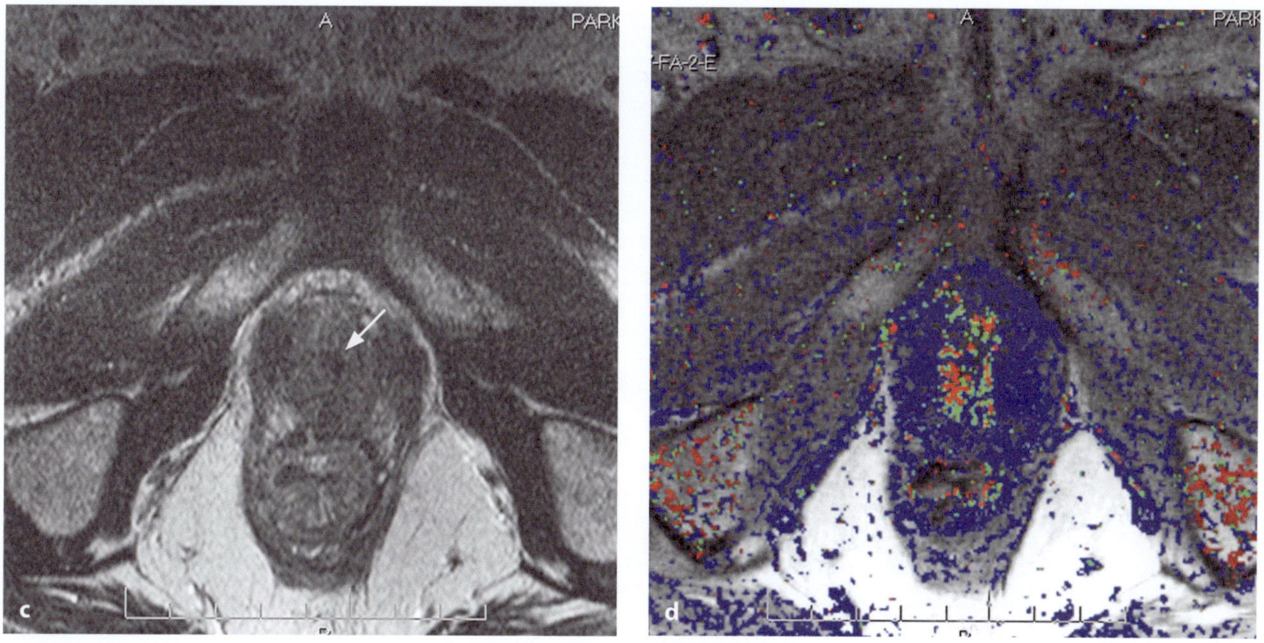

Fig. 10.2 c, d Right midgland carcinoma extending into central gland

Fig. 10.2 e, f

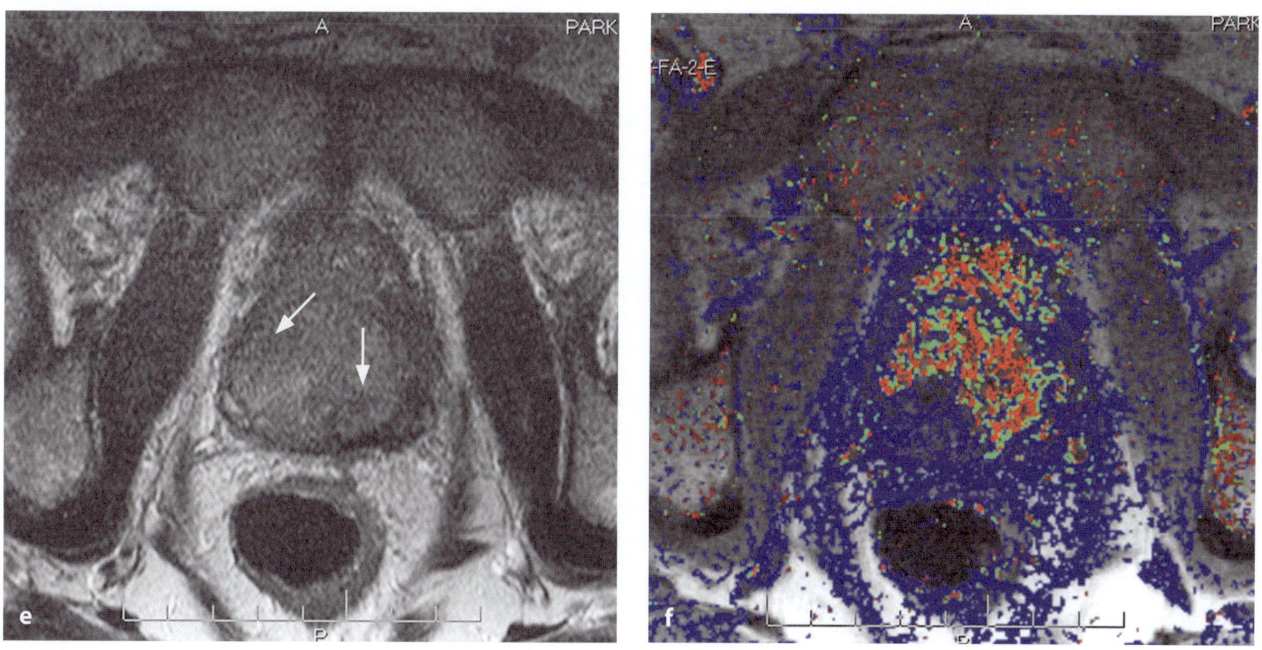

Fig. 10.2 e, f With right and anterior tumor extension

Fig. 10.2 g, h

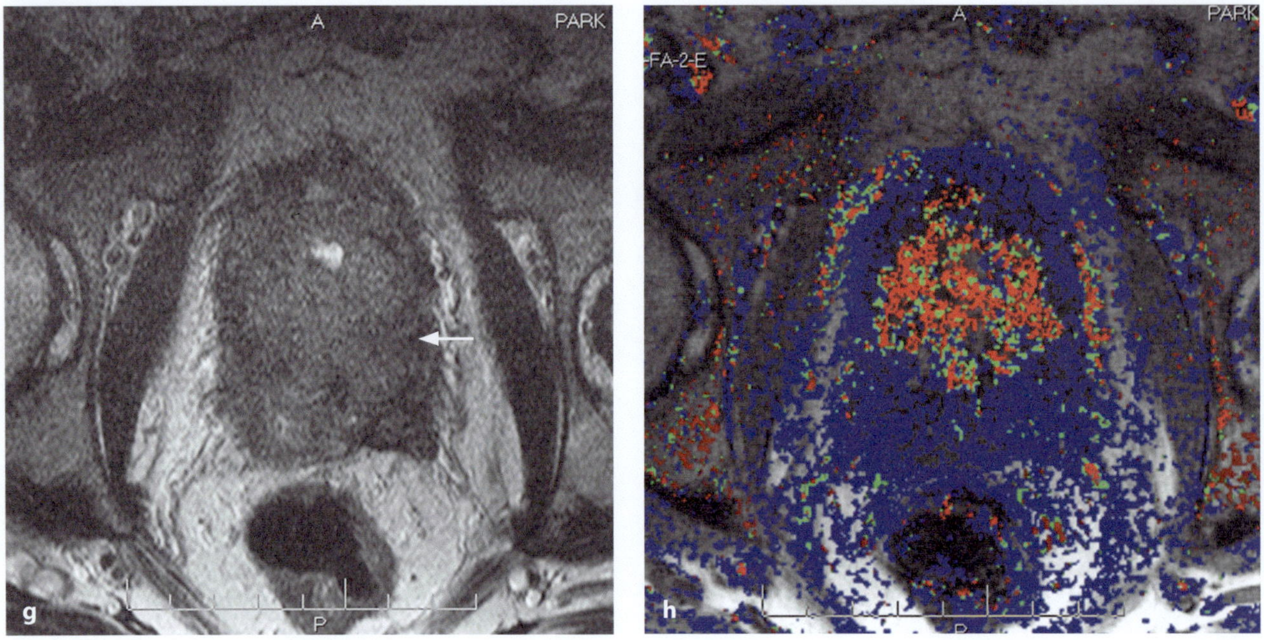

Fig. 10.2 g, h With central gland extension

Fig. 10.2 i, j

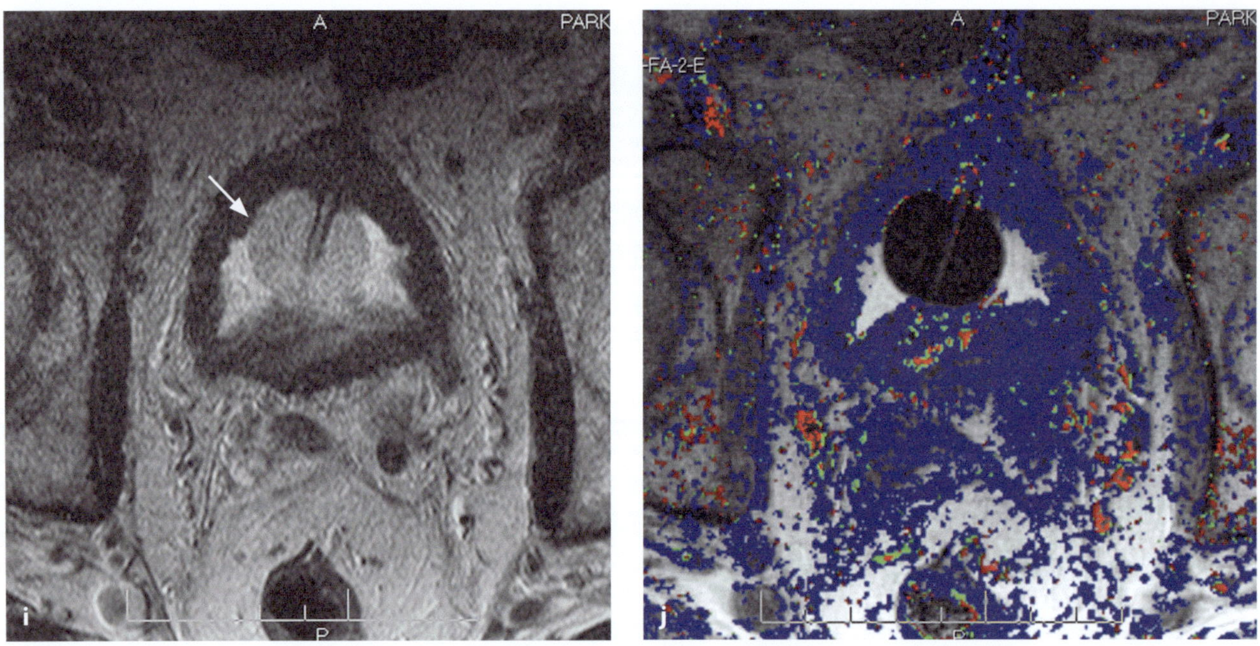

Fig. 10.2 i, j With invasion into bladder-note bladder wall thickening and catheter in position

References

11

1. Aus G, Abbou CC, Bolla M, et al. EAU guidelines on prostate cancer. Eur Urol 2005; 48:546–551
2. Iselin CE, Robertson JE, Paulson DF. Radical perineal prostatectomy: oncological outcome during a 20-year period. J Urol 1999; 161:163–168
3. Zelefsky MJ, Wallner KE, Ling CC, et al. Comparison of the 5-year outcome and morbidity of three-dimensional conformal radiotherapy versus transperineal permanent iodine-125 implantation for early-stage prostatic cancer. J Clin Oncol 1999; 17:517–522
4. Aus G. Current status of HIFU and cryotherapy in prostate cancer: a review. Eur Urol 2000; 50:927–934
5. Ragde H, Blasko JC, Grimm PD, et al. Brachytherapy for clinically localized prostate cancer: results at 7- and 8-year follow-up. Semin Surg Oncol 1997; 13:438–443
6. Poissonnier L, Chapelon JY, Rouviere O, et al. Control of prostate cancer by transectal HIFU in 227 patients. Eur Urol 2007: 51:381–387
7. Bahn DK, Lee F, Badalament R, Kumar A, Greski J, Chernick M. Targeted cryoablation of the prostate: 7-year outcomes in the primary treatment of prostate cancer. Urology 2002; 60:3–11
8. Huber P, Debus J, Jenne J, et al. Therapeutic ultrasound in tumor therapy; principles, applications and new developments [in German]. Radiologe 1996; 36:64–71
9. Colombel M, Gelet A. Principles and results of high-intensity focused ultrasound for localized prostate cancer. Prostate Cancer Prostatic Dis 2004; 7:289–294
10. Rebillard X, Gelet A, Davin JL, et al. Transrectal high-intensity focused ultrasound in the treatment of localized prostate cancer. J Endourol 2005; 19:693–701
11. Gelet A, Chapelon JY, Poissonnier L, et al. Local recurrence of prostate cancer after external beam radiotherapy; early experience of salvage therapy using high-intensity focused ultrasonography. Urology 2004; 63:625–629
12. Rouviere O, Mege-Lechevallier F, Chapelon JY, et al. Evaluation of color Doppler in guiding prostate biopsy after HIFU ablation. Eur Urol 2006: 50:490–497
13. Rouviere O, Lyonnet D, Raudrant A, et al. MRI appearance of prostate following transrectal HIFU ablation of localized cancer. Eur Urol 2001; 40:265–274
14. Susani M, Madersbacher S, Kratzik C, Vingers L, Marberger M. Morphology of tissue destruction induced by focused ultrasound. Eur Urol 1993; 23 [suppl 1]: 34–38
15. Huisman HJ, Engelbrecht MR, Barentsz JO. Accurate estimation of pharmacokinetic contrast-enhanced dynamic MRI parameters of the prostate. J Magn Reson Imaging 2001; 13:607–614
16. Kim CK, Park BK, Kim B. Localization of prostate cancer using 3T MRI: comparison of T2-weighted and dynamic contrast-enhanced imaging. J Comput Assist Tomogr 2006; 30:7–11
17. Engelbrecht MR, Huisman HJ, Laheij RJ, et al. Discrimination of prostate cancer from normal peripheral zone and central gland tissue by using dynamic contrast-enhanced MR imaging. Radiology 2003; 229:248–254
18. Buckley DL, Roberts C, Parker GJ, Logue JP, Hutchinson CE. Prostate cancer: evaluation of

vascular characteristics with dynamic contrast-enhanced T1-weighted MR imaging- initial experience. Radiology 2004; 233:709–715
19. Le Bihan D, Breton E, Lallemand D, Grenier P, Cabanis E, Laval-Jeantet M. MR imaging of intravoxel incoherent motions: application to diffusion and perfusion in neurologic disorders. Radiology 1986; 161:401–407
20. Kim CK, Park BK, Han JJ, Kang TW, Lee HM. Diffusion-weighted imaging of the prostate at 3 T for differentiation of malignant and benign tissue in transition and peripheral zones: preliminary results. J Comput Assist Tomogr 2007; 31:449–454
21. Gibbs P, Pickles MD, Turnbull LW. Diffusion imaging of the prostate at 3.0 Tesla. Invest Radiol 2006; 41:185–188
22. Pickles MD, Gibbs P, Sreenivas M, Turnbull LW. Diffusion-weighted imaging of normal and malignant prostate tissue at 3.0T. J Magn Reson Imaging 2006; 23:130–134
23. Goldberg SN, Grassi CJ, Cardella JF, et al. Image-guided tumor ablation: standardization of terminology and reporting criteria. Radiology 2005; 235:728–739
24. Kim JK, Hong SS, Choi YJ, et al. Wash-in rate on the basis of dynamic contrast-enhanced MRI: usefulness for prostate cancer detection and localization. J Magn Reson Imaging 2005; 22:639–646
25. Futterer JJ, Engelbrecht MR, Huisman HJ, et al. Staging prostate cancer with dynamic contrast-enhanced endorectal MR imaging prior to radical prostatectomy: experienced versus less experienced readers. Radiology 2005; 237:541–549
26. Carriere KC, Roos LL, Dover DC. Across time and space: variations in hospital use during Canadian health reform. Health Serv Res 2000; 35:467–487
27. Landis JR, Koch GG. The measurement of observer agreement for categorical data. Biometrics 1977; 33:159–174
28. Gelet A, Chapelon JY, Bouvier R, et al. Treatment of prostate cancer with transrectal focused ultrasound: early clinical experience. Eur Urol 1996; 26:174–183
29. Thuroff S, Chaussy C, Vallancien G, et al. High-intensity focused ultrasound and localized prostate cancer: efficacy results from the European multi-centric study. J Endourol 2003; 17:673–677
30. Blana A, Walter B, Rogenhofer S, Wieland WF. High-intensity focused ultrasound for the treatment of localized prostate cancer: 5-year experience. Urology 2004; 63:297–300
31. Chaussy C, Thuroff S, Rebillard X, Gelet A. Technology insight: high-intensity focused ultrasound for urologic cancers. Nat Clin Pract Urol 2005; 2:191–198
32. Uchida T, Ohkusa H, Nagata Y, Hyodo T, Satoh T, Irie A. Treatment of localized prostate cancer using high-intensity focused ultrasound. BJU Int 2006; 97:56–61
33. Uchida T, Illing RO, Cathcart PJ, Emberton M. To what extent does the prostate-specific antigen nadir predict subsequent treatment failure after transrectal high-intensity focused ultrasound therapy for presumed localized adenocarcinoma of the prostate? BJU Int 2006; 98:537–539
34. Chen ME, Johnston DA, Tang K, Babaian RJ, Troncoso P. Detailed mapping of prostate carcinoma foci: biopsy strategy implications. Cancer 2000; 89:1800–1809
35. Lee HM, Hong JH, Choi HY. High-intensity focused ultrasound therapy for clinically localized prostate cancer. Prostate Cancer Prostatic Dis 2006; 9:439–443
36. Pound CR, Partin AW, Eisenberger MA, Chan DW, Pearson JD, Walsh PC. Natural history of progression after PSA elevation following radical prostatectomy. JAMA 1999; 281:1591–1597
37. Amling CL Bergstralh EJ Blute ML, Slezak JM, Zincke H. Defining prostate specific antigen progression after radical prostatectomy: what is the most appropriate cut point? J Urol 2001: 165:1146–1151
38. Rogers R, Grossfeld GD, Roach M III, et al. Radiation therapy for the management of biopsy proved local recurrence after radical prostatectomy. J Urol 1998; 160:1748–1753
39. Bott SR. Management of recurrent disease after radical prostatectomy. Prostate Cancer Prostatic Dis 2004; 7:211–216
40. Lightner DI, Lange PH, Reddy PK, Moore L. Prostate specific antigen and local recurrence

after radical prostatectomy. Prostate Cancer Prostatic Dis 2004; 7:211–216

41. Connolly JA, Shinohara K, Presti JC Jr, Caroll PR. Local recurrence after radical prostatectomy: characteristics in size, location, and relationship to prostate-specific antigen and surgical margins. Urology 1996; 47:225–231
42. Saleem MD, Sanders H, Abu El Naser M, El-Galley R. Factors predicting cancer detection in biopsy of the prostatic fossa after radical prostatectomy. Urology 1998; 51:283–286
43. Leventis AK, Shariat SF, Slawin KM. Local recurrence after radical prostatectomy: correlation of US features with prostatic fossa biopsy findings. Radiology 2001; 219:432–439
44. Ornstein DK, Colberg JW, Virgo KS, et al. Evaluation and management of men whose radical prostatectomies failed: results of an international survey. Urology 1998; 52:1047–1054
45. Scattoni V, RoscignoM, Raber M, Consonni P, Da Pozzo L, Rigatti P. Biopsy of the vesico-urethal anastomosis after radical prostatectomy: when and how. Eur Urol 2002; 38 [suppl 1]:89–95
46. Silverman JM, Krebs TL. MR imaging evaluation with a transrectal surface coil of local recurrence of prostatic cancer in men who have undergone radical prostatectomy. AJR 1997; 168:379–385
47. Sella T, Schwartz LH, Swindle PV, et al. Suspected local recurrence after radical prostatectomy: endorectal coil MR imaging. Radiology 2004; 231:379–378
48. Futterer JJ, Engelbrecht MR, Huisman HJ, et al. Staging prostate cancer with dynamic contrast enhanced endorectal MR imaging prior to radical prostatectomy: experienced versus less experienced readers. Radiology 2005; 237:541–549
49. Futterer JJ, Heijmink S, Scheenen T, et al. Prostate cancer localization with dynamic contrast-enhanced MR imaging and proton MR spectroscopic imaging. Radiology 2006; 241:449–458
50. Portalez D, Malavaud B, Herigault G, et al. Predicting prostate cancer with dynamic endorectal coil MR and proton spectroscopic MR imaging [in French]. J Radiol 2005; 85[12 Pt 1]: 1999–2004
51. Buckley DL, Roberts C, Parker GJ, Logue JP, Hutchinson CE. Prostate cancer: evaluation of vascular characteristics with dynamic contrast enhanced T1-weighted MR imaging- initial experience. Radiology 2004; 233:709–715
52. Lange P, Ercole CI, Lightner DI, Fraley EE, Vesella R. The value of serum prostate specific antigen determinations before and after prostatectomy. J Urol 1989; 141:873–879
53. Foster LS, Jajodia P, Fournier G Jr, Shinohara K, Caroll P, Narayan P. The value of prostate specific antigen and transrectal ultrasound guided biopsy in detecting prostatic fossa recurrences following radical prostatectomy. J Urol 1993; 149:1024–1028
54. Scattoni V, Roscigno M, Raber M, et al. Multiple vesico-urethral biopsies following a radical prostatectomy. J Urol 2003 44:407–414
55. Swindle PW, Kattan MW, Scardino PT. Markers and meaning of primary treatment failure. Urol Clin North Am 2003; 30:377–401
56. John H, Hauri D, Maake C. The effect of seminal vesicle-sparing radical prostatectomy on serum prostate-specific antigen level. BJU Int 2003; 92:920–923
57. Sella T, Schwartz LH, Hricak H. retained seminal vesicles after radical prostatectomy; frequency, MRI characteristics, and clinical relevance. AJR 2006; 186:539–546
58. Pucar D, Shukla-Dave A, Hricak H, et al. Prostate cancer: correlation of MR imaging and MR spectroscopywith pathologic findings after radiation therapy- initial experience. Radiology 2005; 236:545–553
59. Coakley FV, The HS, Qayyum A, et al. Endorectal MR imaging and MR spectroscopic imaging for locally recurrent prostate cancer after external beam radiation therapy: preliminary experience. Radiology 2004; 233:441–448
60. Mueller-Lisse UG, Vigneron DB, Hricak H, et al. Localized prostate cancer: effect of hormone deprivation therapy measured by using combined three-dimensional 1H MR spectroscopy and MR imaging- clinicopathologic case-controlled study. Radiology 2001; 221:380–390
61. Siegal JA, Yu E, Brawer MK. Topography of neovascularity in human prostate carcinoma. Cancer 1995; 75:2545–2551

62. Brawer MK, Deerings RE, Brown M, Preston SD, Bigler S. Predictors of pathologic stage in prostate carcinoma: the role of neovascularity. Cancer 1994; 73:678–687
63. Choi YJ, Kim JK, Kim N, et al. Functional MR imaging of prostate cancer. RadioGraphics 2007; 27:63–75
64. Rehman S, Jayson G. Molecular Imaging of Antiangiogenic agents. Oncologist 2005;10:92–103
65. Cosgrove D. Angiogenesis imaging- Ultrasound. Br J Radiol 2003;76:43–9
66. Escudier B, Lassau N, Couanet D et al. Phase II trial of thalidomide in renal-cell carcinoma. Ann Oncol 2002;13:1029–35
67. Eggermont AM. Evolving imaging technology: contrast -enhanced Doppler ultrasound is early and rapid predictor of tumor response. Ann Oncol 2005; 16:995–6
68. Blay JY, Landi B, Bonvalot S, Monges G, Ray-Coquard I, Duffaud F et al. Recommendations for the management of GIST patients. Bull Cancer 2005:92:907–18
69. Jain RK. Normalization of tumor vasculature: an emerging concept in antiangiogenic therapy. Science 2005; 307:58–62
70. Tranquart F. Developpements recents en imagerie ultrasonore de contraste a vise oncologique. J Radiol 2007;88:1759–69
71. Kennedy JE. High-intensity focused ultrasound in the treatment of solid tumours. Nat Rev Cancer 2005;5:321–7
72. Grenier N, Trillaud H, Palussiére J, Mougenot C, Quesson B et al. Thérapies par ultrasons focalizés. J Radiol 2007;88:1787–800
73. Chapelon JY, Margonari J, Theillere Y et al. Effects of high-energy focused ultrasound on kidney tissue in the rat and the dog. Eur Urol 1992;22:147–52
74. Poissonnier L, Gelet A, Chapelon JY et al. [Results of transrectal focused ultrasound for the treatment of localized prostate cancer (120 patients with PSA <or + 10 ng/ml]. Prog Urol 2003;13:60–72
75. Uchida T, Ohkusa H, Yamashita H et al. Five years experience of transrectal high-intensity focused ultrasound using the Sonoblate device in the treatment of localized prostate cancer. Int J Urol 2006;13:228–33
76. Gelet A, Chapelon JY, Bouvier R, Pangaud C, Lasne Y. Local control of prostate cancer by transrectal high intensity focused ultrasound therapy: preliminary results. J Urol 1999;161:156–62
77. Rouviere O, Souchon R, Salomir R, Gelet A, Chapelon JY, Lyonnet D. Transrectal high-intensity focused ultrasound ablation of prostate cancer: Effective treatment requiring accurate imaging. Eur J Radiol 2007;63:317–27
78. Rouviere O, Mege-Lechevallier F, Chapelon JY et al. Evaluation of Color Doppler In Guiding Prostate Biopsy after HIFU Ablation. Eur Urol 2006;50:490–7
79. Girouin N, Mege-Lechevallier F, Tonina Senes A et al. Prostate dynamic contrast-enhanced MRI with simple visual diagnostic criteria: is it reasonable? Eur Radiol 2007;17:1498–509
80. Villers A, Puech P, Mouton D, Leroy X, Ballereau C, Lemaitre L. Dynamic contrast enhanced, pelvic phased array magnetic resonance imaging of localized prostate cancer for predicting tumor volume: correlation with radical prostatectomy findings. J Urol 2006; 176:2432–7
81. Taouli B. Le rôle de la spectroscopie IRM dans l'évaluation du cancer de la prostate. J Radiol 2006;87:222–7
82. Kim JK, Hong SS, Choi YJ et al. Wash-in rate on the basis of dynamic contrast-enhances MRI: usefulness for prostate cancer detection and localization. J Magn Reson Imaging 2005;22:639–46
83. Rouviere O, Valette O, Grivolat S et al. Recurrent prostate cancer after external beam radiotherapy: value of contrast-enhanced dynamic MRI in localizing intraprostatic tumor-correlation with biopsy findings. Urology 2004;63:922–7
84. Sala E, Eberhardt SC, Akin O et al. Endorectal MR imaging before salvage prostatectomy: tumor localization and staging. Radiology 2006;238:176–83
85. Sedelaar JP, Aarnink RG, van Leenders GJ et al. The application of three-dimensional contrast-enhanced ultrasound to measure volume of affected tissue after HIFU treatment for localized prostate cancer. Eur Urol 2000;37:559–68

86. Rouviere O, Lyonnet D, Raudrant A et al. The application of three-dimensional contrast-enhanced ultrasound to measure volume of affected tissue after HIFU treatment for localized cancer. Eur Urol 2001;40:265–74
87. Coakley FV, Teh HS, Qayyum A et al. Endorectal MR imaging and MR spectroscopic imaging for locally recurrent prostate cancer after external beam radiation therapy: preliminary experience. Radiology 2004;233–441–8.
88. Parivar F, Hricak H, Shinohara K et al. Detection of locally recurrent prostate cancer after cryosurgery: evaluation by transrectal ultrasound, magnetic resonance imaging, and three-dimensional proton magnetic resonance spectroscopy. Urology 1996;48:594–9
89. Roy C, Servois V, Sauer B. Les thérapeutiques et la surveillance dans le cancer de la prostate et leurs implications sur l'imagerie. J Radiol 2006;87:244–56
90. Coakley FV, Hricak H, Wefer AE, Speight JL, Kurhanewicz J, Roach M. Brachy-therapy for prostate cancer: endorectal MR imaging of local treatment-related changes. Radiology 2001;219–817–21
91. Singh H, Canto El, Shariat SF et al. Predictors of prostate cancer after initial negative systematic 12 core biopsy. J Urol 2004;171:1850–4
92. Mian BM, Naya Y, Okihara K, Vakar-Lopez F, Troncoso P, Babaian RJ. Predictors of cancer in repeat extended multisite prostate biopsy in men with previous negative extended multisite biopsy. Urology 2002;60:836–40
93. Engelbrecht MR, Huisman HJ, Laheij RJ et al. Discrimination of prostate cancer from normal peripheral zone and central gland tissue by using dynamic contrast-enhanced MR imaging. Radiology 2003;229–248–54
94. Rouviere O, Raudrant A, Ecochard R et al. Characterization of time-enhancement curves benign and malignant prostate tissue at dynamic MR imaging. Eur Radiol 2003;13:931–43
95. Padhani AR, Gapinski CJ, Macvicar DA et al. Dynamic contrast enhanced MRI of prostate cancer: correlation with morphology and tumour stage, histological grade and PSA. Clin Radiol 2000;55:99–109
96. Turnbull LW, Buckley DL, Turnbull LS, Liney GP, Knowles AJ. Differentiation of prostatic carcinoma and benign prostatic hyperplasia: correlation between dynamic Gd-DTPA-enchanced MR imaging and histopathology. J Magn Reson Imaging 1999;9: 311–6
97. Mitterberger M, Pinggera GM, Horninger W et al. Comparison of contrast enhanced color Doppler targeted biopsy to conventional systematic biopsy: impact on Gleason score. J Urol 2007;178:464–468; discussion 468.
98. Rouviere O, Hartman RP, Lyonnet D. Prostate MR imaging at high-field strength: evolution or revolution? Eur Radiol 2006;16:276–284
99. Kim CK, Park BK, Lee HM et al. MRI Techniques for prediction of local tumor progression after high-intensity focused ultrasonic ablation of prostate cancer. AJR 2008;190:1180–1186
100. Casciani E, Polettini E, Carmenini E et al. Endorectal and dynamic contrast-enhanced MRI for detection of local recurrence after radical prostatectomy. AJR 2008;190:1187–1192
101. Lassau N, Brule A, Chami L et al. Évaluation précoce des traitements anti-angiogéniques par échographie dynamique de contraste. J Radiol 2008;89:549–55
102. Cheikh AB, Girouin N, Ryon-Taponnier P et al. Détection par IRM des récidives locales du cancer de prostate après traitement par ultrasons focalizés de haute intensité (HIFU) transrectaux: étude préliminaire. J Radiol 2008;89:571–7
102. Hu JC, Wang Q, Pashos CL, et al: Utilization and outcomes of minimally invasive radical prostatectomy. J Clin Oncol 26:2278–2284, 2008
103. Nelson B, Kaufman M, Broughton G, et al: Comparison of length of hospital stay between radical retropubic prostatectomy and robotic assisted laparoscopic prostatectomy. J Urol 177:929–931, 2007
104. Gettman MT, Blute ML: Critical comparison of laparoscopic, robotic, and open radical prostatectomy: techniques, outcomes, and cost. Curr Urol Rep 7:193–199, 2006
105. Descazeaud A, Peyromaure M, Zerbib M: Will robotic surgery become the gold standard for radical prostatectomy? Editorial. Eur Urol 51:9–11, 2007

106. Vickers AJ, Bianco FJ, Serio AM, et al: The surgical learning curve for prostate cancer control after radical prostatectomy. J Natl Cancer Inst 99:11711177, 2007
107. Magera JS Jr, Inman BA, Slezak JM, et al: Increased optical magnification from 2.5X to 4.3X with technical modification lowers positive margin rate in open radical prostatectomy. J Urol 179:130–135, 2008
108. Thompson RH, Blute ML, Slezak JM, et al: Is the GPSM scoring algorithm for patients with prostate cancer valid in the contemporary era? J Urol 178:459463, 2007
109. Hull GW, Fabbani F, Abbas F, et al: Cancer control with radical prostatectomy done in 1,000 consecutive patients. J Urol 167:528–534, 2002
110. Catalona WJ, Carvalhal GF, Mager DE, et al: Potency, continence, and complication rates in 1,870 consecutive radical retropubic prostatectomies. J Urol 162:433–438, 1999
111. Duchene DA, Moinzadeh A, Gill IS, et al: Survey of residency training in laparoscopic and robotic surgery. J Urol 176:2158–2166, 2006
112. Rassweiler J, Hruza M, Teber D, Su L-M: Laparoscopic and robotic assisted radical prostatectomy-critical analysis of the results. Eur Urol 49:612–624, 2006

MIX
Papier aus verantwortungsvollen Quellen
Paper from responsible sources
FSC® C105338

If you have any concerns about our products,
you can contact us on
ProductSafety@springernature.com

In case Publisher is established outside the EU,
the EU authorized representative is:
Springer Nature Customer Service Center GmbH
Europaplatz 3, 69115 Heidelberg, Germany

Printed by Libri Plureos GmbH
in Hamburg, Germany